FOCUS ON NEUROPSYCHOLOGY RESEARCH

FOCUS ON NEUROPSYCHOLOGY RESEARCH

JOSHUA R. DUPRI
EDITOR

Nova Science Publishers, Inc.
New York

Library of Congress Cataloging-in-Publication Data
Focus on neuropsychology research / Joshua R. Dupri (editor).
    p. cm.
Includes bibliographical references and index.
ISBN 1-59454-779-3
1. Neuropsychology. I. Dupri, Joshua R.
[DNLM: 1. Neuropsychology. 2. Mental Processes--physiology. 3. Brain--physiology. 4. Models, Neurological. WL 103.5 F652 2006]
QP360.F63
612.8'2--dc22

2006
2005030795

Published by Nova Science Publishers, Inc. ✦ *New York*

CONTENTS

PREFACE

Neuropsychology is the study of brain-behavior relationships and examines such domains of cognitive functioning as memory, attention, visual-perceptual abilities, language and intellectual function. It is strongly scientific in its approach and shares an information processing view of the mind with cognitive psychology and cognitive science. It is one of the most eclectic of the psychological disciplines, overlapping at times with areas such as neuroscience, philosophy (particularly philosophy of mind), neurology, psychiatry and computer science (particularly by making use of artificial neural networks).

Executive function has been conceptualized as a set of interrelated cognitive processes that are essential for regulation of cognition, behavior, and emotion. Hypothesized component processes include cognitive flexibility, decision making, inhibitory control, planning and organization, self-monitoring, as well as working memory. Historically, the neurobiological basis of executive functions in humans was largely examined through the administration of performance-based neuropsychological tests to patients with acquired focal brain lesions. Such studies led to the widely held belief that the integrity of the frontal lobes is central to executive functions. However, while lesion studies have been highly informative, they suffer from a number of methodological weaknesses including the inability to investigate the broader neural circuitry that contributes to executive functions. Over the past twenty five years functional neuroimaging techniques, in particular positron emission tomography (PET) and functional magnetic resonance imaging (fMRI), have been increasingly applied in the effort to elucidate the neural circuitry subserving executive functions. In chapter I, the authors review functional neuroimaging research addressing the neural substrates of executive functions in healthy adults, and discuss applications of neuroimaging techniques to the identification of the neural correlates of executive dysfunction in selected psychiatric and neurological illnesses.

Available neurophysiological and neuroimaging studies support the view that attentional processing is carried out by means of the reciprocal communications between distributed neural networks of brain areas including frontal and prefrontal cortex, as well as the occipital-temporal-parietal cortices. In chapter II, ERPs were recorded using a 32 channels whole-head montage while volunteers performed conjoined selection tasks of spatial location and spatial frequency. Target stimuli and distractors were presented within and without attended locations. The data indicate that during spatially directed selective processing, the visual system, although overall increasing processing activation for all stimuli falling within the attended channel of attention, treats the relevant and irrelevant sources of information differently. They also suggest that this occurs not only within the relevant channel of attention, but without it too. Indeed, the present findings suggest that, while enhancing processing of frequency-relevant gratings with respect to frequency-irrelevant ones since the earliest sensory level, as reflected by C1, at the attended location, the system seems also actively to suppress the processing of the latter stimuli with respect to the former ones at the neglected location, already starting at early sensory level, as reflected by P1. As for the prefrontal cortex, ERPs data and their topography suggested that distinct sub-regions of the latter might serve distinct attention functions. In fact, while dorsolateral regions would control the orienting of attention toward relevant space locations, the left-hemisphere inferior posterior prefrontal cortex (PFC) may suppress processing of distractors within an attended channel. Conversely, the dorsal frontal-polar PFC might bust, although in different degrees, the post-perceptual/semantic processing of relevant information by posterior brain areas independent of location relevance.

Unilateral neglect refers to the failure, due to unilateral brain damage, in exploring portion of space contralateral to the side of lesion. It is a largely shared opinion that the deficit could be described with reference to specific spatial co-ordinate systems. Where neglect is referring to the mid-sagittal plane of the patient's body, it has been defined viewer–centred (or egocentric) and within it a variety of components have been distinguished, such as retinotopic-, head-, limb- and trunk-centred. Whereas, were patients show failures in representing stimuli within the extra-personal domain, such as the surrounding 'environment' and the hand-reach visual space, disorder has been specifically defined "allocentric" neglect. Several studies have compared the specific contribution of viewer and allocentric frames of reference on neglect. Some evidence suggests a major contribution of the environment-centred system on neglect. Other data support a viewer-centred predominance when the environmental frame is derived exclusively from gravitational information without using visual cues. In chapter III, the authors wished to learn how neglect allocation is affected by the differential intervention of viewer, environment and array centered spatial representations. Fifteen left-neglect patients were asked to search for visually presented targets. They performed the searching either in an upright position or lying on their right side, in a position orthogonal to the environment. This latter condition was meant to dissociate viewer-centered and environment-centered frames. The visual display, within which stimuli were presented, could be either aligned with the patient's body or rotated of 90° counterclockwise. Finally, they analyzed the effects of stimulus content on neglect severity. Numbers, letters, and drawings of objects or animals were used as stimuli. Patients' spatial neglect was found to be allocated mainly with reference to the viewer's body and, to a lesser degree, to the environment. Moreover, the amount of neglect centered on the environment was found to be enhanced by the alignment of the display with its vertical. The authors interpreted these data as an evidence that environment-centered neglect may be partially due to a mental rotation of viewer-based representations. This phenomenon would very likely be mediated by environmental visual cues as well as the visual display within which patients are searching for targets. Regarding stimulus material, patients manifested more severe neglect with figures, improved with letters and did even better with numbers. This pattern of results is in line with Weintraub and Mesulam's (1988) finding of a less severe neglect with 'verbal' than with 'non verbal' stimuli.

The aim of chapter IV was to determine the impact of neuropsychological parameters on the academic aptitude test (AAT) achievement at the end of high school in 1996 when they should be graduating from high school and on job status carried out six years later during 2002. From a representative sample of 1817 Chilean school-age children (mean age 18.0 ± 0.9 y) graduating from high school in 1996 in Chile's Metropolitan Region, 96 were selected with high (> 120 WAIS-R) and low IQ (< 100 WAIS-R) (1:1), from the high and low socio-economic strata (SES) (1:1) and of both sexes (1:1). AAT scores for university admission were obtained for 84 school-age children from University of Chile records and were divided into two groups: high AAT (≥ median (Md)= score 631) and low AAT (< Md). IQ was determined by the Wechsler Intelligence Scale for Adults (WAIS-R) and the Raven Progressive Matrices Test in the school-age children and their parents. Scholastic achievement (SA) was measured applying the standard Spanish language and mathematics tests. SES was evaluated using Graffar's modified method. Nutritional status was assessed through anthropometric measurements of weight and height to establish the body mass index (BMI) according to Garrow; head circumference (HC) was compared with Tanner, Nellhaus, Roche et al. and Ivanovic et al. tables and was expressed as Z score (Z-HC); body composition parameters such as arm circumference-for-age, triceps skinfold-for-age, arm muscle area-for-age and arm fat area-for-age were calculated using data from Frisancho. Brain morphology was determined by magnetic resonance imaging (MRI). Job status was expressed as: (1) jobless, (2) workers without further schooling, (3) students at institutes and (4) students at universities. Statistical analysis included correlation and logistic regressions using the Statistical Analysis System (SAS). Results showed that students with high AAT score presented IQ, parental IQ, SA, brain volume (BV), Z-HC, maternal schooling, house-hold head occupation and quality of housing significantly higher than their peers that achieved the lowest AAT scores of whom 19% had suffered severe undernutrition in the first year of life (Fisher p< 0.0054). However, logistic regression revealed that student IQ is the best predictor of AAT score and the odds ratio value (1.252) implies that when the IQ score increases by one point, the probability to obtain a high AAT score increases in 25.2%. Students at universities presented AAT, child and maternal IQ, SA, BV, birth weight and birth height, Z-HC and socio-economic conditions significantly higher than their peers from the other three job statuses; however, AAT score at the end of high school was the best predictor of the job status six years later (odds ratio value= 1.025) which indicates that when AAT score increases by one point the probability for university admission and for university graduation increases 2.5%. In a multifactorial approach, these results point out the importance of neuropsychological parameters on children's achievement for university admission and future jobs.

In chapter V, two experiments investigated the reliability of dichotic listening tasks under two conditions of administration: on tape or on a computer. Stimuli in both experiments were words (bower, dower, power, and tower) pronounced with an emotional tone of anger, happiness, neutrality, or sadness. Experiment 1 required participants to detect a target word in each dichotic pair. Accordingly, 40 right-handed participants were randomly assigned to a condition in which the dichotic word recognition task was completed twice either in a taped version or directly on a computer. Experiment 2 involved the detection of a target emotion. A different group of 40 right-handed participants completed the dichotic emotion recognition task twice either on tape or on-computer. In Experiment 1, results showed a large right ear advantage of similar magnitude and test-retest reliability on both versions of the task. In Experiment 2, the laterality effect also had a similar reliability in both versions. However, the magnitude of the observed left ear advantage (LEA) varied as a function of procedure.

Specifically, on computer, the LEA was significant only in females. Implications of these findings for the use of computer tasks to measure functional lateralization in research and applied settings are discussed. Factors responsible for variability in the results obtained in Experiment 2 are also discussed.

Although the power of memory is evident in various daily life experiences (e.g., personal history, knowledge of facts and concepts, and learning of complex skills), memory also has its fallible side. Memory experiences are encoded as separate pieces of a puzzle. At retrieval, this puzzle has to be reconstructed. This reconstruction makes our memory susceptible to distortions. Inspired by ongoing discussions about recovered memories, researchers have studied personality and social factors that make people vulnerable to memory distortions, including pseudo-memories. Recent studies highlight the role of higher cognitive functions in reconstructing our memories. Chapter VI aims to give an overview of the current state of affairs linking executive functions to pseudo-memories. Evidence from aging, lesion, and imaging studies (Positron Emission Tomography and functional Magnetic Resonance Imaging) will be discussed. Studies conducted in our laboratory also suggest that suboptimal inhibition, monitoring and working memory functions contribute to the development of pseudo-memories. Explaining and identifying the neural basis of pseudo-memories can be regarded as a promising and new domain within neuropsychology.

Polyphenols have received particular attention because of their possible beneficial health effects in age-related neurological disorders. In support of this hypothesis, epidemiological studies reported a lower incidence of stroke, Parkinson's disease and dementia in populations that consume beverages or food (i.e. red wine, green tea, fruits, vegetables) enriched in polyphenolic compounds. These findings concur with animal and *in vitro* studies indicating that polyphenols derived from either beverages, fruits (e.g. catechins, resveratrol) or plant extracts (i.e. blueberry, Ginkgo biloba and tea) displayed neuroprotective abilities. For example, the authors' studies and those obtained by other groups indicated that various polyphenols derived from green tea and red wine protected cultured neuronal cells against toxicity induced by free radicals and beta-amyloid (Aß) peptides, whose accumulation likely play a deleterious role in age-related neurological disorders. These effects involved their well-known antioxidant activities, but also their abilities to directly interact with Aß and to modulate intracellular effectors and genes associated with cell death/survival. Chapter VII overviews epidemiologic and pre-clinical studies that support the role of polyphenols in the beneficial effects of diet in human.

The purpose of chapter VIII is to review the recent literature regarding the assessment of biased responding, especially in the context of malingering. It makes the case that biased responding is multifaceted and that clinicians need to be aware of a variety of issues pertaining to effort. The different types of malingering are discussed, as well as the particular situations when patients are likely to feign symptoms. The more common commercially-available tests to assess effort are reviewed, with a discussion of their strengths and weaknesses. Other means of assessing response bias are mentioned, including the use of traditional neuropsychological assessments, as well as the issue of coached malingerers. Finally, specific suggestions for the practicing neuropsychologist are given.

In: Focus on Neuropsychology Research
Editor: Joshua R. Dupri, pp. 1-36

ISBN 1-59454-779-3
© 2006 Nova Science Publishers, Inc.

Chapter 1

NEURAL SUBSTRATES OF EXECUTIVE FUNCTIONS: INSIGHTS FROM FUNCTIONAL NEUROIMAGING

Robert M. Roth, John J. Randolph,*
Nancy S. Koven, and Peter K. Isquith

Neuropsychology Program and Brain Imaging Laboratory
Department of Psychiatry; Dartmouth Medical School

ABSTRACT

Executive function has been conceptualized as a set of interrelated cognitive processes that are essential for regulation of cognition, behavior, and emotion. Hypothesized component processes include cognitive flexibility, decision making, inhibitory control, planning and organization, self-monitoring, as well as working memory. Historically, the neurobiological basis of executive functions in humans was largely examined through the administration of performance-based neuropsychological tests to patients with acquired focal brain lesions. Such studies led to the widely held belief that the integrity of the frontal lobes is central to executive functions. However, while lesion studies have been highly informative, they suffer from a number of methodological weaknesses including the inability to investigate the broader neural circuitry that contributes to executive functions. Over the past twenty five years functional neuroimaging techniques, in particular positron emission tomography (PET) and functional magnetic resonance imaging (fMRI), have been increasingly applied in the effort to elucidate the neural circuitry subserving executive functions. In the present chapter, we review functional neuroimaging research addressing the neural substrates of executive functions in healthy adults, and discuss applications of neuroimaging techniques to the identification of the neural correlates of executive dysfunction in selected psychiatric and neurological illnesses.

---

* Corresponding author: Robert M. Roth, Ph.D., Brain Imaging Laboratory, Dartmouth Medical School/DHMC, 1 Medical center Drive, Lebanon, NH, USA 03756-0001. Phone: 603-650-5824; Fax: 603-650-5842; E-Mail: Robert.M.Roth@Dartmouth.edu

INTRODUCTION

The Executive Function Construct

Executive function may be conceptualized as a collection of interrelated higher level or supervisory cognitive processes involved in the selection, initiation, execution and monitoring of complex domain specific cognitive processes and motor responses, as well as aspects of emotional processing. Stated more broadly, executive functions are concerned with the self-regulation of cognition, behavior and emotion [1-3]. Executive functions have also been conceptualized as exerting regulatory control over the basic, domain-specific neuropsychological functions (e.g., language, visuospatial functions, memory, emotional experience, motor skills) in the service of reaching intended goals.

Executive function is generally considered an umbrella construct that subsumes a collection of related yet at least partially distinct processes that provide for intentional, goal-directed problem solving, as well as organization and direction of cognitive activity, emotional response, and overt behavior. However, the operational definition of executive function and the specific cognitive processes subsumed under this construct have varied somewhat among authors [4, 5, 6]. Theoretical concepts or models such as the *supervisory attention system* [7], the *central executive* [8], or *managerial knowledge units* [9] have been put forth in an effort to explain the structure and role of executive functions, as well as the relationship between executive and other cognitive functions. Processes commonly regarded as executive functions include the ability to initiate behaviors, inhibit competing actions or stimuli, select relevant goals, plan and organize means to solve complex problems, shift problem-solving strategies flexibly when necessary, regulate emotions, and monitor and evaluate behavior [3, 6, 10, 11]. Working memory capacity, whereby information is actively held "online" so that it may be manipulated and transformed in the service of planning and guiding cognition and behavior, is also described as a key aspect of executive function [11, 12].

Developmental Course

The development and maturation of executive functions is considerably more prolonged than that of other cognitive functions such as language [13-18], and differences in the developmental course of specific executive functions may also be observed [19]. This extended developmental course parallels the prolonged pattern of neurodevelopment of the frontal lobes including growth in synaptic connections, myelination, and bioelectric signal coherence [20-22]. The development of executive functions such as the self-regulation of emotion and behavior begins in infancy [23] and continues into the preschool period [24-27] through adolescence and early adulthood [28-30]. Decline in the use of executive functions in later adulthood and old age is also observed, though change tends to be modest and is not found for all executive functions nor for all healthy individuals [31-34]. As with many other dimensions of psychological and neuropsychological functioning, the decline of executive functions varies across individuals in terms of the age of onset, rate of decline, and actual proficiency level at any given age. Several variables have been associated with age-associated decline in executive functions such as changes in the structural integrity of white matter pathways, neurodegenerative changes in frontal lobe grey matter, as well as genetic factors [35-38].

Historical Perspective on the Neuroanatomical Basis

Executive functions were thought to be subserved primarily, if not solely, by the frontal lobe since at least the 19th century when Phineas Gage demonstrated dramatic changes in self-regulatory function after a dynamite tamping rod was propelled through his frontal lobe [39]. Further, more substantial evidence of executive deficits associated with frontal lobe damage came about in the 1940's and 1950's in the context of war related brain injury [e.g., 40]. However, a wealth of evidence has accumulated indicating that while damage to the frontal lobes can indeed result in significant executive dysfunction [41-43], these complex, higher order processes are not solely a product of frontal activity. Executive dysfunction may also be seen in cases of injury or pathology to non-frontal cortical as well as subcortical regions [e.g., 44, 45, 46]. Thus, the historical view of executive functions as subserved *solely* by the frontal lobes is an oversimplification of the complex organization of the brain, leading some authors to caution against attributing executive deficits to frontal lobe pathology except at a hypothesis generating level [47]. Nevertheless, an understanding of the frontal region of the brain is important in any discussion of the executive functions. The frontal lobes are richly and reciprocally interconnected through numerous neuroanatomical pathways with other cortical and subcortical regions of the brain such as the limbic (motivational/mnemonic) system, the reticular activating (arousal) system, the posterior association cortex (perceptual/cognitive processes and knowledge base), and the motor (action) regions [11, 48-51]. This broad connectivity underlies the regulatory control that the frontal brain systems exert over the posterior cortical and subcortical systems.

FUNCTIONAL NEUROIMAGING OF EXECUTIVE FUNCTIONS

Brain-behavior relationships underlying executive functions remain elusive given the challenges inherent in traditional neuropsychological methods. Recent advances in technology, specifically functional neuroimaging, are beginning to provide a more detailed picture of these relationships. In the present chapter we provide a brief description of the functional neuroimaging techniques most commonly employed to study executive functions. We then selectively review functional neuroimaging studies investigating the neural substrates of executive functions in healthy humans. Specifically, we discuss cognitive flexibility, decision making, planning, self-monitoring, response inhibition, organization, and working memory. We then illustrate the utility of functional neuroimaging for studying executive dysfunction in selected psychiatric and neurological disorders.

Some Functional Neuroimaging Basics

By far the most commonly employed functional neuroimaging technologies for studying the neural substrates of executive functions are positron emission tomography (PET) and functional magnetic resonance imaging (fMRI). Briefly, PET is a scanning technique that involves visualizing brain structure and function through the detection of small amounts of radioactively labeled compounds that are injected (e.g., water or glucose) or inhaled (e.g., oxygen) shortly before or during scans/tasks. As the radioactive atoms in the compound decay they release small positively charged particles called positrons. The positrons subsequently collide with negatively charged electrons resulting in the creation of a pair of particles of light called photons that are picked up by detectors in the scanner. Brain regions where the labeled compound has accumulated, and thus it is believed where activated related to a given task was greatest, are identified through computer programs designed to analyze the information and to generate three-dimensional, cross-sectional images that represent the biological activity where the compound has accumulated. PET is increasingly used in combination with computerized tomography and structural magnetic resonance imaging in order to provide more accurate localization of activation.

fMRI is based on the observation that hemodynamic activity is closely related to neural activity [52-54]. About four to six seconds after an electrical burst of neural activity can be detected in a region, a hemodynamic response occurs as active neurons use up oxygen from oxygen-rich blood that is infused into the region. fMRI takes advantage of the different magnetic properties of oxygenated and deoxygenated hemoglobin, each of which gives off a slightly different signal. The MRI scanner detects this slight difference, which is known as the blood oxygen level dependent (BOLD) contrast, and the information is used to generate three-dimensional images.

The two most commonly employed task designs in functional neuroimaging are referred to as *blocked* and *event-related* designs. Blocked designs involve the presentation of different task conditions in separate trains of stimuli called *epochs*. Conditions of interest may involve one or more cognitive, sensory or motor tasks. These conditions are then compared to control conditions in order to facilitate identification of brain regions specifically related to the task condition of interest. Control tasks are usually quite similar to the condition of interest, but exclude demands on the process of interest. For example, an imaging study of response inhibition may use a go/nogo task that has a condition in which 20% of stimuli are nogo and 80% of stimuli are go (i.e., inhibit condition), while another condition may involve only the presentation of only go stimuli without any demand for inhibition (i.e., control condition). Activation related to inhibition is found by subtracting activation to the 100% go condition from that found for the 20% nogo condition. In event-related designs, stimuli of interest are presented in random or pseudorandom order within the same epoch. Using the go/nogo example above, an event-related design could present the nogo and go stimuli in a random order within the same train of stimuli (e.g., go - go - nogo - go - nogo), and thus a direct comparison can be made between activations to the nogo and go stimuli.

Event-related designs have several advantages over blocked designs, such as allowing for greater control over the potential impact of fluctuations in arousal, attention, and mood over the course of an experiment. However, under some circumstances, blocked designs can be more powerful in detecting effects of interest. Several excellent texts are available for readers interested in more detailed explanations of these neuroimaging methods and their limitations, as well as data analytic techniques [55-57].

Cognitive Flexibility

The ability to think flexibly (also referred to as set shifting) is considered an integral component of normal executive functioning. Deficits in cognitive flexibility are often seen in patients with frontal lobe damage, especially when the dorsolateral cortex is involved. Such patients are generally slower to switch between two tasks or concepts, even when they are able to perform each of the two tasks accurately, and have difficulty benefiting from feedback indicating that their current pattern of responding is no longer correct [58].

Trail making tests are often administered to assess cognitive flexibility, and require the respondent to alternate cognitively and motorically between sets of numbers and letters. To examine brain regions activated during this kind of task-switching, Moll and colleagues used a verbal adaptation of a traditional paper-and-pencil trail-making test in an fMRI paradigm, reporting critical roles for the dorsolateral and medial frontal cortex, as well as the intraparietal sulcus [59]. Gurd et al. reported prominent posterior parietal fMRI activation when participants were required to produce triads of words from three semantic categories [60]. This pattern of activation underscores the role of widespread networks involved in set-shifting that extend beyond the frontal lobes and require coordination with posterior areas.

Another popular test of executive functioning, the Wisconsin Card Sorting Test (WCST), has also been examined using neuroimaging techniques to uncover frontal lobe activation correlates. Early PET and fMRI studies reported dorsolateral activation during WCST performance [61, 62], specifically bilateral inferior frontal sulci [63]. However, without further investigation, it is unclear whether this activation represents set-shifting, working memory, error recognition, or some combination of these executive processes, as the WCST is multidimensional in its task demands. To address this, Konishi and colleagues used event-related fMRI to compare patterns of brain activation during a set-shifting task condition of the WCST to those found during a working memory condition [64]. Results showed that activation associated with set-shifting overlapped in the same region of the inferior frontal sulci in which activation was found to be associated with working memory, suggesting that set-shifting and working memory act in concert in the same areas of the frontal cortex. A recent study that further decomposed elements of set-shifting found that right frontal regions were responsive to receipt of negative feedback during the WCST administration whereas analogous left frontal regions were activated during updating of behavior [65]. Given this evidence for hemispheric specialization within the set-shifting domain, it appears that interhemispheric transfer within frontal regions is the key for successful completion of this task. Monchi et al. also reported dissociations between regions activated to different aspects of the WCST [66]. They found that the mid-dorsolateral frontal cortex was activated when participants received either positive or negative feedback likely related to working memory demands; a cortical-basal ganglia circuit involving the mid-ventrolateral frontal cortex, caudate nucleus, and thalamus increased activity only for negative feedback, related to the need to shift response set; and posterior frontal cortex activity to both responding on the task and feedback, interpreted as suggesting a role in the association of specific stimuli to actions.

In summary, dorsolateral cortex is integral for performing aspects of task switching yet acts jointly with posterior brain regions for successful execution. Some evidence suggests frontal laterality with left and right regions specialized for different aspects of set-shifting. Other evidence indicates considerable overlap in frontal lobe regions during both tasks of mental flexibility and working memory, highlighting the multifunctional role of the same tissue.

Decision Making

The ability to make decisions, particularly when faced with novel and/or complex problems, is a fundamental skill for everyday life. Neuropsychologists are commonly confronted with patients who have difficulty making decisions or who make poor decisions that lead to significant difficulties in their lives such as interpersonal, legal, or occupational problems. The contribution that functional neuroimaging can make to our understanding of the neural substrates of decision making is highlighted by evidence that standard neuropsychological tests may be insensitive in some patients who show problems with decision making in everyday life [e.g., 67].

Two neuroimaging studies have employed the "Iowa Gambling Task" originally developed by Bechara and colleagues [68], a task commonly used to assess decision making ability in behavioral studies. On each trial a card is selected from one of four decks and feedback is provided. However, the nature of the feedback is predetermined by the experimenter with a fixed schedule of reward (win money) and punishment (lose money) for each of the decks, but with occasional, unpredictable monetary loss that is higher for the decks that provide higher rewards when selected. An attractive feature of this task is that it reflects aspects of real life decision making such as dealing with uncertainty and modifying future decisions based on positive and negative feedback. Behavioral investigations with this task have shown that poor performance is associated with lesions in the ventromedial aspect of the orbital frontal cortex and amygdala, although not exclusively [69, 70]. Using PET, Ernst et al. demonstrated widespread activations including the orbital and dorsolateral frontal cortex, as well as the anterior cingulate gyrus during the gambling task (71). Fukui and colleagues demonstrated that risky as opposed to safe decisions (based on the card deck selected) during the gambling task were specifically associated with medial frontal fMRI activation [72].

Rogers and colleagues employed PET with participants performing a task that involved predicting which of two computer generated outcomes would occur [73]. Importantly, both a large reward and large penalty were associated with selection of the least likely outcome, while a small reward and small penalty was associated with the most likely outcome. Brain activation related to making decisions was observed in the anterior-lateral part of the middle frontal gyrus, posterior part of the anterior inferior frontal gyrus, and orbital frontal gyrus, as well as areas within the cerebellum and parietal lobes.

Paulus et al. conducted a PET study in which participants had to decide in which of two locations a stimulus would appear [74]. Unbeknownst to participants, 50% of responses were preset to be correct, irrespective of location. Thus feedback was unhelpful in guiding decision making, in contrast to studies in which feedback could be used to increase advantageous decision making. Areas of activation observed included the dorsolateral frontal cortex, cingulate gyrus, parietal lobe, insula, and thalamus. Further research by this group found that error rates and varying predictability of the feedback affected frontal-parietal and cingulate activation in a manner consistent with the idea that these regions are involved in maintaining a representation of the history of responses and their outcomes in order to inform ongoing decision making, as well as playing a role in switching between decision making strategies [75].

Other research suggests that different cognitive components of decision making are associated with at least partially non-overlapping neural circuitry. A PET study investigated brain activation during performance of a task requiring participants to identify, through hypothesis testing and feedback, a rule determining which of two checkerboard stimuli was correct on each trial (although in actuality feedback was arbitrary) [76]. The task was performed with and without the requirement to make an actual choice via a motor response, permitting a dissociation of neural activity associated with hypothesis generation/testing and that related to making a decision based on the hypotheses. During hypothesis generation/testing, activations were noted in the cerebellum, anterior cingulate gyrus, right precuneus, right thalamus, and left inferior frontal gyrus. In contrast, when participants were required to make a decision based on their hypotheses, the left anterior cingulate gyrus and right lateral orbitofrontal cortex were activated. A recent fMRI study reported that the cerebellum appears to play an important role in the use of probabilistic reasoning to inform decision making under conditions of uncertainly (for example, inferring that your boss is angry because you were late for a meeting rather than several other possible causes) [77], consistent with the prior observation of cerebellar activation during hypothesis generation/testing [76].

While research into the neural substrates of decision making is limited, these functional neuroimaging studies have been largely consistent with behavioral work indicating a particularly important role for the frontal cortex. There is some suggestion that different frontal subregions may be preferentially recruited depending on whether decision making can be guided by feedback versus when the relationship between decisions and feedback are random [74]. Furthermore, preliminary evidence suggests that various cognitive operations involved in decision making likely involve at least partially non-overlapping neural circuitry.

Planning

The ability to plan behavior is a critical executive function used in daily life, and involves activities such as thinking ahead, setting goals, determining a course of action, and using relational logic to proceed through a task or problem. Functional imaging studies of planning ability have typically involved use of the Tower of London and Tower of Hanoi paradigms. For the Tower of London, participants view a split screen with a "problem space" and a "goal space." The goal space contains three pegs with an arrangement of colored balls that needs to be matched by manually (using a response glove) or mentally manipulating balls in the problem space. Some studies employ easy and hard conditions, which typically require 2-3 and 4-5 move solutions, respectively. Control conditions typically consist of counting total number of balls of specific colors (see Figure 1 for an illustration). For the Tower of Hanoi paradigm, discs of different sizes are arranged a priori on three pegs, and participants are instructed to move discs so that they are arranged in hierarchical order onto a specified peg.

In general, there do not appear to be significant differences in activation patterns based on response modality (i.e., solving problems mentally or manually), although conceptually, the mentally based paradigm involves a greater working memory component.

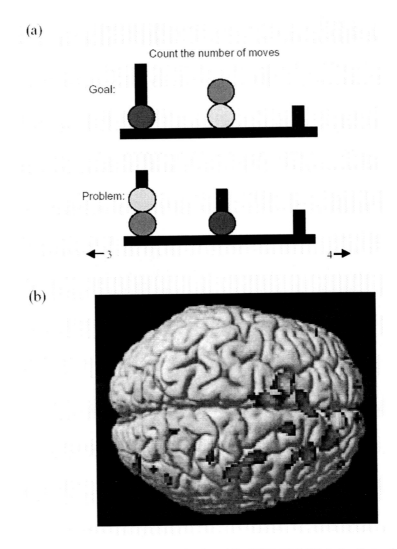

Figure 1. (1a) illustration of a Tower of London task adapted for fMRI; (b) fMRI during the hard condition relative to the easy task condition (difficulty being based on number of moves required to solve problem) in a healthy adult, showing prominent right hemisphere, especially frontal lobe, activation (*from the Brain Imaging Laboratory at Dartmouth Medical School*)

Imaging studies across Tower of London and Tower of Hanoi paradigms have generally found activity in bilateral frontal and striatal regions. In an early study using SPECT, Rezai et al. found that performance on the Tower of London activated left and right mesial frontal cortex (left greater than right) and right parietal cortex, and produced decreased left occipital cortex activation [78]. Morris et al. also investigated Tower of London activation using SPECT, and found increased left frontal cortical activation, particularly when participants took more time to plan their moves and when participants used fewer moves to complete a problem [79]. Baker et al. used PET to examine activation patterns during the Tower of London more broadly, and found that performance was associated with bilateral premotor and dorsolateral frontal cortex, anterior cingulate gyrus, bilateral medial and superior parietal cortex, lateral occipital cortex, left cerebellar hemisphere and cerebellar vermis, right thalamus, and right caudate nucleus [80]. They also found that increasing task difficulty (i.e., using a hard vs. easy condition subtraction) was associated with relative increases in frontal, premotor, and medial parietal cortices and robust activations in right dorsolateral frontal and bilateral premotor cortex. Decreased activation in the posterior cingulate gyrus, bilateral hippocampus and insula, and left cerebellum was associated with increased task difficulty. In another early PET study using the Tower of London paradigm, Owen et al. found increased activation in left dorsolateral frontal cortex and the head of the left caudate nucleus when comparing a difficult planning condition (4-5 move solution) to a control condition [81]. Contrasting simple from difficult conditions revealed increased activation in left caudate nucleus and right thalamus. Dagher et al. used five levels of problem complexity (1-5 move solutions) to examine PET activation on a modified Tower of London task [82]. These authors found that increasing task complexity correlated with increased activation in bilateral premotor, dorsolateral frontal, and rostral anterior cingulate cortex, and right dorsal caudate nucleus.

In recent years, increasingly sophisticated experimental designs have allowed for additional levels of analysis and enhanced spatial resolution of brain activation patterns in response to planning; these studies have primarily used fMRI. In the first fMRI study of Tower of London activation, Lazeron et al. found increased activity in bilateral dorsolateral frontal cortex, left anterior cingulate cortex, left insula, and bilateral cuneus and precuneus, and left angular gyrus [83]. In contrast to previous work, they did not find activation differences across easy and hard conditions. Rowe et al. examined activation patterns associated with planning and executing Tower of London moves versus merely imagining necessary moves without actually solving problems [84]. Activations associated with planning, executing, and imagining moves were in dorsal frontal, parietal, and premotor cortex as well as the cerebellum, with no dissociable activation for specific conditions, suggesting that the dorsal frontal cortex is involved in multiple aspects of planning. Employing the Tower of Hanoi paradigm, Fincham et al trained participants extensively to use a specific strategy ("perceptual subgoaling") to solve the Tower of Hanoi problems, thereby clarifying active circuitry during use of a specific strategy [85]. Using event-related fMRI, they found a functional dissociation pattern between working memory task demands in right frontal and parietal regions, and planning of task subgoals associated with left posterior frontal activity.

More recently, van den Heuvel et al. used a parametric, event-related fMRI Tower of London task to examine brain activation patterns associated with planning. Such a design enabled analysis not only of performance based on task complexity, but also based specifically on correct responses by "binning" such responses for functional analyses [86]. Planning was associated with activation in right dorsolateral frontal cortex, left caudate nucleus, bilateral precuneus, bilateral inferior parietal cortex, bilateral premotor cortex, right globus pallidus, and right insular cortex. Task complexity was positively correlated with left dorsolateral frontal cortex, left insular cortex, right globus pallidus, and right caudate nucleus activity. Newman et al. employed multiple analytic strategies, including fMRI, functional connectivity analysis, and computational modeling to examine activation patterns associated with Tower of London performance [87]. Their findings indicated that bilateral frontal cortical activation was associated with moderate and difficult Tower of London items, with attenuated right frontal activation on easy problems. Functional connectivity analyses showed increased and correlated right frontal and superior parietal activity when task demands increased.

In summary, activation patterns on tasks of strategic planning in healthy adults generally involve bilateral frontal and striatal regions. Recruitment of parietal and selected other regions are also observed and appear to depend on the nature of the task design and paradigm employed.

Response Inhibition

Response inhibition, the ability to withhold responding to task irrelevant information, stop one's behavior at the appropriate time or to a stimulus, or terminate specific thoughts, is considered by some as a core executive function [88]. Functional neuroimaging research on the neural substrates of response inhibition has commonly relied upon adaptations of tests well known in the clinical neuropsychology literature, most often variations on the classic go/nogo and Stroop tasks. Other studies have used adaptations of less widely used tests, while still others have employed more experimental tasks in the scanner.

Konishi and colleagues conducted two studies using event-related fMRI to evaluate the neural correlates of response inhibition using a simple two stimulus go/nogo task. Results revealed that inhibition was associated with right posterior inferior frontal cortex activation irrespective of the hand used to respond to the go stimulus [64, 89]. Other studies using basic go/nogo tasks have observed nogo-related activations in other regions including bilateral middle frontal cortex, left dorsal premotor, dorsolateral frontal, striatum, parietal lobe and the occipital-temporal area [90-92].

Several investigations have used continuous performance type tasks to study inhibitory control. For example, Garavan and colleagues required participants to press a button whenever target letters (X and Y) were presented. However, they were to alternate responding to these target letters such that if any one of them was presented twice in a row, the second presentation would require withholding responding (i.e., become a nogo stimulus on that trial) [93, 94]. Results indicated that successful inhibition was associated with activation of the several predominantly right hemisphere regions including the inferior and middle frontal gyri, insula, and the inferior parietal lobule.

Numerous studies have employed adaptations of the Stroop task to study response inhibition, or interference control as it is often referred to in such studies. Several PET studies have been conducted with most showing that the interference effect is most strongly associated with activation of the anterior cingulate gyrus [95-98]. Blocked and event-related fMRI studies have also observed anterior cingulate gyrus activation with a fair degree of consistency [99-101] (see Figure 2 for an illustration). Some negative findings have however been reported for the cingulate [102], and interference effect related activations have also been reported for several other regions in PET and fMRI studies including the inferior frontal gyrus, insula, parietal lobe, striatum, thalamus, as well as the frontopolar and occipital-temporal regions [e.g. 97, 98, 101, 102]. In addition, the precise role of the anterior cingulate gyrus in Stroop task performance is a matter of considerable debate, with some authors arguing for a role in cognitive processes other than response inhibition [103].

(a)

Neutral Condition	Congruent Condition	Incongruent Condition
XXXX	TWO	TWO
XXXX	TWO	TWO
XXXX		TWO
XXXX		

(b)

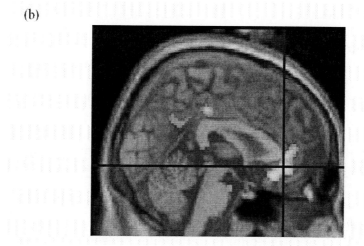

Figure 2. (a) illustration of a Counting Stroop task adapted for fMRI; (b) fMRI during the incongruent condition relative to the congruent condition in a group of 13 healthy adults, showing prominent activation of the anterior cingulate gyrus (*from the Brain Imaging Laboratory at Dartmouth Medical School*)

These investigations demonstrate that response inhibition involves distributed neural circuitry including several frontal lobe subregions and other cortical and subcortical areas. The variability noted in regions activated is consistent with the idea that the specific cognitive operations underlying successful inhibition will likely differ to some extent depending on the nature of the task and task parameters employed, such as stimulus duration, demands placed on working memory, and frequency of nogo stimuli within the train of go stimuli. For example, the Stroop task requires inhibition of a competing response (i.e., word) in order to provide a response to the target stimulus (i.e., color). In contrast, in a simple two stimulus go/nogo task, one must inhibit responding to a specific single stimulus and no alternate response is required. Furthermore, while neuropsychological tests and functional neuroimaging tasks have generally focused on inhibition of motor or cognitive responses, the neural circuitry observed likely differs to some extent from that required for the inhibition of emotional responses [e.g., 104, 105]. Finally, although lesion studies have often suggested a role for the orbitofrontal cortex in response inhibition [106], few neuroimaging studies have observed activation in this region association with inhibition [107, 108]. This discrepancy is likely due in part to the difficulty imaging the orbitofrontal region secondary to current technical limitations.

Self-Monitoring

Self-monitoring is an important yet historically overlooked aspect of executive functioning. It is a multi-faceted concept that involves not only the ability to monitor ongoing behaviors, but also to identify and acknowledge personal characteristics, perspectives, and tendencies. Fortunately, neuroimaging of neural substrates of self-monitoring, as assessed using self-reflection tasks, has received considerable attention in recent years. Self-reflection studies typically ask participants to rate statements that apply to self-related or other-related judgments. Activation patterns associated with self-reflection often include anterior and posterior cingulate cortex and bilateral frontal regions, with additional areas of activity depending on the task paradigm. Although some authors specifically reference the right frontal cortex as a seat of self-related processing [109], others dispute this notion [110].

An early functional imaging study used PET to determine brain activation correlated with rating relevance of trait adjectives to self versus others [111]. Findings indicated that processing of self-related adjectives activated right anterior cingulate and left frontal regions. Using fMRI, Kircher et al. investigated activation patterns associated with self-descriptive adjectives from a list that were previously rated by participants as reflecting their core personality characteristics [112]. Activation on this task was primarily in the left hemisphere and included left inferior frontal, left anterior cingulate, and left parietal cortex, and as well as bilateral precuneus regions. Using a unique paradigm, Vogeley et al. asked participants to read brief stories or hypothetical situations and then ascribe responsibility in these passages to themselves (self condition) or to others (Theory of Mind condition) [113]. Activation in self conditions was found in bilateral anterior cingulate cortex, right premotor cortex, bilateral precuneus, and the right temporal-parietal junction. Gusnard et al. found that ratings of self-referential versus non-self referential pictures were associated with increases in dorsal medial frontal cortex activity and relative decreases in ventral medial frontal activity [114]. These authors posited that dorsal medial frontal is associated with attention-demanding processing generally, and self-referential processing specifically. Using fMRI, Johnson et al. asked participants to rate self-reflective (e.g., "I'm a good friend") and semantic (e.g., "You need water to live") statements with yes/no responses [115]. They found that self-reflection was associated with activity in anterior medial frontal and posterior cingulate cortex, thalamus, bilateral inferior temporal gyrus, and bilateral cerebellum.

Initial studies examining neural correlates of self-reflection generally used blocked fMRI designs and few secondary analyses. More recent studies have employed event-related designs, functional connectivity analyses, and higher spatial resolution secondary to use of more sophisticated imaging magnets, and theoretical perspectives from convergent disciplines. For example, using event-related fMRI, Kelley et al. asked participants to rate trait adjectives relative to themselves or another person (President George W. Bush), or a control task involving judging whether a word was in upper or lowercase letters [116]. Ratings of self or another person, compared to the control task, were associated with inferior left frontal and anterior cingulate activity. Activation specific to self ratings was associated with medial frontal cortex and posterior cingulate activity. Kjaer et al. used PET and connectivity analyses to examine self-reflection [117]. In contrast to previous studies using only brief periods of self-reflective thought, these authors had participants "think intensely" for two minutes during four separate conditions: own personality traits, own physical appearance, other's personality traits (i.e., the Danish Queen; the study was conducted in Denmark), and other physical appearance. They found that reflection on personal characteristics was associated activation in precuneus, angular gyri bilaterally, and anterior cingulate cortex. Connectivity analyses indicated correlated activity between the anterior cingulate gyrus, precuneus, and cerebellum during self-reflection as well as connectivity between the precuneus and frontal, temporal, and parietal regions. Using fMRI, Schmitz et al. examined activation patterns in response to trait adjectives that described participants or significant others relative to a control condition where participants rated the positive valence of the same adjectives [118]. Results indicated that in self- or other-referential conditions, increased activation was observed in anterior medial frontal and retrosplenial cortex relative to the control condition. When comparing self-evaluation to other-evaluation conditions, activation was specific to right dorsolateral frontal cortex, again indicating the critical role of this region in self-reflection.

Building on social cognitive theory, Lieberman et al. recently attempted to dissociate evidence-based versus intuition-based self-knowledge systems [119]. Participants rated adjectives related to areas in which they had high or low experience (soccer and acting); the authors hypothesized that the process of rating adjectives in areas where participants had high levels of experience would more likely activate brain regions associated with intuitive self-reflection compared to regions activated by rating low-experience activities. Results indicated that this was indeed the case, with high experience ratings activating ventromedial frontal cortex, basal ganglia, and amygdala, regions previously thought to be associated with intuitive self-reflective thought. Ratings in low experience areas were associated with regions believed to be involved in evidence-based, episodic self-reflection including lateral frontal cortex, posterior parietal cortex, and the hippocampus.

One additional area of research relative to self-reflection is sleep, which is known to be associated with decreased self-awareness [120]. During rapid eye movement sleep (which is associated with dreaming), in particular, reduced brain activity has been noted in precuneus, orbital and dorsolateral frontal, parietal, and posterior cingulate cortex [121], that is, the very areas that tend to show activation during self-reflective tasks. Similarly, during slow-wave sleep, reduced activity occurs in precuneus, orbitofrontal cortex, and anterior cingulate cortex [122]. In general, brain activation on tasks of self-reflection tends to occur primarily in medial and dorsolateral frontal and parietal regions, although due to moderate variability in task design, patterns tend to vary across most studies.

Organization

The ability to organize information, thoughts or behaviors in a logical sequence or grouping can considerably facilitate task completion or recall of information from memory. Some work has specifically examined activation patterns related to spontaneous or trained use of cognitive strategies in executive and memory tasks. This work has relevance for the majority of functional neuroimaging research, as variable strategy use tends to be associated with differential patterns of brain activity. Elfgren and Risberg examined activation patterns associated with use of verbal and visual strategies during verbal and design fluency tasks [123]. Findings indicated that during a verbal fluency task, participants who used a verbal strategy to recall words showed increased left frontal activation relative to a control condition. Those reporting use of both verbal and visual strategies did not show similar changes. For a design fluency condition, participants using a visuospatial strategy showed bilateral frontal and right orbital and dorsolateral activation. Those using mixed verbal and visual strategies on this task showed primarily left frontal activation including dorsolateral, orbital, and superior frontal regions. In terms of behavioral performance, participants using a verbal strategy generated more words than those using mixed strategies; no performance differences were found based on differential strategy use on the design fluency task. Supporting this work was a study by Reichle et al. who examined differences in neural activity in participants using primarily verbal or visuospatial strategies during a sentence-picture verification task [124]. These authors found expected increases in left frontal regions, particularly Broca's area, during employment of verbal strategies, and parietal activity during visuospatial strategy use. Mediating these patterns, however, were individual differences in cognitive skills; participants with better reading span performance showed less activation in Broca's area when using a verbally mediated strategy, and those with better spatial reasoning skill showed less left parietal activity. These findings suggest that activation patterns are not only a function of strategy employed, but also baseline cognitive abilities.

Burbaud et al. examined activation patterns associated with spontaneous cognitive strategy on a serial subtraction task [125]. Participants using a verbal strategy primarily showed activation in left dorsolateral frontal cortex; those using a visually mediated strategy displayed bilateral frontal and left inferior parietal activation. In an attempt to better understand the neural underpinnings of episodic memory encoding, Savage et al. used PET to examine the ability to organize information from a word list by semantic category [126]. Findings indicated that overt attempts to semantically encode information were associated with left inferior and left dorsolateral frontal activation relative to covert or absent semantic encoding. Further, these effects were significantly moderated by orbitofrontal blood flow in that participants with increased perfusion in this region tended to spontaneously use semantic strategies during free recall. A study by Fink et al. indicated that differential strategy use on a line bisection judgment task was associated with overlapping but generally distinct activation patterns [127]. Specifically, when participants were asked to compare length of left and right line segments, they activated left superior posterior parietal cortex. When asked to determine whether a mark represented the center of a line, participants activated the lingual gyrus bilaterally and anterior cingulate cortex.

Training of cognitive strategies has also been found to alter brain activity or neurochemistry. For example, Valenzuela et al. found evidence of positive changes in hippocampal neurochemistry after training of multiple verbal and visual memory strategies in healthy older adults [128]. Olesen et al. examined activation changes secondary to training of working memory and found increased activity after training in right middle frontal gyrus, right inferior parietal cortex, and bilaterally in the intraparietal cortex [129]. Overall, activation patterns secondary to strategy use involve increased frontal and parietal activity, tend to vary across studies and paradigms, and differ based on factors such as baseline cognitive ability, task employed, and spontaneous versus experimenter-generated strategy.

Working Memory

Working memory involves the retention and manipulation of information in memory "online" over time. This executive function has received by far the most empirical attention in the neuroimaging literature, in part due to its hypothesized involvement in several illnesses, and due to its central role in many theories of cognitive functioning [11, 88, 130, 131].

In one of the first functional neuroimaging studies examining working memory, Jonides and colleagues used PET and a spatial working memory dot-probe task in which participants were presented with a spatial configuration of dots over a brief time delay and asked to identify whether a subsequently presented probe coincided with a dot location [132]. Results revealed prominent activation of the inferior frontal gyrus. Other PET and fMRI neuroimaging studies have also utilized various delayed-response tasks that place demands on working memory for spatial [e.g., 133, 134, 135] or verbal stimuli [136-139], with most studies providing additional support for the role of the frontal lobes, particularly the dorsolateral frontal cortex, in active maintenance processes.

In addition to delayed-response paradigms, many neuroimaging studies have utilized n-back tasks to examine neural networks involved in working memory [e.g., 140, 141-143]. In the n-back task (see Figure 3 for an illustration), stimuli such as letters are presented consecutively and participants are required to respond to any letter that is identical to the letter presented one, two, or three trials back. Investigations using the n-back have most commonly reported that the dorsolateral and ventral frontal cortical regions are associated with sustained active maintenance processes while the ventral region is also activated during more transient working memory processes. Similar findings have been found using non-visual stimuli [144, 145], highlighting the substantial overlap in areas of activation within the frontal cortex seen when demand is placed on working memory.

During working memory tasks, bilateral frontal lobe as well as bilateral parietal lobe activations are frequently noted. However, there is evidence to suggest some degree of modality specificity with respect to regions of the frontal cortex activated during working memory tasks, with the verbal task showing greater left [144, 146] and spatial tasks [136, 147] showing greater right activation in homologous regions, although this hemispheric asymmetry has not been reported consistently [142]. Other studies have begun to suggest that different subregions within the frontal lobe may play unique roles in various aspects of working memory. For example, Petrides has posited a dissociation between the dorsolateral and ventral frontal cortex, with ventral regions being associated with active maintenance of information in working memory, and dorsal regions recruited only when active manipulation/monitoring of information within working memory is required [148]. D'Esposito and colleagues found support for this dorsal/ventral dissociation using working memory tasks that required the manipulation of information (e.g., n-back tasks) and tasks that required maintenance of information over time (e.g., delayed-response tasks) [136]. Several other PET and fMRI studies have also found support for the dorsal/ventral dichotomy [e.g., 137, 149, 150-153; although some inconsistent findings have also been reported [142, 154, 155].

Although much of the focus has been on identifying the specific subregions with the frontal cortex involved in aspects of working memory, several other brain regions also appear to be involved in this cognitive function, consistent with the evidence for distributed networks underlying other executive functions. These regions include most prominently the posterior parietal cortex, anterior cingulate gyrus, and basal ganglia [156-158]. Further research will likely provide additional evidence for the heterogeneity of frontal subregions and their associated cortical and subcortical circuitry with respect to their role in specific components of working memory processes.

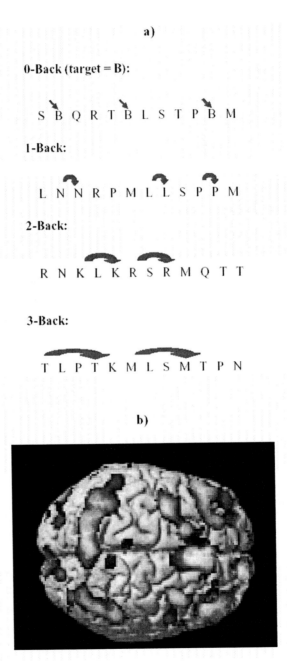

Figure 3. (a) illustration of an auditory-verbal n-back task adapted for fMRI; (b) fMRI during the 3-back condition relative to a 0-back vigilance control condition in a healthy adult, showing prominent bilateral frontal and parietal activation (*from the Brain Imaging Laboratory at Dartmouth Medical School*)

FUNCTIONAL IMAGING OF EXECUTIVE FUNCTIONS IN SELECTED PSYCHIATRIC AND NEUROLOGICAL DISORDERS

As noted above, executive dysfunction is observed in numerous psychiatric, neurological and systemic disorders. For many such disorders the specific nature and course of executive dysfunction, its impact on daily functioning, and its etiological correlates and treatment are the subject of considerable empirical research. A comprehensive review of the literature on executive functions in these disorders is beyond the scope of the present chapter. Here we briefly review research evaluating brain activation during the performance of executive function tasks in selected disorders to illustrate the potential for functional neuroimaging to help elucidate the neural substrates of executive dysfunction. Specifically, we discuss literature on attention-deficit/hyperactivity disorder, schizophrenia, multiple sclerosis, and traumatic brain injury.

Attention-Deficit/Hyperactivity Disorder (ADHD)

Executive dysfunction in ADHD has been observed on a variety of clinical and experimental neuropsychological tests that require executive functions for adequate performance [159-162]. Furthermore, executive dysfunction in children with ADHD may also be recognized by parents and teachers in naturalistic settings [163]. Executive dysfunction in ADHD is found in both children and adults with the disorder, is not limited to a given subtype, cannot be readily accounted for by comorbid psychopathology, and may improve with stimulant medications such as methylphenidate [162, 164-166].

Among the executive functions, deficits in working memory and response inhibition have been posited as being core cognitive difficulties in ADHD [88]. Functional neuroimaging studies have found abnormalities in patients with ADHD during the performance of tasks involving working memory or response inhibition. Schweitzer et al. used PET in 6 adults with ADHD and 6 healthy participants performing a Paced Auditory Serial Addition Test (PASAT). Results revealed that while the healthy group activated the expected frontal and temporal lobe regions, adults with ADHD showed prominent parietal-occipital activations [167]. The presence of more prominent posterior activations in the ADHD group was interpreted as possibly reflecting greater reliance on visual skills to compensate for frontal impairment. Valera and colleagues studied working memory in 20 unmedicated adults with ADHD and 20 healthy participants using a 2-back verbal working memory fMRI task [168]. While the groups did not differ with respect to behavioral performance, the ADHD group showed significantly reduced activation in cerebellar and occipital regions, as well as a trend towards less activation of the frontal lobe relative to the healthy group. Together, these studies support the involvement of frontal lobe abnormality in working memory deficits seen in ADHD, while findings for other regions are inconsistent.

Response inhibition has been studied in ADHD using Stroop, Stop Signal, and go/nogo tasks. Bush and colleagues demonstrated reduced anterior cingulate gyrus activation but abnormally increased frontal-striatal-insular activation in adults with ADHD during performance of an fMRI Counting Stroop Task [169]. Durston et al. observed decreased caudate nucleus and globus pallidus activation, as well as increased right parietal and posterior cingulate activation, in children with ADHD relative to a healthy comparison group when required to inhibit responding during a go/nogo task [170]. Two other fMRI studies of inhibitory control using go/nogo and stop signal tasks in children and adolescents with ADHD also reported reduced striatal activation [171, 172]. Striatal activation has also been reported to increase following treatment with methylphenidate for ADHD [172]. Findings for frontal lobe changes have been inconsistent, with some studies reporting decreased activation [170, 171] while others report increased activation [172, 173].

Overall, functional neuroimaging studies indicate that executive dysfunction in ADHD is related to abnormality of frontal-striatal and cerebellar circuitry. Furthermore, during the performance of executive tasks, other frontal and non-frontal regions may be recruited to compensate for abnormal regions. The finding of abnormal frontal, striatal and cerebellar activation in studies of ADHD appears to be consistent with evidence of structural abnormalities in these regions [174-177], although the precise relationship between structural and functional abnormalities remains to be elucidated.

Schizophrenia

A large literature on cognitive functioning in schizophrenia suggests that individuals with this illness display deficits across numerous neuropsychological domains, including deficits in sensory-motor skills, language functioning, affective processing, intellectual abilities, memory, visual-spatial skills, attention, and executive functioning [for review see, 178]. The magnitude of the cognitive deficit in schizophrenia can remain relatively stable over time despite fluctuations in other symptoms, and the degree of dysfunction has high predictive value for long-term disability [179].

Early functional neuroimaging research on schizophrenia used PET while patients performed the Wisconsin Card Sorting Task (WCST). Results generally showed decreased activation most prominently in the dorsolateral frontal cortex [180-182]. More recent fMRI research using the WCST replicated the PET findings, showing reduced frontal, temporal, and cerebellar activation [183, 184]. Despite some negative findings, reduced frontal activation during WCST performance remains one of the most consistent findings in the schizophrenia literature [185]. The abnormality observed with WCST performance in schizophrenia has been argued to reflect deficits in cognitive flexibility and/or working memory. Abnormal brain activation in schizophrenia has also been noted on several different verbal and visual tasks of working memory such as the Sternberg Item Recognition Task [186, 187] and the n-back task [188-192] using either PET or fMRI.

Furthermore, patients with schizophrenia have been demonstrated to have abnormal brain activation on tasks tapping other executive functions such as planning, response inhibition and decision making. Andreasen and colleagues used PET in a study of Tower of London performance in neuroleptic-naïve and chronic patients with schizophrenia [193]. Both patient groups showed lower left medial frontal and right parietal activation relative to a healthy comparison group. Also using PET, Yucel et al. noted decreased activity in the anterior cingulate gyrus in patients with schizophrenia during a Stroop task [194]. fMRI has also been used to investigate response inhibition in schizophrenia. Rubia et al. reported that relative to a comparison group, patients with schizophrenia show decreased activation in left anterior cingulate during both a go/nogo and stop signal task, with reduced left dorsolateral frontal and increased thalamus and putamen activations also seen during a stop signal task [195]. Perlstein et al. observed that patients with schizophrenia have reduced right dorsolateral frontal cortex activation when required to inhibit responding during a continuous performance test [196]. Decision making deficits in schizophrenia have been found to be associated with abnormally decreased fMRI activation of the inferior and medial frontal and superior temporal gyrus, as well as increased activation of the parietal cortex [197].

It is clear from the confluence of data that brain activation is abnormal in schizophrenia during the performance of tasks evaluating a variety of executive functions. However, inconsistency in the patterns of activation has been noted. For example, different studies have reported that frontal lobe activation in schizophrenia is normal, increased or decreased, may be spatially extended, and abnormalities have been lateralized to both the left and right hemispheres. The reasons for these discrepancies remain to be determined but likely include differences in the nature of the tasks used and study design, patient sample characteristics, as well as brain scanning parameters. Furthermore, it remains uncertain whether dysfunction arises from neural abnormalities primarily in frontal regions or as a result of dysregulation of the frontal lobe by other structures such as anterior cingulate, parietal cortex, basal ganglia, hippocampus, or thalamus. The application of higher-order multivariate statistical techniques to the analysis of functional activation connectivity patterns likely will prove helpful in characterizing the relationships between regional abnormalities [e.g., 198, 199].

Multiple Sclerosis

Cognitive dysfunction has been observed in 43-65% of patients with multiple sclerosis (MS) [200], and executive functions are among the most commonly impaired cognitive abilities [201, 202]. Only recently has research focused on the neural correlates of executive function and dysfunction in MS.

The majority of studies examining neural correlates of executive function in MS have focused on working memory. Staffen et al. used fMRI to investigate brain activation associated with working memory by using a visual form of the Paced Auditory Serial Addition Test (PASAT) in early-stage MS patients [203]. Despite similar behavioral performance relative to controls, MS patients showed differential brain activation relative to controls, primarily in terms of increased right dorsolateral frontal activity, interpreted as evidence of neural plasticity. Mainero et al. examined activation associated with the original PASAT task in MS patients, and found that patients' expanded brain activation in bilateral frontal, parietal, and temporal regions became less significant as task performance declined [204]. In a recent study, Wishart et al. examined brain activation patterns associated with working memory in MS using the n-back task [205]. They found that, although behavioral performance on the task was similar between patients and matched controls, patients showed decreased activation in traditional areas of working memory circuitry (i.e., frontal and parietal regions), and increased activation in medial frontal, bilateral middle temporal, and occipital regions. These findings were interpreted as representing compensatory patterns of brain activation that were associated with intact performance in the face of ongoing neurological disease. Sweet et al. also employed the n-back task in MS patients [206]. These authors found that patients' activation patterns were relatively consistent with previously documented working memory circuitry, although enhanced activation was noted in left hemispheric regions including sensorimotor, anterior cingulate, dorsolateral, and orbitofrontal cortex. Au Duong et al. investigated effective connectivity based on early-stage MS patients' performance on the PASAT [207]. Results indicated that, relative to matched controls, MS patients showed significantly altered connectivity throughout a hypothesized working memory network involving bilateral frontal and anterior cingulate cortex.

Other studies have examined neural correlates of inhibitory processing and planning in MS. For example, Parry et al. investigated inhibitory control in MS using the counting Stroop task, and found that patients showed increased left medial frontal and decreased right frontal and basal ganglia activation relative to controls, despite comparable task performance [208]. This difference in activation was also correlated with brain parenchyma volume in patients, indicating that increasingly atypical activation was associated with greater brain atrophy. Curiously, this pattern of activation normalized when rivastigmine, a cholinergic agonist, was administered to patients. These findings suggest that in the absence of medical intervention, medial frontal cortex may serve to compensate for reduced activity in frontal and other regions in MS during executive task performance. Lazeron et al. used the TOL task to examine brain activation associated with strategic planning in patients with moderately advanced MS [209]. Findings indicated a similar pattern of activation in patients relative to matched controls in the cerebellum and bilateral frontal and parietal cortex, despite the fact that patients' behavioral task performance was significantly worse. These results were interpreted to indicate that MS patients with moderate disease severity may have exhausted potentially adaptive brain plasticity, resulting in weaker behavioral planning ability.

Research into functional imaging correlates of executive functions in MS is in its infancy. Studies have shown that MS patients with normal cognitive performance generally display more distributed brain activation patterns than healthy participant groups, suggesting that patients may recruit additional brain regions to maintain adequate performance despite advancing disease [205]. Evidence also suggests that lesion burden may play a critical role in the intensity and spatial extent of brain activation patterns associated with cognition in MS [204, 210]. Future functional imaging studies will likely benefit from evaluating the impact of depression on neural activity associated with executive functions, given the elevated rate of depression in the illness and the negative impact that depression has on cognition in MS [211, 212].

Traumatic Brain Injury

Traumatic brain injury (TBI), even when relatively mild, may be associated with deficits on tests of executive functions [for review see 213]. Functional neuroimaging research in TBI to date has largely focused on working memory given the common report by patients of problems with short-term memory, speed of information processing, and concentration. McAllister and colleagues have used fMRI and the n-back task to evaluate working memory in adults with mild TBI. In a first study, patients with mild TBI within one month of injury and healthy comparison participants completed an auditory 2-back task [214]. Results revealed that the TBI group had significantly less activation in frontal-parietal circuitry than the comparison group when comparing the 1-back to the 0-back condition (i.e., low working memory load). However, the patient group showed significantly more extensive activation than the healthy group as working memory load increased. In a follow-up study, brain activation was evaluated during an auditory 3-back task in patients with mild TBI within 1 month of injury and healthy comparison participants [215]. Although the comparison group maintained their ability to activate frontal-parietal working memory circuitry with each increase in working memory load, the patient group displayed abnormally increased activation during the moderate processing load condition (i.e., 2-back), but very little increase in activation associated with the highest processing load condition (i.e., 3-back). These findings were interpreted as suggesting that patients with mild TBI may have difficulty recruiting or modulating working memory resources, an abnormality that the authors have argued may be related to disturbances in catecholamine systems [216].

Christodoulou et al. also investigated working memory but in patients with moderate to severe TBI and healthy comparison participants, using a modified version of the PASAT [217]. Both groups showed patterns of activation that included similar regions within the frontal, parietal, and temporal lobes. However, the TBI group showed a more diffuse pattern of activation and greater lateralization to the right hemisphere, especially in the frontal lobe. Perlstein and colleagues studied a small group of patients with moderate to severe TBI about 12 months post-injury and a group of healthy comparison participants [218]. Participants completed a visual sequential-letter memory N-back task that varied working memory load from zero to three letters, similar to the auditory-verbal n-back employed in the McAllister et al. studies [214, 215]. Results indicated that the patient group generally showed lesser working memory load-related increases in activation than the comparison group in frontal-parietal regions. Furthermore, with increasing load the patients showed greater right dorsolateral frontal cortex activation, while this load effect was observed for the left dorsolateral region in the healthy group.

Taken together, these findings indicate that fMRI is a promising tool to help identify the neural correlates of cognitive deficits commonly seen in patients with TBI across the range of severity. In addition, while the above studies have varied in methodology and sample characteristics, the results suggest that TBI may be characterized not only by reduced brain activation, but also by disturbances in the ability to modulate processing resources according to cognitive demands.

CONCLUSION

The present review of functional neuroimaging studies shows a general concordance with the information obtained from the long history of lesion studies in human neuropsychology. Regardless of whether PET or fMRI is used, performance on executive function tasks is most commonly associated with activation of one or more subregions within the frontal lobes. The specific frontal subregions activated appear to vary to some extent with the nature of the executive function being evaluated, as well as the specific executive task demands, but there is clearly some overlap. For example, Konishi and colleagues observed that inhibiting responses during a go/nogo task and cognitive flexibility on a WCST both activated the right inferior frontal cortex [64]. Duncan and Owen noted that across many different cognitive demands (e.g., working memory, inhibition, and even episodic memory tasks) clusters of activation tend to be seen in common frontal lobe subregions including the mid-dorsolateral and mid-ventrolateral areas, as well as the dorsal anterior cingulate gyrus [219]. These investigations indicate that it is imprudent at this time to attribute dysfunction in a specific executive subdomain, or on a specific test of executive function, to a narrowly defined region of the frontal lobe. Furthermore, functional neuroimaging studies have provided a wealth of evidence supporting the idea that executive functions are subserved by distributed neural networks that include several cortical and subcortical regions. This latter observation is in accord with many clinical neuropsychological studies that have noted executive deficits in patients with non-frontal focal lesions.

Functional neuroimaging investigations of executive functions in patients with psychiatric and neurological illnesses have begun to shed light on the complexity of brain-behavior relationship. In patient populations such as MS, TBI, schizophrenia, and others, neuroimaging studies have observed a complex pattern of changes that include areas of increased and decreased peak activations, as well as abnormalities in the spatial extent of activations. Whether these changes are purely functional, or related at least in part to structural changes [220], remains to be fully elucidated. Furthermore, while some of these changes may represent alterations specifically related to the disease process, others have been interpreted as potentially reflecting the brain's attempt to compensate for structural or functional abnormalities, or are due to the effects of interventions such as medications.

It is likely that some of the inconsistencies in the functional neuroimaging literature are related to the methodological limitations of current studies. Sample sizes in most studies have been modest secondary to various logistical factors, including but not limited to the high cost of scanner use. Technological limitations in fMRI studies, such as poor signal-to-noise ratio in some brain regions such as the orbitofrontal cortex, have impeded the determination of the role that these regions may play in executive functions. Fortunately, improvements in technology are beginning to result in better spatial and temporal resolution [221].

In addition to the necessity for further technological advancements, there are multiple possibilities for enhancing functional neuroimaging paradigms. As in neuropsychological practice and research, an emphasis on ecological and external validity of fMRI tasks and findings will likely occur. For example, in addition to using experimental tasks of planning such as the Tower of London, virtual reality goggles will be capable of creating an environment where the participant may be asked to plan spatially the most efficient route in a fictitious (or real) city. A more general goal for scanner tasks will be to develop normative brain activation data for standardized tasks that are commonly used. Such data will allow for more meaningful analyses and conclusions and open the door for multiple clinical applications. For example, neuropsychological evaluations may begin to include functional neuroimaging to delineate appropriate, compensatory, or reduced activation in response to tasks on which a patient shows significant impairment during cognitive testing. Furthermore, we anticipate an extension of the work described earlier related to strategy use [85]. Participant-generated and experimenter-guided strategy use will become a critical variable in understanding more effectively individual differences in activation patterns, not to mention promoting the emergence of functional neuroimaging informed development of cognitive remediation techniques designed to target specific neural circuitry.

It should be noted, however, that while functional neuroimaging is providing important new information on the neural basis of executive functions, no methodology is sufficient in isolation, nor should findings exist in a vacuum. Instead, functional neuroimaging may be seen as adding a critical *localization* component to structured observations of behavior via laboratory or clinical neuropsychological assessment, both in terms of brain regions involved in a deficit and preserved regions being recruited in the attempt to compensate for abnormalities. Thus, at least a basic understanding of the functional neuroimaging literature on executive functions (as well as other functions), including methodological issues and appropriate data interpretation, will likely continue to grow in importance as a part of the knowledge base of neuropsychologists.

REFERENCES

[1]   Barkley RA. The executive functions and self-regulation: an evolutionary neuropsychological perspective. *Neuropsychology Review.* 2001;11(1):1-29.

[2]   Gioia GA, Isquith PK, Guy SC. Assessment of executive function in children with neurological impairments. In: Simeonsson R, Rosenthal S, editors. *Psychological and developmental assessment.* New York: The Guilford Press; 2001. p. 317 to 356.

[3]   Stuss DT, Alexander MP. Executive functions and the frontal lobes: a conceptual view. *Psychological Research.* 2000;63(3-4):289-298.

[4]   Lezak MD. Neuropsychological assessment. 3 ed. New York: Oxford University Press; 1995.

[5]   Stuss DT, Benson DF. Neuropsychological studies of the frontal lobes. *Psychological Bulletin* 1984;95:3-28.

[6]   Tranel D, Anderson SW, Benton AL. Development of the concept of 'executive function' and its relationship to the frontal lobes. In: Boller F, Grafman J, editors. *Handbook of neuropsychology.* Amsterdam: Elsevier Science; 1994. p. 125-148.

[7]   Norman DA, Shallice T. Attention to action: Willed and automatic control of behavior. In: Davidson RJ, Schwartz GE, Shapiro D, editors. Consciousness and self-regulation: Advances in research and theory. New York: Plenum; 1986. p. 1-18.

[8]   Baddeley A. The central executive: a concept and some misconceptions. *Journal of the International Neuropsychological Society* 1998;4(5):523-6.

[9]   Grafman J. Plans, actions, and mental sets: Managerial knowledge units in the frontal lobes. In: Perecman E, editor. Integrating theory and practice in clinical neuropsychology. Hillsdale, NJ: Erlbaum; 1989. p. 93-138.

[10]   Burgess PW. Theory and methodology in executive function research. In: Rabbitt P, editor. *Methodology of frontal and executive function.* Hove, U.K.: Psychology Press; 1997. p. 81-116.

[11]   Goldman-Rakic P. Circuitry of primate prefrontal cortex and regulation of behavior by representational memory. In: Mountcastle V, Plum F, Geiger S, editors. *Handbook of physiology - the nervous system.* Bethesda, MD: American Physiological Society; 1987. p. 373-417.

[12]   Baddeley A. Working memory: looking back and looking forward. Nature Reviews Neuroscience 2003;4(10):829-839.

[13]   Anderson P. Assessment and development of executive function (EF) during childhood. *Child Neuropsychology* 2002;8(2):71-82.

[14]   Brocki KC, Bohlin G. Executive functions in children aged 6 to 13: a dimensional and developmental study. *Developmental Neuropsychology* 2004;26(2):571-93.

[15] Carlson SM. Executive function in context: development, measurement, theory, and experience. *Monographs of the Society for Research in Child Development* 2003;68(3):138-51.

[16] Pennington BF, Ozonoff S. Executive functions and developmental psychopathology. *Journal of Child Psychology & Psychiatry & Allied Disciplines* 1996;37(1):51-87.

[17] Segalowitz SJ, Davies PL. Charting the maturation of the frontal lobe: an electrophysiological strategy. *Brain & Cognition* 2004;55(1):116-33.

[18] Zelazo PD. The development of conscious control in childhood. *Trends in Cognitive Sciences* 2004;8(1):12-7.

[19] Anderson V. Assessing executive functions in children: biological, psychological, and developmental considerations. *Pediatric Rehabilitation.* 2001;4(3):119-136.

[20] Krasnegor NA, Lyon GR, Goldman-Rakic PS. Development of the prefrontal cortex: Evolution, neurobiology and behavior. Baltimore: Paul H. Brookes Publishing Co.; 1997.

[21] Miller CA. Gross morphology and architectonics of the frontal lobes. In: Miller BL, Cummings JL, editors. *The human frontal lobes.* New York: The Guilford Press; 1999.

[22] Thompson PM, Giedd JN, Woods RP, MacDonald D, Evans AC, Toga AW. Growth patterns in the developing brain detected by using continuum mechanical tensor maps. *Nature* 2000;404(6774):190-3.

[23] Dawson G, Panagiotides H, Klinger LG, Hill D. The role of frontal lobe functioning in the development of infant self-regulatory behavior. *Brain & Cognition* 1992;20(1):152-75.

[24] Diamond A, Taylor C. Development of an aspect of executive control: development of the abilities to remember what I said and to "do as I say, not as I do". *Developmental Psychobiology* 1996;29(4):315-34.

[25] Espy KA, Stalets MM, McDiarmid MM, Senn TE, Cwik MF, Hamby A. Executive functions in preschool children born preterm: application of cognitive neuroscience paradigms. *Child Neuropsychology* 2002;8(2):83-92.

[26] Kerr A, Zelazo PD. Development of "hot" executive function: the children's gambling task. *Brain & Cognition* 2004;55(1):148-57.

[27] Zelazo PD, Muller U, Frye D, Marcovitch S, Argitis G, Boseovski J, et al. The development of executive function in early childhood. *Monographs of the Society for Research in Child Development* 2003;68(3):vii-137.

[28] Span MM, Ridderinkhof KR, van der Molen MW. Age-related changes in the efficiency of cognitive processing across the life span. *Acta Psychologica* 2004;117(2):155-83.

[29] van der Molen MW. Developmental changes in inhibitory processing: evidence from psychophysiological measures. *Biological Psychology* 2000;54(1-3):207-39.

[30] Zelazo PD, Craik FI, Booth L. Executive function across the life span. *Acta Psychologica* 2004;115(2-3):167-83.

[31] Daigneault S, Braun CM, Whitaker HA. Early effects of normal aging on perseverative and non-perseverative prefrontal measures. *Developmental Neuropsychology* 1992;8:99-114.

[32] De Luca CR, Wood SJ, Anderson V, Buchanan JA, Proffitt TM, Mahony K, et al. Normative data from the CANTAB. I: development of executive function over the lifespan. *Journal of Clinical & Experimental Neuropsychology* 2003;25(2):242-54.

[33] Verhaeghen P, Cerella J. Aging, executive control, and attention: a review of meta-analyses. *Neuroscience & Biobehavioral Reviews* 2002;26(7):849-57.

[34] Wecker NS, Kramer JH, Wisniewski A, Delis DC, Kaplan E. Age effects on executive ability. *Neuropsychology* 2000;14(3):409-14.

[35] Carmelli D, Swan GE, DeCarli C, Reed T. Quantitative genetic modeling of regional brain volumes and cognitive performance in older male twins. *Biological Psychology* 2002;61(1-2):139-55.

[36] Jernigan TL, Archibald SL, Fennema-Notestine C, Gamst AC, Stout JC, Bonner J, et al. Effects of age on tissues and regions of the cerebrum and cerebellum. *Neurobiology of Aging* 2001;22(4):581-94.

[37] O'Brien JT, Wiseman R, Burton EJ, Barber B, Wesnes K, Saxby B, et al. Cognitive associations of subcortical white matter lesions in older people. Annals of the New York Academy of Sciences 2002;977:436-444.

[38] Valenzuela MJ, Sachdev PS, Wen W, Shnier R, Brodaty H, Gillies D. Dual voxel proton magnetic resonance spectroscopy in the healthy elderly: subcortical-frontal axonal N-acetylaspartate levels are correlated with fluid cognitive abilities independent of structural brain changes. *Neuroimage* 2000;12(6):747-56.

[39] Damasio H, Grabowski T, Frank R, Galaburda AM, Damasio AR. The return of Phineas Gage: clues about the brain from the skull of a famous patient. *Science.* 1994;264(5162):1102-5.

[40] Luria AR. Higher cortical functions in man. Second ed. New York: Plenum Press; 1981.

[41] Miller BL, Cummings JL. The human frontal lobes. New York: Guilford Press; 1999.

[42] Robbins TW. Dissociating executive functions of the prefrontal cortex. Philosophical Transactions of the Royal Society of London - Series B: Biological Sciences 1996;351(1346):1463-1470.

[43] Stuss DT, Knight RT. Principles of frontal lobe function. New York: Oxford University Press; 2002.

[44] Gottwald B, Wilde B, Mihajlovic Z, Mehdorn HM. Evidence for distinct cognitive deficits after focal cerebellar lesions. *Journal of Neurology, Neurosurgery & Psychiatry* 2004;75(11):1524-31.

[45] Van Der Werf YD, Weerts JG, Jolles J, Witter MP, Lindeboom J, Scheltens P. Neuropsychological correlates of a right unilateral lacunar thalamic infarction. *Journal of Neurology, Neurosurgery & Psychiatry* 1999;66(1):36-42.

[46] Wang PY. Neurobehavioral changes following caudate infarct: a case report with literature review. *Chung Hua i Hsueh Tsa Chih - Chinese Medical Journal.* 1991;47(3):199-203.

[47] Denkla MB. A theory and model of executive function: A neuropsychological perspective. In: Lyon GR, Krasnegor NA, editors. *Attention, memory and executive function.* Baltimore: Brookes; 1996. p. 263-278.

[48] Alexander GE, Crutcher MD, DeLong MR. Basal ganglia-thalamocortical circuits: parallel substrates for motor, oculomotor, "prefrontal" and "limbic" functions. *Progress in Brain Research* 1990;85:119-146.

[49] Barbas H. Connections underlying the synthesis of cognition, memory, and emotion in primate prefrontal cortices. *Brain Research Bulletin* 2000;52(5):319-330.

[50] Cummings JL. Anatomic and behavioral aspects of frontal-subcortical circuits. Annals of the New York Academy of Sciences 1995;769:1-13.

[51] Thierry AM, Gioanni Y, Dégénétais E, Glowinski J. Hippocampo-prefrontal cortex pathway: Anatomical and elctrophysiological characteristics. *Hippocampus* 2000;10:411-419.

[52] Arthurs OJ, Boniface S. How well do we understand the neural origins of the fMRI BOLD signal? *Trends in Neurosciences.* 2002;25(1):27-31.

[53] Kwong KK, Belliveau JW, Chesler DA, Goldberg IE, Weisskoff RM, Poncelet BP, et al. Dynamic magnetic resonance imaging of human brain activity during primary sensory stimulation. Proceedings of the National Academy of Sciences of the United States of America 1992;89(12):5675-9.

[54] Logothetis NK. The neural basis of the blood-oxygen-level-dependent functional magnetic resonance imaging signal. Philosophical Transactions of the Royal Society of London - Series B: Biological Sciences 2002;357(1424):1003-37.

[55] Friston KJ, Holmes AP, Worsley KJ, Poline JP, Frith CD, Frackowiak RSJ. Statistical parametric maps in functional imaging: A general linear approach. *Human Brain Mapping* 1995;2:189-210.

[56] Jezzard P, Matthews PM, Smith SM. Functional MRI; an introduction to methods. New York: Oxford University Press; 2001.

[57] Ogawa S, Menon RS, Kim SG, Ugurbil K. On the characteristics of functional magnetic resonance imaging of the brain. *Annual Review of Biophysics & Biomolecular Structure.* 1998;27:447-74.

[58] Banich MT. Neuropsychology: The neural bases of mental function. Boston: Houghton-Mifflin Co.; 1997.

[59] Moll J, de Oliveira-Souza, R., Tovar Moll, F., Bramati, I. E., & Andreiuolo, P. A. The cerebral correlates of set-shifting. *Arquivos de Neuro-Psiquiatria* 2005;60(4).

[60] Gurd JM, Amunts K, Weiss PH, Zafiris O, Zilles K, Marshall JC, et al. Posterior parietal cortex is implicated in continuous switching between verbal fluency tasks: an fMRI study with clinical implications. *Brain* 2002;125(Pt 5):1024-38.

[61] Berman KF, Ostrem JL, Randolph C, Gold J, Goldberg TE, Coppola R, et al. Physiological activation of a cortical network during performance of the Wisconsin Card Sorting Test: a positron emission tomography study. *Neuropsychologia* 1995;33(8):1027-46.

[62] Nagahama Y, Fukuyama, H., Yamaguchi, H., Matsuzaki, S., Konishi, J., Shibasaki, H., Kimura, J. Common inhibitory mechanism in human inferior prefrontal cortex revealed by event-related functional MRI. *Brain* 1996;122:981-991.

[63] Konishi S, Nakajima, K., Uchida, I., Kameyama, M., Nakahara, K., Sekihara, K., & Miyashita, Y. Transient activation of inferior prefrontal cortex during cognitive set shifting. *Nature Neuroscience* 1998;1(1):80-84.

[64] Konishi S, Nakajima K, Uchida I, Kikyo H, Kameyama M, Miyashita Y. Common inhibitory mechanism in human inferior prefrontal cortex revealed by event-related functional MRI. *Brain* 1999;122(Pt 5):981-91.

[65] Konishi S, Hayashi T, Uchida I, Kikyo H, Takahashi E, Miyashita Y. Hemispheric asymmetry in human lateral prefrontal cortex during cognitive set shifting. Proceedings of the National Academy of Sciences of the United States of America. 2002;99(11):7803-8.

[66] Monchi O, Petrides M, Petre V, Worsley K, Dagher A. Wisconsin Card Sorting revisited: distinct neural circuits participating in different stages of the task identified by event-related functional magnetic resonance imaging. *Journal of Neuroscience* 2001;21(19):7733-41.

[67] Eslinger PJ, Damasio AR. Severe disturbance of higher cognition after bilateral frontal lobe ablation: patient EVR. *Neurology* 1985;35(12):1731-41.

[68] Bechara A, Damasio AR, Damasio H, Anderson SW. Insensitivity to future consequences following damage to human prefrontal cortex. *Cognition* 1994;50:7-15.

[69] Bechara A, Damasio H, Damasio AR, Lee GP. Different contributions of the human amygdala and ventromedial prefrontal cortex to decision-making. *Journal of Neuroscience* 1999;19(13):5473-81.

[70] Manes F, Sahakian B, Clark L, Rogers R, Antoun N, Aitken M, et al. Decision-making processes following damage to the prefrontal cortex. *Brain* 2002;125(Pt 3):624-39.

[71] Ernst M, Bolla K, Mouratidis M, Contoreggi C, Matochik JA, Kurian V, et al. Decision making in a risk-taking task: a PET study. *Neuropsychopharmacology* 2002;26:682–691.

[72] Fukui H, Murai T, Fukuyama H, Hayashi T, Hanakawa T. Functional activity related to risk anticipation during performance of the Iowa gambling task. *NeuroImage* 2005;24:253-259.

[73] Rogers RD, Owen AM, Middleton HC, Williams EJ, Pickard JD, Sahakian BJ, et al. Choosing between small, likely rewards and large, unlikely rewards activates inferior and orbital prefrontal cortex. *Journal of Neuroscience* 1999;19(20):9029-38.

[74] Paulus MP, Hozack N, Zauscher B, McDowell JE, Frank L, Brown GG, et al. Prefrontal, parietal, and temporal cortex networks underlie decision making in the presence of uncertainty. *NeuroImage* 2001;13(1):91-100.

[75] Paulus MP, Hozack N, Frank L, Brown GG. Error rate and outcome predictability affect neural activation in prefrontal cortex and anterior cingulate during decision making. *NeuroImage* 2002;15(4):836-846.

[76] Elliott R, Dolan RJ. Activation of different anterior cingulate foci in association with hypothesis testing and response selection. *Neuroimage* 1998;8(1):17-29.

[77] Blackwood N, Ffytche D, Simmons A, Bentall R, Murray R, Howard R. The cerebellum and decision making under uncertainty. *Cognitive Brain Research* 2004;20(1):46-53.

[78] Rezai K, Andreasen N, Alliger R, Cohen G, Swayze V, O'Leary D. The neuropsychology of the prefrontal cortex. *Archives of Neurology* 1993;50:636-642.

[79] Morris R, Ahmed S, Syed G, Toone B. Neural correlates of planning ability: Frontal lobe activation during the Tower of London test. *Neuropsychologia* 1993;31:1367-1378.

[80] Baker S, Rogers R, Owen A, Frith C, Dolan R, Frackowiak R, et al. Neural systems engaged by planning: a PET study of the Tower of London task. Neuropsychologia 1996;34:515-526.

[81] Owen A, Doyon J, Petrides M, Evans A. Planning and spatial working memory: a Positron Emission Tomography study in humans. *European Journal of Neuroscience* 1996;8:353-364.

[82] Dagher A, Owen A, Boecker H, Brooks D. Mapping the network for planning: a correlational PET activation study with the Tower of London task. *Brain* 1999;122:1973-1987.

[83] Lazeron R, Rombouts S, Machielsen W, Scheltens P, Witter M, Uylings H, et al. Visualizing brain activation during planning: The Tower of London test adapted for functional MR imaging. *Am J Neuroradiol* 2000;21:1407-1414.

[84] Rowe J, Owen A, Johnsrude I, Passingham R. Imaging the mental components of a planning task. *Neuropsychologia* 2001;39:315-327.

[85] Fincham J, Carter C, V vV, Stenger V, Anderson J. Neural mechanisms of planning: A computational analysis using event-related fMRI. Proceedings of the National Academy of Science 2002;99:3346-3351.

[86] van den Heuvel O, Groenewegen H, Barkhof F, Lazeron R, van Dyck R, Veltman D. Frontostriatal system in planning complexity: a parametric functional magnetic resonance version of the Tower of London task. Neuroimage 2003;18:367-374.

[87] Newman S, Carpenter P, Varma S, Just M. Frontal and parietal participation in problem solving in the Tower of London: fMRI and computational modeling of planning and high-level perception. *Neuropsychologia* 2003;41:1668-1682.

[88] Barkley RA. Behavioral inhibition, sustained attention, and executive functions: constructing a unifying theory of ADHD. *Psychological Bulletin* 1997;121(1):65-94.

[89] Konishi S, Nakajima K, Uchida I, Sekihara K, Miyashita Y. No-go dominant brain activity in human inferior prefrontal cortex revealed by functional magnetic resonance imaging. *European Journal of Neuroscience* 1998;10:1209-1213.

[90] Menon V, Adleman NE, White CD, Glover GH, Reiss AL. Error-related brain activation during a Go/NoGo response inhibition task. *Human Brain Mapping* 2001;12(3):131-43.

[91] Mostofsky SH, Schafer JG, Abrams MT, Goldberg MC, Flower AA, Boyce A, et al. fMRI evidence that the neural basis of response inhibition is task-dependent. *Cognitive Brain Research.* 2003;17(2):419-30.

[92] Watanabe J, Sugiura M, Sato K, Sato Y, Maeda Y, Matsue Y, et al. The human prefrontal and parietal association cortices are involved in NO-GO performances: an event-related fMRI study. *Neuroimage* 2002;17(3):1207-16.

[93] Garavan H, Ross TJ, Stein EA. Right hemispheric dominance of inhibitory control: an event-related functional MRI study. Proceedings of the National Academy of Sciences of the United States of America. 1999;96(14):8301-6.

[94] Kelly AM, Hester R, Murphy K, Javitt DC, Foxe JJ, Garavan H. Prefrontal-subcortical dissociations underlying inhibitory control revealed by event-related fMRI. European *Journal of Neuroscience* 2004;19(11):3105-12.

[95] Bench CJ, Frith CD, Grasby PM, Friston KJ, Paulesu E, Frackowiak RS, et al. Investigations of the functional anatomy of attention using the Stroop test. *Neuropsychologia* 1993;31(9):907-22.

[96] Carter CS, Mintun M, Cohen JD. Interference and facilitation effects during selective attention: an H215O PET study of Stroop task performance. *Neuroimage* 1995;2(4):264-72.

[97] Pardo JV, Pardo PJ, Janer KW, Raichle ME. The anterior cingulate cortex mediates processing selection in the Stroop attentional conflict paradigm. Proceedings of the National Academy of Sciences of the United States of America 1990;87(1):256-9.

[98] Ravnkilde B, Videbech P, Rosenberg R, Gjedde A, Gade A. Putative tests of frontal lobe function: a PET-study of brain activation during Stroop's Test and verbal fluency. *Journal of Clinical & Experimental Neuropsychology* 2002;24(4):534-47.

[99] Bush G, Whalen PJ, Rosen BR, Jenike MA, McInerney SC, Rauch SL. The counting Stroop: an interference task specialized for functional neuroimaging--validation study with functional MRI. *Human Brain Mapping* 1998;6(4):270-82.

[100] Carter CS, Macdonald AM, Botvinick M, Ross LL, Stenger VA, Noll D, et al. Parsing executive processes: strategic vs. evaluative functions of the anterior cingulate cortex. Proceedings of the National Academy of Sciences of the United States of America 2000;97(4):1944-8.

[101] Leung HC, Skudlarski P, Gatenby JC, Peterson BS, Gore JC. An event-related functional MRI study of the stroop color word interference task. *Cerebral Cortex* 2000;10(6):552-60.

[102] Zysset S, Muller K, Lohmann G, von Cramon DY. Color-word matching stroop task: separating interference and response conflict. *Neuroimage* 2001;13(1):29-36.

[103] Carter CS, Botvinick MM, Cohen JD. The contribution of the anterior cingulate cortex to executive processes in cognition. *Reviews in the Neurosciences* 1999;10(1):49-57.

[104] Beauregard M, Levesque J, Bourgouin P. Neural correlates of conscious self-regulation of emotion. *Journal of Neuroscience.* 2001;21(18):RC165.

[105] Levesque J, Eugene F, Joanette Y, Paquette V, Mensour B, Beaudoin G, et al. Neural circuitry underlying voluntary suppression of sadness. *Biological Psychiatry.* 2003;53(6):502-10.

[106] Stuss DT, Levine B. Adult clinical neuropsychology: lessons from studies of the frontal lobes. *Annual Review of Psychology* 2002;53:401-433.

[107] de Zubicaray GI, Zelaya FO, Andrew C, Williams SC, Bullmore ET. Cerebral regions associated with verbal response initiation, suppression and strategy use. *Neuropsychologia* 2000;38(9):1292-304.

[108] Horn NR, Dolan M, Elliott R, Deakin JF, Woodruff PW. Response inhibition and impulsivity: an fMRI study. *Neuropsychologia* 2003;41(14):1959-66.

[109] Keenan J, Wheeler M, Gallup G, Pascual-Leone A. Self-recognition and the right prefrontal cortex. *Trends in Cognitive Sciences* 2000;4:338-344.

[110] Morin A. Right hemispheric self-awareness: A critical assessment. *Consciousness and Cognition* 2002;11:396-401.

[111] Craik F, Moroz T, Moscovitch M, Stuss D, Winocur G, Tulving E, et al. Search of the self: A positron emission tomography study. *Psychological Science* 1999;10:26-34.

[112] Kircher T, Senior C, Phillips M, Benson P, Bullmore E, Brammer M, et al. Towards a functional neuroanatomy of self processing: effects of faces and words. *Cognitive Brain Research* 2000;10:133-144.

[113] Vogeley K, Bussfeld P, Newen A, Herrmann S, Happe F, Falkai P, et al. Mind reading: Neural mechanisms of theory of mind and self-perspective. *Neuroimage* 2001;14:170-181.

[114] Gusnard D, Akbudak E, Shulman G, Raichle M. Medial prefrontal cortex and self-referential mental activity: Relation to a default mode of brain function. Proceedings of the National Academy of Science 2001;98:4259-4264.

[115] Johnson S, Baxter L, Wilder L, Pipe J, Heiserman J, Prigatano G. Neural correlates of self-reflection. *Brain* 2002;125:1808-1814.

[116] Kelley W, Macrae C, Wyland C, Caglar S, Inati S, Heatherton T. Finding the self? An event related fMRI study. *Journal of Cognitive Neuroscience* 2002;14:785-794.

[117] Kjaer T, Nowak M, Lou H. Reflective self-awareness and conscious states: PET evidence for a common midline parietofrontal core. *Neuroimage* 2002;17:1080-1086.

[118] Schmitz T, Kawahara-Baccus T, Johnson S. Metacognitive evaluation, self-relevance, and the right prefrontal cortex. *Neuroimage* 2004;22:941-947.

[119] Lieberman MD, Jarcho, J.M., & Satpute, A.B. Evidence-based and intuition-based self-knowledge: An fMRI study. Journal of Personality and Social Psychology 2004;87:421-435.

[120] Kahan T, La Berge S, Levitan L, Zimbardo P. Similarities and differences between dreaming and waking cognition: An exploratory study. Consciousness and Cognition 1997;6:132-147.

[121] Braun A, Balkin T, Wesensten N, Gwardry F, Carson R, Varga M, et al. Dissociated pattern of activity in visual cortices and their projections during human rapid eye movement sleep. *Science* 1998;279:91-95.

[122] Marquet P, Degueldre C, Aerts J, Peters J, Luxen A, Franck G. Functional neuranatomy of human slow wave sleep. *Journal of Neuroscience* 1997;17:2807-2812.

[123] Elfgren C, Risberg J. Lateralized frontal blood flow increases during fluency tasks: influence of cognitive strategy. *Neuropsychologia* 1998;36:505-512.

[124] Reichle E, Carpenter P, Just M. The neural bases of strategy and skill in sentence-picture verification. *Cognitive Psychology* 2000;40:261-295.

[125] Burbaud P, Camus O, Guehl D, Bioulac B, Caille J-M, Allard M. Influence of cognitive strategies on the pattern of cortical activation during mental subtraction: A functional imaging study in human subjects. *Neuroscience Letters* 2000;287:76-80.

[126] Savage CR, Deckersbach T, Heckers S, Wagner AD, Schacter DL, Alpert NM, et al. Prefrontal regions supporting spontaneous and directed application of verbal learning strategies: Evidence from PET. *Brain* 2001;124:219-231.

[127] Fink G, Marshall J, Weiss P, Toni I, Zilles K. Task instructions influence the cognitive strategies involved in line bisection judgments: evidence from modulated neural mechanisms revealed by fMRI. *Neuropsychologia* 2002;40:119-130.

[128] Valenzuela M, Jones M, Win W, Rae C, Graham S, Shnier R, et al. Memory training alters hippocampal neurochemistry in healthy. *Neuroreport* 2003;14:1333-1337.

[129] Olesen P, Westerberg H, Klingberg T. Increased prefrontal and parietal activity after training of working memory. *Nature Neuroscience* 2004;7:75-79.

[130] Baddeley A. Working memory. *Science* 1992;255(5044):556-9.

[131] Fuster JM. Executive frontal functions. *Experimental Brain Research.* 2000;133(1):66-70.

[132] Jonides J, Smith EE, Koeppe RA, Awh E, Minoshima S, Mintum M. Spatial working memory in humans as revealed by PET. *Nature* 1993;33:623-625.

[133] Goldberg TE, Herman KF, Randolph C, Gold JM, Weinberger DR. Isolating the mnemonic component in spatial delayed response: A controlled PET ISO-labeled water regional cerebral blood flow study in normal humans. *NeuroImage* 1996;3:69-78.

[134] Mecklinger A, Bosch V, Gruenewald C, Bentin S, von Cramon DY. What have klingon letters and faces in common? An fMRI study on content-specific working memory systems. *Human Brain Mapping* 2000;11:146-161.

[135] Sweeney JA, Minlun MA, Kwee S, Wiseman MB, Brown DL, Rosenburg DR, et al. Positron emission tomography study of voluntary saccadic eye movements and spatial working memory. *Journal of Neurophysiology* 1996;75:454-468.

[136] D'Esposito M, Aguirre GK, Zarahn E, Ballard D, Shin RK, Lease J. Functional MRI studies of spatial and nonspatial working memory. *Cognitive Brain Research* 1998;7:1-13.

[137] D'Esposito M, Postle BR, Ballard D, Lease J. Maintenance versus manipulation of information held in working memory: An event-related fMRI study. *Brain & Cognition* 1999;41:66-86.

[138] Owen AM, Lee ACH, Williams EJ. Dissociating aspects of verbal working memory within the human frontal lobe: Further evidence for a "process specific" model of lateral frontal organization. *Psychobiology* 2000;28:146-155.

[139] Walter H, Bretschneider V, Gron G, Zurowski B, Wunderlich AP, Tomczak R, et al. Evidence for quantitative domain dominance for verbal and spatial working memory in frontal and parietal. *Cortex* 2003;39:897-911.

[140] Honey GD, Bullmore ET, Sharma T. Prolonged reaction time to a verbal working memory task predicts increased power of posterior parietal cortical activation. *Neuroimage.* 2000;12(5):495-503.

[141] Jansma JM, Ramsey NF, Coppola R, Kahn RS. Specific versus nonspecific brain activity in a parametric N-back task. *Neuroimage* 2000;12(6):688-97.

[142] Nystrom LE, Braver TS, Sabb FW, Delgado MR, Noll DC, Cohen JD. Working memory for letters, shapes, and locations: fMRI evidence against stimulus-based regional organization in human prefrontal cortex. *Neuroimage* 2000;11(5 Pt 1):424-46.

[143] Ragland JD, Turetsky BI, Gur RC, Gunning-Dixon F, Turner T, Schroeder L, et al. Working memory for complex figures: An fMRI comparison of letter and fractal n-back tasks. *Neuropsychology* 2002;16:370-379.

[144] Awh E, Jonides J, Smith EE, Schumacher EH, Koeppe RA, Katz S. Dissociation of storage and rehearsal in verbal working memory: Evidence from positron emission tomography. *Psychological Science* 1996;7:25-31.

[145] Klingberg T, Kawashima R, Roland PE. Activation of multi-modal cortical areas underlies short-term memory. *European Journal of Neuroscience* 1996;8:1965-1971.

[146] Fiez JA, Raichle ME, Balota DA, Tallal P, Petersen SE. PET activation of posterior temporal regions during auditory word presentation and verb generation. *Cerebral Cortex* 1996;6:1-10.

[147] Reuter-Lorenz PA, Jonides J, Smith EE, Hartley A, Miller A, Marshuetz C, et al. Age differences in the frontal lateralization of verbal and spatial working memory revealed by PET. *Journal of Cognitive Neuroscience* 2000;12:174-187.

[148] Petrides M. Specialized systems for the processing of mnemonic information within the primate frontal cortex. Philosophical Transactions of the Royal Society of London - Series B: *Biological Sciences.* 1996;351(1346):1455-61.

[149] Bunge SA, Klingberg T, Jacobsen RB, Gabrieli JD. A resource model of the neural basis of executive working memory. Proceedings from the National Academy of Science 2000;97:3573-3578.

[150] Owen AM, Evans AC, Petrides M. Evidence for a two-stage model of spatial working memory processing within the lateral frontal cortex: a positron emission tomography study. *Cerebral Cortex.* 1996;6(1):31-8.

[151] Owen AM, Herrod NJ, Menon DK, Clark JC, Downey SP, Carpenter TA, et al. Redefining the functional organization of working memory processes within human lateral prefrontal cortex. *European Journal of Neuroscience.* 1999;11(2):567-74.

[152] Postle BR, Berger JS, D'Esposito M. Functional neuroanatomical double dissociation of mnemonic and executive control processes contributing to working memory performance. Proceedings from the National Academy of Science 1999;96:12959-12964.

[153] Rypma B, Prabhakaran V, Desmond JE, Gabrieli JD. Load-dependent roles of frontal brain regions in the maintenance of working memory. NeuroImage 1999;9:216-226.

[154] Wagner AD, Maril A, Bjork RA, Schacter DL. Prefrontal contributions to executive control: fMRI evidence for functional distinctions within lateral Prefrontal cortex. *Neuroimage* 2001;14(6):1337-47.

[155] Wager TD, Smith EE. Neuroimaging studies of working memory: a meta-analysis. *Cognitive, Affective & Behavioral Neuroscience* 2003;3(4):255-74.

[156] Collette F, Van der Linden M. Brain imaging of the central executive component of working memory. *Neuroscience & Biobehavioral Reviews* 2002;26(2):105-25.

[157] Petit L, Courtney SM, Ungerleider LG, Haxby JV. Sustained activity in the medial wall during working memory delays. *Journal of Neuroscience* 1998;18(22):9429-37.

[158] Postle BR, D'Esposito M. Dissociation of human caudate nucleus activity in spatial and nonspatial working memory: an event-related fMRI study. *Cognitive Brain Research* 1999;8(2):107-15.

[159] Barkley RA. ADHD and the nature of self-control. New York: Guilford Press; 1997.

[160] Hervey AS, Epstein JN, Curry JF. Neuropsychology of adults with attention-deficit/hyperactivity disorder: A meta-analytic review. *Neuropsychology* 2004;18(3):485-503.

[161] Seidman LJ, Biederman J, Faraone SV, Weber W, Ouellette C. Toward defining a neuropsychology of attention deficit-hyperactivity disorder: performance of children and adolescents from a large clinically referred sample. *Journal of Consulting & Clinical Psychology* 1997;65(1):150-60.

[162] Woods SP, Lovejoy DW, Ball JD. Neuropsychological characteristics of adults with ADHD: a comprehensive review of initial studies. *Clinical Neuropsychologist* 2002;16(1):12-34.

[163] Gioia GA, Isquith PK, Kenworthy L, Barton RM. Profiles of everyday executive function in acquired and developmental disorders. *Child Neuropsychology* 2002;8(2):121-137.

[164] Aron AR, Dowson JH, Sahakian BJ, Robbins TW. Methylphenidate improves response inhibition in adults with attention-deficit/hyperactivity disorder. *Biological Psychiatry.* 2003;54(12):1465-8.

[165] Murphy KR, Barkley RA, Bush T. Executive functioning and olfactory identification in young adults with attention deficit/hyperactivity disorder. *Neuropsychology* 2001;15(2):211-220.

[166] Roth RM, Saykin AJ. Executive dysfunction in attention-deficit/hyperactivity disorder: cognitive and neuroimaging findings. *Psychiatric Clinics of North America* 2004;27:83-96.

[167] Schweitzer JB, Faber TL, Grafton ST, Tune LE, Hoffman JM, Kilts CD. Alterations in the functional anatomy of working memory in adult attention deficit hyperactivity disorder. *American Journal of Psychiatry* 2000;157(2):278-80.

[168] Valera EM, Faraone SV, Biederman J, Poldrack RA, Seidman LJ. Functional neuroanatomy of working memory in aduls with attention-deficit/hyperactivity disorder. *Biological Psychiatry* 2005;57:439-447.

[169] Bush G, Frazier JA, Rauch SL, Seidman LJ, Whalen PJ, Jenike MA, et al. Anterior cingulate cortex dysfunction in attention-deficit/hyperactivity disorder revealed by fMRI and the Counting Stroop. *Biological Psychiatry* 1999;45(12):1542-52.

[170] Durston S, Tottenham NT, Thomas KM, Davidson MC, Eigsti I-M, Yang Y, et al. Differential patterns of striatal activation in young children with and without ADHD. *Biological Psychiatry* 2003;53(10):871-878.

[171] Rubia K, Overmeyer S, Taylor E, Brammer M, Williams SC, Simmons A, et al. Hypofrontality in attention deficit hyperactivity disorder during higher-order motor control: a study with functional MRI. *American Journal of Psychiatry* 1999;156(6):891-6.

[172] Vaidya CJ, Austin G, Kirkorian G, Ridlehuber HW, Desmond JE, Glover GH, et al. Selective effects of methylphenidate in attention deficit hyperactivity disorder: a functional magnetic resonance study. Proceedings of the National Academy of Sciences of the United States of America 1998;95(24):14494-9.

[173] Schulz KP, Fan J, Tang CY, Newcorn JH, Buchsbaum MS, Cheung AM, et al. Response inhibition in adolescents diagnosed with attention deficit hyperactivity disorder during childhood: an event-related FMRI study. American *Journal of Psychiatry* 2004;161(9):1650-1657.

[174] Castellanos FX, Giedd JN, Eckburg P, Marsh WL, Vaituzis AC, Kaysen D, et al. Quantitative morphology of the caudate nucleus in attention deficit hyperactivity disorder. *American Journal of Psychiatry* 1994;151(12):1791-6.

[175] Castellanos FX, Giedd JN, Marsh WL, Hamburger SD, Vaituzis AC, Dickstein DP, et al. Quantitative brain magnetic resonance imaging in attention-deficit hyperactivity disorder. *Archives of General Psychiatry* 1996;53(7):607-16.

[176] Kates WR, Frederikse M, Mostofsky SH, Folley BS, Cooper K, Mazur-Hopkins P, et al. MRI parcellation of the frontal lobe in boys with attention deficit hyperactivity disorder or Tourette syndrome. Psychiatry Research: *Neuroimaging* 2002;116(1-2):63-81.

[177] Mostofsky SH, Reiss AL, Lockhart P, Denckla MB. Evaluation of cerebellar size in attention-deficit hyperactivity disorder. Journal of Child Neurology 1998;13(9):434-9.

[178] Heinrichs RW, Zakzanis KK. Neurocognitive deficit in schizophrenia: A quantitative review of the evidence. *Neuropsychology* 1998;12:426-445.

[179] Weinberger DR, Gallhofer B. Cognitive function in schizophrenia. *International Clinical Psychopharmacology* 1997;12:29-36.

[180] Weinberger DR, Berman KF, Illowsky BP. Physiological dysfunction of dorsolateral prefrontal cortex in schizophrenia. III. A new cohort and evidence for a monoaminergic mechanism. *Archives of General Psychiatry* 1988;45(7):609-15.

[181] Berman KF, Zec RF, Weinberger DR. Physiologic dysfunction of dorsolateral prefrontal cortex in schizophrenia. II. Role of neuroleptic treatment, attention, and mental effort. *Archives of General Psychiatry* 1986;43(2):126-35.

[182] Weinberger DR, Berman KF, Zec RF. Physiologic dysfunction of dorsolateral prefrontal cortex in schizophrenia. I. Regional cerebral blood flow evidence. *Archives of General Psychiatry* 1986;43(2):114-24.

[183] Riehemann S, Volz HP, Stutzer P, Smesny S, Gaser C, Sauer H. Hypofrontality in neuroleptic-naive schizophrenic patients during the Wisconsin Card Sorting Test--a fMRI study. *European Archives of Psychiatry & Clinical Neuroscience* 2001;251(2):66-71.

[184] Volz HP, Gaser C, Hager F, Rzanny R, Mentzel HJ, Kreitschmann-Andermahr I, et al. Brain activation during cognitive stimulation with the Wisconsin Card Sorting Test--a functional MRI study on healthy volunteers and schizophrenics. *Psychiatry Research* 1997;75(3):145-57.

[185] Weinberger DR, Berman KF. Prefrontal function in schizophrenia: confounds and controversies. Philosophical Transactions of the Royal Society of London - Series B: *Biological Sciences.* 1996;351(1346):1495-503.

[186] Manoach DS, Press DZ, Thangaraj V, Searl MM, Goff DC, Halpern E, et al. Schizophrenic subjects activate dorsolateral prefrontal cortex during a working memory task, as measured by fMRI. *Biological Psychiatry.* 1999;45(9):1128-37.

[187] Manoach DS, Gollub RL, Benson ES, Searl MM, Goff DC, Halpern E, et al. Schizophrenic subjects show aberrant fMRI activation of dorsolateral prefrontal cortex and basal ganglia during working memory performance. *Biological Psychiatry.* 2000;48(2):99-109.

[188] Callicott JH, Bertolino A, Mattay VS, Langheim FJ, Duyn J, Coppola R, et al. Physiological dysfunction of the dorsolateral prefrontal cortex in schizophrenia revisited. *Cerebral Cortex.* 2000;10(11):1078-92.

[189] Carter CS, Perlstein W, Ganguli R, Brar J, Mintun M, Cohen JD. Functional hypofrontality and working memory dysfunction in schizophrenia. *American Journal of Psychiatry* 1998;155(9):1285-7.

[190] Honey GD, Bullmore ET, Sharma T. De-coupling of cognitive performance and cerebral functional response during working memory in schizophrenia. *Schizophrenia Research.* 2002;53(1-2):45-56.

[191] Jansma JM, Ramsey NF, van der Wee NJ, Kahn RS. Working memory capacity in schizophrenia: a parametric fMRI study. *Schizophrenia Research* 2004;68(2-3):159-71.

[192] Thermenos HW, Goldstein JM, Buka SL, Poldrack RA, Koch JK, Tsuang MT, et al. The effect of working memory performance on functional MRI in schizophrenia. *NeuroImage* 2005;74(2-3):179-194.

[193] Andreasen NC, Rezai K, Alliger R, Swayze VW, 2nd, Flaum M, Kirchner P, et al. Hypofrontality in neuroleptic-naive patients and in patients with chronic schizophrenia. Assessment with xenon 133 single-photon emission computed tomography and the Tower of London. *Archives of General Psychiatry.* 1992;49(12):943-58.

[194] Yucel M, Pantelis C, Stuart GW, Wood SJ, Maruff P, Velakoulis D, et al. Anterior cingulate activation during Stroop task performance: a PET to MRI coregistration study of individual patients with schizophrenia. *American Journal of Psychiatry.* 2002;159(2):251-4.

[195] Rubia K, Russell T, Bullmore ET, Soni W, Brammer MJ, Simmons A, et al. An fMRI study of reduced left prefrontal activation in schizophrenia during normal inhibitory function. *Schizophrenia Research* 2001;52(1-2):47-55.

[196] Perlstein WM, Dixit NK, Carter CS, Noll DC, Cohen JD. Prefrontal cortex dysfunction mediates deficits in working memory and prepotent responding in schizophrenia. *Biological Psychiatry* 2003;53(1):25-38.

[197] Paulus MP, Hozack NE, Zauscher BE, Frank L, Brown GG, McDowell J, et al. Parietal dysfunction is associated with increased outcome-related decision-making in schizophrenia patients. *Biological Psychiatry.* 2002;51(12):995-1004.

[198] Meyer-Lindenberg A, Poline JB, Kohn PD, Holt JL, Egan MF, Weinberger DR, et al. Evidence for abnormal cortical functional connectivity during working memory in schizophrenia. *American Journal of Psychiatry* 2001;158(11):1809-17.

[199] Schlosser R, Gesierich T, Kaufmann B, Vucurevic G, Hunsche S, Gawehn J, et al. Altered effective connectivity during working memory performance in schizophrenia: a study with fMRI and structural equation modeling. *Neuroimage* 2003;19(3):751-63.

[200] Rao S. Neuropsychology of multiple sclerosis: A critical review. *Journal of Clinical and Experimental Neuropsychology* 1986;8:503-542.

[201] Rao S, Leo G, Bernardin L, Unverzagt F. Cognitive dysfunction in multiple sclerosis. Frequency, patterns, and predictions. *Neurology* 1991;41:685-691.

[202] Wishart HA, Sharpe D. Neuropsychological aspects of multiple sclerosis: A quantitative review. *Journal of Clinical & Experimental Neuropsychology* 1997;19:810-824.

[203] Staffen W, Mair A, Zauner H, Unterrainer J, Niederhofer H, Kutzelnigg A, et al. Cognitive function and fMRI in patients with multiple sclerosis: evidence for compensatory cortical activation during an attention tas. *Brain* 2002;125:1275-1282.

[204] Mainero C, Caramia F, Pozzilli C, Pisani A, Pestalozza I, Borriello G, et al. fMRI evidence of brain reorganization during attention and memory tasks in multiple sclerosis. *Neuroimage* 2004;21:858-867.

[205] Wishart HA, Saykin AJ, McDonald BC, Mamourian AC, Flashman LA, Schuschu KR, et al. Brain activation patterns associated with working memory in relapsing-remitting MS. *Neurology* 2004;62(2):234-238.

[206] Sweet LH, Rao SM, Primeau M, Mayer AR, Cohen RA. Functional magnetic resonance imaging of working memory among multiple sclerosis patients. *Journal of Neuroimaging* 2004;14(2):150-7.

[207] Au Duong MV, Boulanouar K, Audoin B, Treseras S, Ibarrola D, Malikova I, et al. Modulation of effective connectivity inside the working memory network in patients at the earliest stage of multiple sclerosis. *NeuroImage* 2005;24:533-538.

[208] Parry A, Scott R, Palace J, Smith S, Matthews P. Potentially adaptive functional changes in cognitive processing for patients with multiple sclerosis and their acute modulation by rivastigmine. *Brain* 2003;126:2750-2760.

[209] Lazeron R, Rombouts S, Scheltens P, Polman C, Barkhof F. An fMRI study of planning-related brain activity in patients with moderately advanced multiple sclerosis. *Multiple Sclerosis* 2004;10:549-555.

[210] Filippi M, Rocca M. Disturbed function and plasticity in multiple sclerosis as gleaned from functional magnetic resonance imaging. *Current Opinion in Neurology* 2003;16:275-282.

[211] Arnett PA, Higginson CI, Voss WD, Randolph JJ, Grandey AA. Relationship between coping, cognitive dysfunction and depression in multiple sclerosis. *Clinical Neuropsychologist* 2002;16(3):341-55.

[212] Arnett PA, Higginson CI, Randolph JJ. Depression in multiple sclerosis: relationship to planning ability. Journal of the International *Neuropsychological Society* 2001;7(6):665-74.

[213] McDonald BC, Flashman LA, Saykin AJ. Executive dysfunction following traumatic brain injury: neural substrates and treatment strategies. *Neurorehabilitation.* 2002;17(4):333-44.

[214] McAllister TW, Saykin AJ, Flashman LA, Sparling MB, Johnson SC, Guerin SJ, et al. Brain activation during working memory 1 month after mild traumatic brain injury: a functional MRI study. *Neurology* 1999;53(6):1300-8.

[215] McAllister TW, Sparling MB, Flashman LA, Guerin SJ, Mamourian AC, Saykin AJ. Differential working memory load effects after mild traumatic brain injury. *Neuroimage* 2001;14(5):1004-12.

[216] McAllister TW, Flashman LA, Sparling MB, Saykin AJ. Working memory deficits after traumatic brain injury: catecholaminergic mechanisms and prospects for treatment - a review. *Brain Injury* 2004;18(4):331-50.

[217] Christodoulou C, DeLuca J, Ricker JH, Madigan NK, Bly BM, Lange G, et al. Functional magnetic resonance imaging of working memory impairment after traumatic brain injury. *Journal of Neurology, Neurosurgery & Psychiatry* 2001;71(2):161-8.

[218] Perlstein WM, Cole MA, Demery JA, Seignourel PJ, Dixit NK, Larson MJ, et al. Parametric manipulation of working memory load in traumatic brain injury: behavioral and neural correlates. *Journal of the International Neuropsychological Society* 2004;10(5):724-41.

[219] Duncan J, Owen AM. Common regions of the human frontal lobe recruited by diverse cognitive demands. *Trends in Neurosciences* 2000;23:475-483.

[220] Johnson SC, Saykin AJ, Baxter LC, Flashman LA, Santulli RB, McAllister TW, et al. The relationship between fMRI activation and cerebral atrophy: comparison of normal aging and alzheimer disease. *Neuroimage* 2000;11(3):179-87.

[221] Di Salle F, Esposito F, Elefante A, Scarabino T, Volpicelli A, Cirillo S, et al. High field functional MRI. *European Journal of Radiology.* 2003;48(2):138-45.

In: Focus on Neuropsychology Research
Editor: Joshua R. Dupri, pp. 37-88

ISBN 1-59454-779-3
© 2006 Nova Science Publishers, Inc.

Chapter 2

ERP Signs of Frontal and Occipital Processing of Visual Targets and Distractors Within and Without the Channel of Spatial Attention

Alberto Zani[1] and Alice Mado Proverbio[2]

[1]Institute of Molecular Bioimaging and Physiology (IBFM),
National Research Council (CNR), Via Fratelli Cervi 93,
20090 Segrate (MI), Italy, alberto.zani@ibfm.cnr.it
[2]Department of Psychology, University of Milano-Bicocca,
Via dell'Innovazione 10, 20126 Milan, Italy.

ABTRACT

Available neurophysiological and neuroimaging studies support the view that attentional processing is carried out by means of the reciprocal communications between distributed neural networks of brain areas including frontal and prefrontal cortex, as well as the occipital-temporal-parietal cortices. In this study ERPs were recorded using a 32 channels whole-head montage while volunteers performed conjoined selection tasks of spatial location and spatial frequency. Target stimuli and distractors were presented within and without attended locations. The data indicate that during spatially directed selective processing, the visual system, although overall increasing processing activation for all stimuli falling within the attended channel of attention, treats the relevant and irrelevant sources of information differently. They also suggest that this occurs not only within the relevant channel of attention, but without it too. Indeed, the present findings suggest that, while enhancing processing of frequency-relevant gratings with respect to frequency-irrelevant ones since the earliest sensory level, as reflected by C1, at the attended location, the system seems also actively to suppress the processing of the latter stimuli with respect to the former ones at the neglected location, already starting at early sensory level, as reflected by P1. As for the prefrontal cortex, ERPs data and their topography suggested that distinct sub-regions of the latter might serve distinct attention functions. In fact, while dorsolateral regions would control the orienting of attention toward relevant space locations, the left-hemisphere inferior posterior prefrontal cortex (PFC) may suppress processing of distractors within an attended channel. Conversely, the dorsal frontal-polar PFC might bust, although in different degrees, the post-perceptual/semantic processing of relevant information by posterior brain areas independent of location relevance.

Keywords: Object and space conjoined attention, ERPs, visual cortex and enhanced processing of relevant stimuli within the focus of attention at C1 level, visual cortex and suppression of processing of irrelevant stimuli without the focus of attention at P1 level, prefrontal cortex and suppression of semantic processing of distractors within the channel of attention, suppression and left hemisphere asymmetry

INTRODUCTION

Selective attention has to be deployed in presence of multiple sources of information competing for processing resources, as in most of the cases whenever attending to the external world. Attention functions to permit selectively attending to the relevant source of information so that the processing of the latter is preferentially enhanced compared with others present in the surrounding environment. Without it, in fact, all stimuli would be processed at the same level (Hillyard *et al.*, 1999; Aston-Jones *et al.*, 1999; Reynolds *et al.*, 2003). Importantly, attention also functions to suppress or "inhibit" the irrelevant source, besides controlling the recruitment of functional circuits suitable for performing a given task. This second, executive type, function is added to cognitive control functions, such as decision-making and control processes that the individual possesses vis-à-vis his own behaviour and the external environment (Posner and Petersen, 1990; Aston-Jones *et al.*, 1999; Gehring and Knight, 2000; Smith and Jonides, 2003). The aforementioned functional distinction is crucial since, from the conceptual and methodological viewpoints, in most of the studies of selective attention using different experimental paradigms it cannot be told whether attention, inhibition, or both are at work.

Neurophysiological research based on recordings of single cell units (Desimone and Duncan, 1995) in animals, as well as haemodynamic and electro-functional imaging studies of human brain, have provided converging evidence on the cortical and subcortical nervous circuits underlying these selection mechanisms (Hillyard *et al.*, 1998, 1999; Corbetta, 1999; Corbetta and Shulman, 1999; Haxby *et al.*, 1999). These data provide direct support for the view that attentional selection of visual inputs is carried out by means of the parallel activation of a distributed neural network in the brain, made up of so-called anterior and posterior attentional systems, whose centers and pathways play different but synergic roles in the selection itself (Posner and Petersen, 1990; La Berge, 1995).

THE POSTERIOR ATTENTION SYSTEM

This system includes the parietal and occipital-temporal cortex, the pulvinar and the superior colliculus, and it is actively involved in the selective processing of visual information. The selective processing strongly depends on the modulated activity of two parallel streams, which from the primary visual cortex (or V1) project to the posterior parietal area (the so-called *dorsal stream*) or to the inferior temporal area (the so-called *ventral stream*), first proposed by Ungerleider and Mishkin (1982), and which were later subjected to intense investigation (for example, see Merigan and Maunsell, 1993; Webster and Ungerleider, 1999). The dorsal stream, which receives both contra- and ipsi-lateral collicular afferents, manages information on stimulus spatial location and movement. Conversely, the ventral stream analyzes stimulus features such as orientation, color, spatial frequency[1], texture, etc.

The two streams of the posterior system involved in the selection and analysis of visual inputs project from the visual cortex on to the posterior parietal (*dorsal stream*) and the inferior temporal (*ventral strea*m) areas, respectively. Evidence has accumulated to indicate that the dorsal stream handles information on stimuli spatial position and motion, as it possesses (also ipsilateral) collicular afferents, while the ventral system analyses physical features such as orientation, color, spatial frequency, texture, etc. (Ungerleider, Mishkin, 1982; Webster and Ungerleider, 1999). While the former mostly receive afferent fibers from large magnocellular gangliar cells, the latter receive afferences from small parvocellular cells. There is also further evidence that these two systems are related to scotopic and peripheral vision, as opposed to photopic and foveal vision, to the vision of low as opposed to high spatial frequencies and, more generally, to the visual attention mechanisms based on space rather than on the object (Fink *et al.,* 1997).

Haemodynamic functional anatomical studies have clearly shown that visual attention modulates the activity of both systems (Cabeza and Nyberg, 2000; Dupont *et al.*, 1998). This modulation has been observed also by measuring changes in amplitude, latency and scalp topography of event-related potentials (ERPs) of the brain to visual stimuli as a function of task relevance and attention condition (e. g., Annlo-Vento and Hillyard, 1996; Martin-Loeches *et al.*, 1999; Previc, 1990; Zani and Proverbio, 1995). Attention mechanisms based on spatial location have been extensively reviewed by Mangun *2003*. Moreover, several previous recent reviews on these mechanisms can be found (e. g., Hillyard *et al.,* 1995; Martinez *et al.*, 1999; Luck *et al.*, 2000).

A bulk of robust electrophysiological evidence is available to indicate that space-based information selection influences the extrastriate visual areas (i.e., Brodmann's areas 18 and 19 of the hemisphere contralateral to the attended field) as early as 70-80 ms post-stimulus (e. g., Mangun *et al.*, 1997; 2001; Martinez *et al.*, 1999).

As for non-spatial features, there are manifold findings that the attentional selection takes place through different neural mechanisms directly affecting the analysis of the specific feature (color, spatial frequency, etc.) (see Proverbio and Zani, 2005). As far as temporal onset is concerned, the attentional effect is believed to be starting at around 60-70 ms,

---

[1] Object recognition is known to occur in the very early stages of processing by means of spatial frequency analysis of the luminance configuration. This is made possible by the presence in visual cortex of specific frequency analyzers in the form of neurons sensitive to a given range of frequencies and organized on the basis of preferences for orientation and color also. The spatial frequency channels vary in sensitivity from 0.8 to 3 octaves approximately, increasing this sensitivity on average to 1.8 octaves in parafovea and 1.4-1.6 octaves in fovea. An octave is the interval between a given spatial frequency (e. g., 1° 30') and double the frequency (in this case 3°). For example, a spatial frequency channel with a sensitivity bandwidth of 1 octave will respond significantly to the preferred frequency (e. g., 2° 15') and to a lesser degree to limiting frequencies within the octave.

corresponding in all probability to the activation of the primary visual area or V1 (see Zani and Proverbio, 2005). For example, the selection of checkerboard patterns based on their check-size produces an increase in amplitude of the sensory responses P1 and N115 recorded at electrodes O1 and O2 corresponding to the primary visual areas (Zani and Proverbio, 1995). Likewise, selecting gratings on the basis of their spatial frequency (Zani and Proverbio, 1997a, 1997b, 1997c, 1997d, 1997e) and orientation (Karayanidis and Michie, 1997), or else selecting alphanumeric characters on the basis of their shape (Skrandies, 1983) produces an increase in the evoked response at the sensory level. This means that the attentional strategy adopted by the observer to identify as rapidly and effectively as possible an interesting object in the visual environment is able to enhance the response of the visual system to that object's features by setting an early selection sensory filter.

This type of filter is seen, as well as in the attentional modulation of P1, also in increases in amplitude of a preceding response, prominent on the hemisphere ipsilateral to stimulation, known as P-N80, as it is called on the basis of its average latency of 80 ms. It has a positive or negative polarity according to the type of stimulus (for example, increasing negativity with increasing spatial frequency), of the hemifield (polarity is reversed on going from the inferior hemifield to the upper hemifield) and of retinal eccentricity. The P-N80 is also known as C1 (acronym of *Component 1*, Jeffreys and Axford, 1972) and its inversion in polarity depends strongly on the crossed retinotopic organization of visual pathways and calcarine fissure in the occipital striate cortex, described as the *cruciform model*. According to this model, based on the organization of visual pathways, stimuli falling beneath the horizontal meridian of the visual field are projected to the superior lip of the calcarine fissure in the hemisphere contralateral, across the vertical meridian, to the area of the visual field affected by the stimuli themselves. Conversely, stimuli falling above the horizontal meridian end up finding their representation in the lower lip of the same fissure with the same hemispheric logistics. The neural generator of this potential was identified in the calcarine fissure of the striate cortex using both *scalp current density* (SCD) mapping (see Proverbio *et al.*, 1996), and the combining of spatio-temporal dipole modelling, with cortical anatomy provided by magnetic resonance (Clark and Hillyard, 1996).

Indeed, independent of the polarity of this component in passive gazing conditions, ERP data indicated that spatially directed selective attention is able to modulate the amplitude of this potential, generally in the direction of increased positivity (Zani and Proverbio, 1997c; 2005). This attentional modulation of P-N80 accounted in human observers engaged in attention tasks is consistent with the neurophysiological evidence obtained using cats and monkeys (see, for instance Motter, 1993, and Lamme and Spekreijse, 2000) on the modulation of neuronal populations of V1, as well as of V2 and V4 during the selection of non spatial features. More recently, several different neurophysiological studies carried out on macaques indicated a clear-cut attentional modulation of V1 for the selection of orientation (Press and Van Essen, 1997; Vanduffel *et al.*, 1997), of movement (Watanabe *et al.*, 1998), of spatial frequency and colour (Metha *et al.*, 1997), as well as of shape (Roelfsema *et al.*, 1997, 1998). Interestingly enough, Ito and Gilbert (1999) found that the firing rate of cells in the primary visual cortex of alert monkeys was significantly modulated by attentional set during a spatial attention task. Overall, these neurophysiological findings provided evidence that attentional modulation of sensory responses can be observed in most areas of the visual cortex, including V1 (see Treue, 2001, for a review), and perhaps earlier in the lateral geniculate nucleus of the thalamus (Vanduffel, Tootell and Orban, 2000). Conflicting evidence concerning V1 modulation for spatial attention has been found, however, by Luck *et al.* (1997), in a macaque study in which different spatial visual attention tasks were used. While finding V2 and V4 modulation, this study did not reveal any modulation of response of the neurons in visual area V1. Noteworthy, the authors correctly stressed that since stimuli attended or ignored by the animal fell in the receptive fields of different neurons, it was impossible to determine whether their firing rate would also have been modulated by attention if both stimuli had fallen in their receptive field.

Again, the study of Aine *et al.* (1995), who combined MRI measures and MEG measures, and the meta-analysis by Shulmann *et al.* (1997) performed by making a comparative survey of a large number of studies carried out using this method, consistently indicate a modulation of visual area 17 during a large number of active tasks involving the discrimination of features. Likewise, some electrophysiological studies (Zani and Proverbio, 1995, 1997; Zani *et al.*, 1999; Proverbio *et al.*, 1998) on healthy volunteers have shown an attentional modulation of early P90 and N115 evoked responses selectively recorded at O1 and O2 scalp sites of mesial occipital areas, which might reflect the activity of intracranial neural generators located in the primary visual area. Consistent findings of a modulation of P1 component have been found by Proverbio *et al.* (1993) in an selective attention task to spatial frequency. In particular, the study by Proverbio *et al.* (1998), using hierarchical alphanumeric stimuli that are either congruent or incongruent at local/global level, demonstrated that whenever a stimulus attended at the local level has the same shape as the global configuration (congruent condition) it elicits a greater N115 response over the mesial occipital area compared with the incongruent condition.

Consistent with the viewpoint that spatially directed attention can modulate the activity of the primary, besides the most championed secondary and tertiary, visual cortices, several relatively recent fMRI studies in humans too have provided evidence of the attentional modulation of V1 activity (Brefcynski and DeYoe, 1999; Gandhi *et al.*, 1999; Somers *et al.*, 1999; Kastner *et al.*, 1999).

Unlike the electrophysiological findings reviewed above, some combined ERPs-fMRI studies have failed to find ERPs evidence for early latency selection effects, notwithstanding the finding of anatomically localized effects at the primary areas of the visual streams (Martinez *et al.*, 1999; 2001a). To explain this conflicting late timing ERPs, but early-level anatomical-functional, evidence, the authors argued that V1 modulation is actually reflecting feedback processes from the extrastriate cortices picked up by fMRI because of its low temporal resolution. In the literature, experimental findings based on different method measures can be found both in support and against this proposal. A recent critical discussion of these multi-methodical findings can be found in Zani and Proverbio, 2005.

Noteworthy here is, however, that against this argument data had been presented (La Berge and Buchsbaum, 1990), and have been recently repeatedly reconfirmed, that attention also modulates the functionality of subcortical structures such as the superior colliculus, the lateral geniculate body, and the pulvinar of the thalamus (see Kastner *et al.*, 2005, for an up-to-date review of these findings), which receive and transmit retinotopically-organized projections to the striate and prestriate cortex. Most interestingly, the enhanced activation of these structures could well account for the increase in visual evoked potentials recorded as early as 40 ms post-stimulus in a spatial attention task by Oakley and Eason (1990). All in all, these results strongly supports the view that visual information might be subjected to a sensory filter controlled and monitored by superior centres such as the dorsolateral frontal areas, which might be capable of modulating the earliest analysis at cortical and subcortical level.

Feature Directed Attention

Research on features selection has traditionally concerned also orientation[2] (Harter and Guido, 1980; Kenemans *et al.*, 1993). Still, due to the use of a single channel recording (e.g., Oz) none of these studies led to knowledge of the scalp topography or localization of the electrocortical orientation selection.

A recent whole-head topographic mapping study by Proverbio, Esposito and Zani (2002) revealed an interesting effect of early modulation of the temporal P1, with a strong lateralization over the left hemisphere, reflecting the attentional selection of grating orientation. In this study, participants were foveally stimulated using a random series of isoluminant black-and-white gratings (3 cpd) having an orientation of 50°, 70°, 90° (vertical), 110° and 130° of visual angle, and a size of 2°. The task consisted in selectively attending and responding to one of the five grating orientations, while ignoring the others. Difference waves obtained by subtracting ERPs to irrelevant from those to relevant orientations showed that the selection of this feature modulated neural processing at an early post-stimulus latency within the P1 latency range. In addition, ERP mapping procedures yielded a focus for this effect over the posterior temporal regions.

It is worth noting that this area was indicated in both neurophysiological and haemodynamic studies as the area of final cortical projection of the ventral visual system having the function of analysing the non-spatial features (*What* system), and thus appears to be preferentially involved in this type of task. Indeed, Vogels and Orban (1994) and Tanaka (2000) found that cells of the inferior temporal cortex in monkey are strongly activated during orientation and/or object discrimination, while the PET study by Kawashima (1998) showed a specific activation of the left inferior temporal cortex during object discrimination in humans.

Besides the left-sided hemispheric asymmetry for the early attention effect, we found similar asymmetries for the attention effects concerning the later N150 and P300 components, as well as a left generator for the extrastriate posterior N150 regardless of grating relevance. All in all, these findings support the hypothesis of a predominant involvement of the left hemisphere in object features discrimination, as also supported by very recent neuroimaging studies (Dupont *et al.*, 1998; Georgopoulos *et al.*, 2001), as well as some ERP attention studies (Eimer, 1996; Martinez *et al.*, 2001b; Zani and Proverbio, 1995).

---

[2] Orientation is a visual attribute analysed at the primary level by visual cortex neurons organized into columns. Campbell and Maffei (1970) provided electrophysiological evidence of the existence of spatial frequency channels sensitive to stimulus orientation, and determined the amplitude of the sensitivity bandwidth in humans by measuring the amplitudes of the evoked potentials as a function of adaptation to high contrast gratings. They showed that when the test stimulus differed in orientation at least 20° or more with respect to the adaptation grating, the amplitude of evoked potentials dramatically increased compared to when they were elicited by stimuli closer in orientation to the adaptation gratings. These findings demonstrated that the orientation sensitivity bandwidth in humans is about 10-20° (varying as a function of stimulus spatial frequency).

Features Conjunction and Object Perception

Neural mechanisms of attentional selection for the manifold features of visual objects, although in part functionally and anatomically distinct, strongly interact with one another, as is also suggested by comparatively recent behavioral findings obtained in brain-lesioned patients. Based on ERP findings, it is further suggested that this interaction begins at an early sensory stage of processing.

In a pioneering ERPs study by Previc and Harter (1982) the participants had to attend and respond to target gratings having each time a given frequency and a given orientation. Spatial frequency was foveally projected and could be high or low and the orientation vertical or horizontal. The results indicated that the amplitude of N2 - i.e., the timing of the first sign of attentional filtering - for target stimuli was greater than the sum of the two responses to the single feature, thus demonstrating a non-additive nature and a close interaction between the mechanisms of selection of frequency and orientation.

In a later ERP study, we investigated the conjoined attentional selection of spatial frequency and spatial location using isoluminant gratings laterally presented in the inferior and superior quadrants of the left and right visual hemifields (Zani and Proverbio, 1997b). Subjects were administered four sinusoidal gratings randomly flashed to the inferior and superior quadrants of the visual field when relevant and irrelevant. The gratings produced stimulation at spatial frequencies of 0.75, 1.5, 3, and 6 cycles per degree (cpd) of visual angle. In different runs, the volunteers selectively attended and responded motorically either to 0.75 or 6 cpd at a relevant location (i. e., one of the visual quadrants) while ignoring all the other gratings and locations. In this way, while the physical stimuli remained unchanged, attention shifted across spatial frequency and spatial location. Thus, as graphically depicted in Figure 1, in separate attention conditions, one and the same stimulus could be (1) relevant both in spatial location and spatial frequency (i.e., L+F+), (2) relevant in location but irrelevant in frequency (L+F−), (3) irrelevant in location but relevant in frequency (L−F+), and (4) irrelevant in both features (L−F−).

ERPs were recorded from homologous mesial-occipital O1 and O2 and lateral-occipital OL and OR electrode sites.

ERP waveforms indicated that a much earlier selection of the frequency occurred than previously believed, that is, within 60-130 ms post-stimulus. More specifically, the two features influenced both the amplitude of the P1 evoked sensory response, even though the effect of frequency relevance was felt only when the stimuli fell in the attended quadrant. The latter findings suggest that the selection mechanisms of the two features operate in parallel right from the earliest stages of analysis, and that object or feature selection, rather than being preceded by a space selection, is centered "on line" on precise coordinates of the attended space. This view is supported in by many studies in the literature.

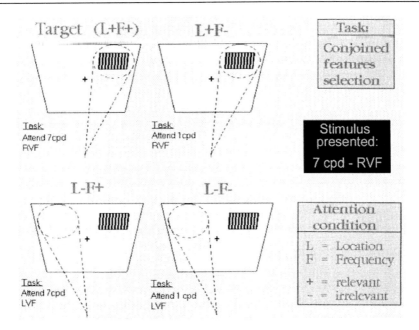

Figure 1. Graphical depiction of the different attentional conditions deriving from the visual conjoined selection tasks used in Zani's and Proverbio's study in (1997a). These tasks required to pay heed to one spatial frequency (F), out of the four randomly presented, at one spatial location (L), that is one of the four quadrants (i.e., ULQ, URQ, LLQ, and LRQ) of the visual field at which the frequencies were flashed, while ignoring all the other locations and all the other frequencies. In different runs, the location and the spatial frequency to pay heed to varied. The examples reported here hold for 7 cpd in the upper right quadrant (URQ), but, with the due adjustments, they hold for 1 cpd too, besides for all the other quadrants. The four sketchy upside-down polygons represent the computer monitor used to present the gratings to the volunteers. The black-and-white grating drawn in the upper right region of these polygons represent the 7 cpd spatial frequency grating flashed in the URQ. The dashed, tilted cones represent the covert orienting, in different experimental runs, of the focus of visual attention toward one of the spatial locations tested. In the two upper conditions drawn, volunteers directed attention toward the upper right location, whereas in the lower conditions they addressed it toward the upper left space location (ULQ). In the upper left condition 7 cpd resulted relevant both in location (L+) and in frequency (F+), because it was the frequency to be attended under the focus of attention. Conversely, in the upper right condition, this same grating, although being still relevant in location (L+) because the focus of attention was directed to the URQ, resulted irrelevant in frequency (F-), because this time 1 cpd was the relevant frequency. In the lower left condition, the 7cpd grating was irrelevant in location (L-), since the focus of attention was oriented to the ULQ, but relevant in frequency (F+), since the same frequency was now relevant at that quadrant. Finally, the lower right condition resulted in 7cpd being irrelevant both in location (L-) and frequency (F-), since attention was directed to 1 cpd at the ULQ.

The visual system is able to process and attentionally select one or more visual features (spatial frequency, depth, stereopsis, colour, orientation, texture, luminance) of the objects in the surrounding environment. Of course, in actual fact, we perceive a unitary environment and not a separate series of objects or individual attributes (Previc, 1990). This perception of the unitary nature derives from the interaction between the "Where" and "What" systems, which, although partially anatomically and functionally distinct, operate in parallel and in very close coordination. Clear evidence of this interdependence comes from neuropsychological and neuroimaging literature. For example, the clinical neuropsychological study by Friedman-Hill et al. (1995) indicated that patients with focused bilateral lesions of the parietal cortex are unable to correctly combine colour and shape of stimuli presented in the two visual hemifields. This suggests that the integrity of the Where system is absolutely essential for the correct recognition of objects. On the other hand, a large body of neuropsychological, neurophysiological and behavioural findings (see Olson and Gettner, 1996 for a review of these data) indicates that the spatial and non-spatial attention mechanisms are probably not separated at all because of the existence of specific selection mechanisms centered on the object at a given spatial location (i.e., *object-centered space receptive fields*). In our view, our electrophysiological data on conjoined selection of spatial frequency and space location (Zani and Proverbio, 1997b, 1997e) reported above are in line with this view of object-based space selection derived from several other research lines in cognitive neuroscience.

The extensive available neurophysiological and psychophysical literature has shown that the perceptual construction of objects takes place through the simultaneous analysis of a complex series of cues (namely luminance, color, texture, motion and binocular disparity) at very early processing stages (Mountcastle, 1998; Regan, 2000). Selective attention is able to modulate (that is, to optimise or ignore) the perception of objects thus constructed, as it results also from studies on the selection of the so-called illusory contours subjective figures. The illusory contours are known to be perceived edges that exist in the absence of local borders and that determine the perception of subjective figures, such as the universally known Kanizsa square or triangle (1976). They are based on the peculiar boundary alignment of inducers (simple geometric shapes in striking contrast with the homogenous background luminance) which elicit the response of edge detectors in area 18 (Hirsch *et al.*, 1995; Larsson *et al.*, 1999) and perhaps 17 (Grosof *et al.*, 1993; Lee and Nguyen, 2001; Olson, 2001), giving rise to the subjective perception of an object with partially illusory boundaries.

In a study carried out on healthy young controls we investigated the brain mechanisms underlying the perception of illusory contours and determined the time course of sensory and perceptual processing in the boundary completion process, analyzing the timing of ERP responses (Proverbio and Zani, 2002). The task consisted in paying attention and respond to the illusory squares while ignoring the other configurations. The object to be detected and attentionally selected thus did not actually exist for retinal photoreceptors, but was really seen by the visual cortex with the same clarity as a real object. ERPs showed that the occurrence of illusory contours was associated with a strong bilateral activation of lateral occipital areas at about 145 ms post-stimulus as indexed by N1 component, followed by a left-sided activation of the same region at about 250 ms of latency. Overall, our data support the view that the integration of contours arises at early stages of visual processing, as proposed by Hess and Field (1999). Moreover, our data also indicate that object-based attention is able to affect illusory contour binding by somewhat enhancing ERPs to the illusory percepts at lateral occipital sites.

Together with other experimental data reviewed so far, our findings indicate that the dorsal and ventral streams of the visual system, although partially anatomically segregated, may be activated in parallel and in an independent or conjoined mode depending on the attentional demands and task requirements. Last, but not least, there is evidence that the perception of multidimensional objects in the visual field is accomplished through a unitary active binding process of spatial and non-spatial features. This mechanism is believed not to be based on hierarchically organized independent processes, but rather to reflect the horizontal processing of visual cells that takes place at very early stages of input analysis. This view seems to be consistent with models assuming that different stimulus attributes may be initially conjoined in a single representation, while at the same time being separately analysed in parallel, dimension by dimension (*Cf.* Treisman, 1999 for a review of these models).

The present review of findings on the functions of posterior regions of the brain in visual attention indicates that attention to space and object-features can modulate neural processing of visual areas, very likely involving the primary striate cortex, as well as sub-cortical thalamic structures, with modalities that are still not clearly known and need to be further investigated. In addition, this literature suggests that attention: (1) enhances processing for all stimuli in an attended channel, and (2), finely modulates activation of the visual regions so that relevant sources of information receive a further activation burst with respect to irrelevant stimuli, with changes apparent as early as 60 ms after delivery of the to-be attended visual stimulus. This implies that attention-dependent neural activation elicited by the irrelevant source of information within the attended channel has somehow to be inhibited through some mechanisms regulated by the anterior attention system. These mechanisms, as well as the timing of their activation, are still not clearly understood, although the bulk of knowledge deriving from both human and animal studies at present available. Below, a review, far from being exhaustive, follows of this knowledge.

The Anterior Attention System

This system includes the frontal and prefrontal areas, the anterior cingulate gyrus, and the baso-ganglia. It is thought to be responsible for the functional recruitment and control of the cerebral areas having the function of carrying out selective information processing across all sensory modalities and complex cognitive tasks (Desimone and Duncan, 1995). Several neuroimaging and clinical studies reported in the literature confirm the crucial role played by this functional system. In particular, it has been shown that the prefrontal cortex (PFC) is involved in all kinds of top-down selective processing, when behavior must be guided by internal states or intentions (Gehring and Knight, 2000; Miller and Cohen, 2001).

Prior to the massive increase in these neuroimaging studies, a bulk of evidence supporting the view of the executive control played by the anterior system derived from patient-based observations. In general, the discoveries made in clinical practice have shown how the above-mentioned deficits are linked to an important disorder of the capacity to maintain a mental representation of stimulus-response mapping strategy or of the stimulus set. In other words, a combined disorder of the working memory system and the attentional system (Shimamura, 2002).

In this regard, evidence is available to show that patients with lesions of the dorsolateral pre-frontal (D-L/P-F) cortex suffer from a set of primary (e. g., deficits of the inhibitory control of response to, or difficulties in detection of, novelty), secondary (e. g., distractibility, reduced attention, etc.), and tertiary (e. g., reduced memory and organizational planning, problems in ordering past, present, and future events) symptoms, linked to a frontal syndrome (Stuss *et al.*, 1994; Knight and Grabowecky, 1995; Swick and Knight, 1999). A body of experimental evidence to support this model has emerged from studies on patients with focal brain lesions subjected to ERP recording. Changes in the amplitude and latency of the most studied component of the ERPs, the P3 wave, have been described in several neurologic and psychiatric disorders (Polich and Herbst, 2001) as well as in some brain lesional syndromes (Deouelle and Knight, 2005; Verleger, 2003).

The P3 component, also indicated as late positive complex (LPC), is a positive potential associated with a number of psychological constructs, including context updating, information contribution, stimulus categorization, memory, checking the correspondence of stimulus information with an internal representation, voluntary orientation and attention allocation (Coles, 1989). Robust evidence has accumulated to show that this complex embodies different sub-components. The most renown, P3b, shows a topographical distribution greatest at central-posterior locations of the scalp, and may be observed when the observer is requested to detect task-relevant infrequent stimuli (Donchin, 1981; Polich, 1998) during signal detection tasks (Sutton et al., 1965), whenever the relevant stimulus corresponds to an internal model (Gomer et al., 1976), and more generally during attentional (Proverbio et al., 1994) and coding tasks as well as mnemonic tasks (Fabiani et al., 1986). Unlike P3b, the P3a is elicited by new rare stimuli, irrelevant to the task, and is associated with automatic voluntary attentional orientation processes (Proverbio and Mangun, 1994), arousal and response to novelty. It has its maximum at more fronto-central regions and it is also about 50 ms earlier than the P3 proper (Squires et al., 1975; Knight, 1996).

Recording of these brain potentials in D-L/P-F patients has shown that, compared with healthy controls, these patients displayed a dramatic reduction in P3a amplitude in the case of 'novel' stimuli (that is, deviant stimuli included in a sequence of irrelevant and relevant stimuli, with the patients instructed to respond to the latter by pressing a button). This reduction was greatest at the anterior electrode sites for all the sensory modes – visual, auditory, and somatosensory - of the stimuli used in these studies (e. g., Knight, 1991; Knight and Grabowecky, 1995). Very interesting is that this specific reduction in frontal P3a was found to be typical of these patients only. Patients with damaged parietal and temporal lobes actually displayed P3as with amplitudes comparable to those obtained in healthy control subjects (Knight, 1991; Knight and Grabowecky, 1995).

In general, these discoveries show how crucial the prefrontal cortex is in the detection of changes in the external environment and in distinguishing derived models of the world both internally and externally (Knight, 1991; Knight and Grabowecky, 1995; Shimamura, 2002). More recent ERP data indicate that what is perhaps the most important deficit linked to a lesion of the D-L/P-F cortex consists in the inability to reject or suppress irrelevant information within all sensory systems, while the major deficit linked to a lesion of the medial prefrontal cortex is impairment of the ability to monitor behavior to guide and compensate possible behavioral errors and conflicts. These two deficits indicate that critical functions of sub-areas of the prefrontal cortex are the control of neural information processing through the modulation of activation of sensory systems, as recently shown by Barcelo and coauthors (2000) for visual extrastriate cortex, and the monitoring of behavior through direct connections to the cingulate cortex (Gehring and Knight, 2000).

It is interesting, in this regard, that more recent studies on patients with prefrontal lesions engaged in goal-directed tasks (see Knight et al., 1999; Hermann and Knight, 2001; and Deouell and Knight, 2005, for reviews of these studies) show that, besides the late P3 component, both the relatively early P1 and N1 components are modulated too by excitatory and inhibitory mechanisms. Based on these findings, the conclusions advanced by the authors are that, on the one hand, this damage disrupts inhibitory modulation of irrelevant inputs to primary sensory cortex, and on the other, results in multi-modal decreases in neural activity in the posterior association cortex in the hemisphere ipsilateral to damage.

Measures of the LPC obtained in normal volunteers too support the view that D-L/P-F areas might be involved in exerting a function of inhibitory filtering of visual task-irrelevant information (Zani and Proverbio, 1995). In this study a group of volunteers was foveally presented with random sequences of checkerboard patterns with check sizes of 5, 6 and 40", 10, 20, 40 and 60 min of arc, respectively. In different experimental sessions, the volunteers were instructed to pay heed and motorically respond to one check size, each time varying, and to ignore all the others. ERPs were recorded from the anterior frontal F7 and F8, besides the posterior mesial-occipital O1 and O2, and lateral-occipital OL and OR, homologous scalp sites falling over the two hemispheres of the brain. At the anterior sites, a late positivity (latency range: 300-480 ms) was recorded being of greater amplitude for irrelevant no-go than for relevant go checks. This finding is consistent with those of previous studies based on both simple (Pfefferbaum et al., 1985; Verleger and Berg, 1991; Roberts et al., 1994), and complex go/no-go tasks requiring the information to be stored in the working memory (e.g., Gevins and Cutillo, 1993), which reported a larger and more anteriorly distributed P3 for no-go than go stimuli in situations in which these two kinds of stimuli are equally probable. It is also strictly consistent with the ERP results of a study by Proverbio and Mangun (1994) robustly suggesting that our finding, rather than reflecting at the scalp the mere suppression of motor activation, was most likely associated with attentional control of processing of irrelevant stimuli. In that study, green squares subtending 1 degree of visual angle were flashed to the left and right visual hemifields under different conditions of covert spatial attention. In different blocks, volunteers were instructed to allocate attention primarily to either the left or to the right stimulus locations, or, in a neutral condition, to divide attention equivalently between the two locations. Regardless of attention condition, however, speeded motor responses were required to all stimuli in both visual fields. Although somewhat earlier than in our study (latency range: 280-380 ms), the P3 revealed to be larger in amplitude to the unattended than the attended stimuli at anterior as well as posterior electrode sites. In addition, at frontal, central and parietal electrode sites P3 was larger to the unattended than to the neutral.

Most interestingly, unlike all these studies in Zani and Proverbio (1995) the ERPs elicited at F7 and F8 sites by stimuli of different check sizes displayed a clear-cut amplitude gradient as a function of attended size, as it was larger for irrelevant stimuli more similar to the relevant target (i.e., one or more octave(s) within the frequency band - and thus more difficult to ignore; e.g. 40 min of arc when 60 min of arc was relevant) and decreasing as the check-sizes became more unlike the target (i.e., more octaves outside the frequency band - and thus easier to ignore; e.g. 5 min of arc when 60 min of arc was relevant). Our findings extended those made in these previous studies, in that they indicate that the larger frontal effect for no-go or irrelevant stimuli does not index inhibition in a simply "all-or-none" fashion, thus enabling more than one binary separation between "irrelevant" and "relevant" stimuli. Rather, to the extent that this larger frontal positivity is indexing a suppressive process, the view is advanced that the extent of process modulation is a function of the degree of similarity of irrelevant stimuli to relevant one(s). In other words, it is a function of the greater or lesser processing interference during the task of the former with the latter, and, as a consequence, of the stronger or weaker need to suppress neural response to irrelevant stimuli within the attentional and motor channels so to avoid processing overload and/or possible incorrect motor responses (i.e., *false alarms*).

To the extent that the suppression of a response represents a gap in the primary mapping strategy between stimulus and response, the anterior distribution of this specific potential seems to be consistent with the role of the frontal lobes in the structuring of temporal events, in the mediation of preparatory processes, of programming and control on the allocation of the individual's attentional resources. It is also consistent with the hypothesis of the frontal lobes being extensively involved in the working memory, as suggested by neurophysiological studies (Goldman-Rakic, 1987), and neuroimaging and clinical ones (Smith and Jonides, 2003).

To further investigate the functionality of frontal regions in attentional control, we carried out a further study in normal volunteers (Zani and Proverbio, 1997a) founded on the selective processing of multidimensional stimuli varying in the conjoined and separate relevance of their spatial location and spatial frequency features. The same stimuli as in the study by Zani and Proverbio (1997b) discussed above were used. However, besides the conjoined selective attention tasks, the volunteers also engaged in a passive gazing of the gratings, and ERPs were recorded from homologous mesial frontal F3 and F4 electrode sites, besides the occipital sites.

ERP measures indicated that, regardless of the spatial frequency attended, within the 300-600 msec post-stimulus latency range, stimuli irrelevant in one (i.e., L+F− and L−F+) or in both features (L-F-) elicited a larger P3 at anterior, compared to posterior, sites. The reverse was true for the targets (L+F+).

Regardless of electrode site, the P3 to targets was larger than to gratings sharing spatial location with them (L+F−). Again, the latter condition yielded larger P3s than did stimuli not sharing spatial location (L−F+) or neither feature (L−F−) with targets, whereas the latter two conditions did not differ from each another. Noteworthy, although at anterior sites the latter two conditions were much larger in amplitude, compared to the passive gazing condition, at posterior sites they were not.

All in all, these findings indicated that, independent of spatial frequency relevance, cognitive processing by the occipital system of stimuli falling outside the focus of spatial attention (i.e., L-F+, L-F-) was suppressed at some previous stage of processing. ERPs pointed to a positive activation occurring with a mean latency of 190 msec within the latency range of 160–260 ms post-stimulus as the timing of this supposed suppression. In actual fact, at frontal sites, P190 was larger for both frequency-relevant and frequency-irrelevant stimuli irrelevant in location (i.e., L−F+ and L−F−) than to neutral stimuli. In turn, neutral stimuli yielded a larger P190 than did stimuli relevant in location (i.e., both L+F+ and L+F−). Conversely, at occipital sites, P190 was largest for passively gazed stimuli (i.e., neutral), and decreased as a gradient from gratings irrelevant in both features to those irrelevant in one feature only, and, finally, to those relevant in both features.

Noteworthy, we obtained the consistent finding that P190 to both L-F+ and L-F- was larger at the frontal electrode site ipsilateral with the attended visual field, in support of the view that the frontal P190 might index an inhibition of processing of both frequency-relevant and frequency-irrelevant stimuli falling outside the focus of attention (see Figure 2).

Overall, the present findings confirmed that inhibition of task-irrelevant stimuli is not a simply "all-or-none" phenomenon, but enables more than one binary separation between "irrelevant" and "relevant" stimuli. More importantly, they indicated a rather complex pattern of functional activation for prefrontal regions. Indeed, these data imply that, unlike in the passive task, during active selection tasks, prefrontal regions differentially are activated to control the selective processing of stimuli falling within or without the focus of spatial attention by the posterior areas of the brain. Consistent with this view, anterior P190 would index an early activation of prefrontal cortex to actively inhibit processing of both relevant and irrelevant sources of information falling *outside* the focus of spatial attention. Unlike this earlier modulation, the later anterior P3 might prove to be a sensitive indicator of a prefrontal belated inhibition of higher level processing of irrelevant stimuli falling *within* the focus of attention.

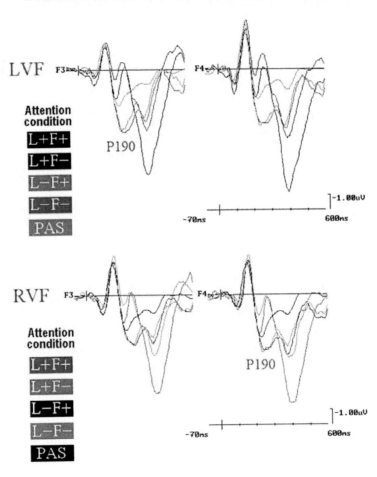

Figure 2. Grand-average ERPs recorded form homologous F3-F4 dorsolateral sites as a function of spatial attention direction (LVF or RVF), and of attention condition: L+F+=location relevant-frequency relevant; L+F-=location relevant-frequency irrelevant; L-F+=location irrelevant-frequency irrelevant; L-F-=both features irrelevant; PAS=passive gazing. Noteworthy, both location irrelevant conditions elicited a prominent P190 much larger than both location relevant conditions, as well as than the passive gazing one. Remarkably, this prominent response to both the location irrelevant conditions was larger at the site ipsilateral to the attention direction.

At this regard, it is worth reporting that several blood-flow imaging studies on normal young volunteers point at an involvement of D-L/P-F cortex in inhibitory processes. Overall, these studies have been mainly founded on four different experimental paradigms derived from cognitive psychology. They have in common a competition between two or more sources of information and, for this reason, elicit attention and inhibition processes due to this competition for control over responses. These are the Stroop task (MacLeod, 1991; Taylor *et al.*, 1997), the stimulus-response compatibility task (Kornblum *et al.*, 1990), the flanker task (Eriksen and Eriksen, 1974; Hazeltine *et al.*, 2000), and the go/no-go task (Casey *et al.*, 1997; Carter *et al.*, 1998).

Although these blood flow studies showed variations in regions of activation as a function of task, they also showed a common activation across tasks of two broad regions of the frontal cortex: namely, the anterior cingulate cortex and the D-L/P-F cortex (Taylor *et al.*, 1997; Casey *et al.*, 1997; Hazeltine *et al.*, 2000). These common regions of activation, among several others, have been, rather recently, confirmed by means of a meta-analytic examination of 15 blood flow studies found in the literature carried out by Jonides *et al.* (2002) with the aim to identify the Brodmann areas interested.

Another line of attractive PET data indicating activation of lateral prefrontal regions *ipsilateral* to the direction of spatially-directed attention deserves to be discussed here because these data were interpreted as a sign of inhibition of stimulus processing in the ignored visual field. Inhibiting attentional demands by non-targets represented a significant component of the task used during PET scanning, and on each experimental trial a display containing two circular patches of grating was presented. From one trial to another, each grating varied randomly in two attributes, orientation (clockwise or counterclockwise) and exact location (above or below the fixation point). In different attention conditions, volunteers were instructed to identify patch orientation or location, or any combination of these features. Among other several findings, most relevant to the theme of this chapter, was the finding of an activation of the lateral prefrontal region greater on the side ipsilateral to attention. The interpretation was advanced that a left frontal activation might be associated with inhibition of the concurrent irrelevant stimuli in the right contralateral field, and vice versa for right frontal activation (Vandenberghe *et al.*, 1997, 2000; Duncan, 2001).

Most interestingly, there is close consistency between these PET findings and our ERP reflections of the activation of prefrontal regions ipsilateral to the direction of spatial attention notwithstanding the differences in stimulation modalities across these studies. This implies that prefrontal regions activate to send signals to the posterior regions on the same brain side for inhibiting processing of both relevant and irrelevant information falling at the contralateral unattended visual field independent of the fact that these stimuli are concurrently or sequentially present in the visual field. In our view, this implication provides further support to the view that this ipsilateral activation reflects an inhibitory function carried out by the prefrontal regions of the brain.

Briefly, the converging results of neuropsychological clinical and electrophysiological studies suggest that the maintenance of short-term behavior control strategies, together with the capacity to inhibit the processing of irrelevant stimuli or events, are among the more important functions performed by prefrontal areas of the anterior attentional system. These two functions are closely related and can account for many of the behavioural disorders deriving from lesions of the prefrontal cortex, which is part of this system.

Functional Hemispheric Asymmetry

Despite the bulk of important insights into the functioning of DL/PF cortex offered by the systematic patient-based analyses reviewed above, up-to-date very scant are the clinical observations of possible functional differences across the left and the right DL/PF cortices. Actually, no systematic search for such asymmetries has been carried out in frontal- and prefrontal-lesioned patients, and the recent scant observations found in the neuropsychological literature have been made almost serendipitously.

In investigating attention and inhibition in patient R.C. whose middle and inferior gyri of the PFC, including the left hemisphere ventrolateral prefrontal area (BA 45), were identified to be damaged by PET scans, Thompson-Schill *et al.* (2002) used an item recognition task with low- and high-conflict conditions. A group of brain lesioned controls having PFC damage sparing BA 45/46 was also tested. The authors found that there were no relevant differences across patient R.C. and the controls for the low-conflict condition. In contrast, R.C. showed a remarkable impairment in response time and accuracy in the high-conflict condition. These findings are consistent with the view that BA 45 is critical for attention control and inhibitory demands.

More recently, Gehring and Knight (2002) investigated the effects of damage to the lateral PFC recording choice reaction times (RTs) in a letter discrimination task that required attention switching and processing selection. Six PFC patients and three parietal patients were compared with age-matched and young controls. PFC patients did not show any significant impairment in switching attention from one condition to another. They, however, displayed a significant increase of the effects of distractor stimuli, implicating the lateral PFC in processing selection. Noteworthy, when carrying out a more detailed analysis of their data searching for possible individual differences, Gehring and Knight (2002) found that three out of the six PFC patients exceeded a "confidence interval" for the raw distracter compatibility effect and the corrected compatibility effect performance measures, denoting a significantly impaired performance relative to the controls. Most interestingly, all these three PFC patients had lesions in the left posterior inferior prefrontal cortex. Based on these findings, the authors concluded that the left PFC, in particular a relatively inferior region, is most critical for modulating the effects of distracting inputs. They, however, cautiously wondered whether the linguistic nature of their stimuli might have contributed to the left-sided localization results.

Recent functional neuroimaging findings in normal young individuals also indicate the involvement of the left PFC in inhibitory processing. Jonides *et al.* (1998) PET scanned a group of normal volunteers while they performed an item recognition task with low- and high-conflict conditions. When comparing between these two conditions, the authors found that a portion of the left hemisphere ventrolateral PFC (BA 45) was the only significant focus of activation, implying that this area is critically involved in attentional and inhibitory processing.

A later er-fMRI study by D'Esposito *et al.* (1999) testing the high-conflict condition only of the item recognition task, reported a similar greater activation of BA 45. Again, Milham *et al.* (2001) with an er-fMRI study based on a Stroop-like task and comparing neural activity during incongruent trials that produced conflict at different response and non-response levels of processing, found an activation of left prefrontal cortex (BA 9/6 and BA 44/45) when conflict raised at non-response level, and the activation of anterior cingulate and right prefrontal cortex when conflict raised at response level. To the extent that the suppression of a response may represent a gap in the maintenance of a mental representation of stimulus-response mapping strategy requiring a control on the allocation of the individual's attentional resources, in other words a combined activation of the working memory and of the attentional systems (see Shimamura, 2000; 2002), then some previous fMRI signs of left IFG activity during retrieval of verbal semantic knowledge (Thompson-Schill *et al.*, 1997) are also much relevant to the present chapter. Indeed, varying the degree of semantic processing independently of selection demands, these authors found that it is not retrieval of semantic knowledge *per se* that was associated with left IFG activation but rather selection of information among competing alternatives from semantic memory.

A likely implication deriving from all these studies is that the left-sided activation reflects inhibiting interfering information and selectively attending to relevant information when a response is being selected. This implication seems plausible although the use of verbal stimulus material in all these studies still casts some doubts of contribution of the latter to the left-sided activation.

Notwithstanding ERPs limitations in localization capacity due to their scarce spatial resolution, some findings of our study on foveal selective attention to check-size in neurologically-intact volunteers (Zani and Proverbio, 1995) also suggested a left-sided lateralization for attentional inhibition. Indeed, post-hoc analyses for a significant ANOVA interaction of the attention and hemisphere factors for the frontal positivity revealed that this component was larger at the left (F7) than at the right (F8) frontal inferior-lateral site for irrelevant patterns only (see Figure 3). This finding, together with the one that at occipital sites the late positivity for the latter stimuli was instead much smaller than the one to the relevant patterns, hints at the left prefrontal regions being strictly involved in the active suppression of cognitive processing of irrelevant sources of information by the occipital-temporal regions of the brain. Thank to their high-temporal resolution, in the order of the millisecond, ERPs indicated the timing of this left hemisphere suppression of cognitive processing of the irrelevant source of information being in the range of 300-480 ms post-stimulus. Quite consistently, when subtracting ERPs to inconspicuous stimuli (F-) flashed at the irrelevant location (L-) from ERPs to distracting stimuli (F-) falling at the attended location (L+) in our spatial frequency and spatial location conjoined selection study (Zani and Proverbio, 1997a), we found that in the P3 latency range this difference was larger at the left (F3) than the right (F4) prefrontal site independent of the direction of spatially-directed attention.

Our P3 findings are in broad agreement with the ERP results of Proverbio and Mangun (1994). Indeed, independent of stimulus hemifield, their P3 showed to be larger in amplitude to the unattended than the attended stimuli over the left hemisphere at all electrode sites, and roughly equivalent in amplitude over the right hemisphere. Thus, while the P3 was larger over the right hemisphere, attention control effects (i.e., unattended − attended) were greatest over the left hemisphere. Time-series isocontour voltage maps computed on the difference waves obtained subtracting ERPs to the attended stimuli from ERPs to the unattended stimuli (Proverbio, *Doctoral thesis*, 1993) revealed that this attention control effects started at the left dorsolateral scalp site around 280 ms post-stimulus and slowly spread, afterward, within 360 ms post-stimulus, first toward the posterior regions of the scalp over the left hemisphere, and, later on, toward the right side of the scalp (see Figure 4).

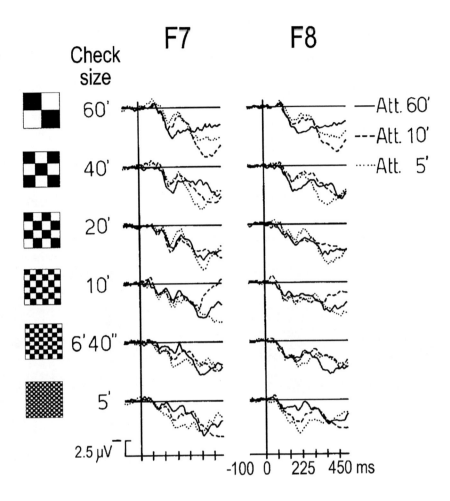

Figure 3. Examples of grand-average ERPs recorded at homologous inferior-lateral frontal sites (F7 and F8) as a function of check size (in minutes of arc) while volunteers paid heed to 60', 10', or 5', respectively. Besides an enhanced frontal positivity peaking at about 225 ms to relevant patterns and the ones that more looked alike the latter (e.g., 5' when 10' was relevant), another notable ERP sign of frontal selective processing consisted in a later P3 greater to the irrelevant patterns that were more unlike the relevant ones (e.g., 5' when 60' was relevant). This later P3 probably reflected an active suppression of the late cognitive processing of hardly-interfering irrelevant stimuli at brain occipital sites since, at these sites, the latter stimuli attained lower ERP amplitudes than relevant ones. (Reprinted from *Electroencephalography and Clinical Neurophysiology*, 95, Zani and Proverbio, ERP signs of early selective attention effects to check size, 277-292. Copyright (1995) with permission of Elsevier Science.)

In concluding this section, it has to be underlined that being our attentional tasks and those by Proverbio and Mangun (1994) based on the selection of nonverbal material, it does not hold the objection that the left-sided asymmetry might simply depend on stimulus material *per se*, as in the most of the studies reviewed above because of their use of verbal stimuli. Rather, this asymmetry seems to be a specific functional property of the left prefrontal cortex.

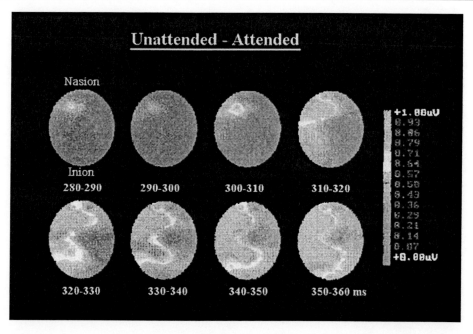

Figure 4. Time series of isocolour voltage maps computed on difference waves obtained subtracting ERPs to spatially-attended stimuli from ERPs to the same stimuli whenever spatially-unattended between 280 and 360 ms post-stimulus. In this latency range the maps suggest attention control effects subserved by an asymmetric activation of the left-sided regions of the brain, with an earlier starting at the left medial dorsolateral prefrontal areas and a later spreading to the central sensory-motor and parietal regions of the brain on the same side (Reproduced and modified from A. M. Proverbio's Doctoral Thesis).

RATIONALE FOR THE PRESENT STUDY

Goals of the present study were manifold. First, we sought to further investigate the timing of the attentional modulation of visual information processing at occipito-temporal regions of the brain. Besides reconfirming the discriminative function between salient and distracting sensory inputs from an attended location served by these regions already at an early P1 processing level, we sought to investigate whether this function might be starting as earliest as at the post-stimulus sensory processing level, as reflected by ERPs C1 response. Second, we sought to further tap prefrontal attentional control and inhibition functions, as well as their hemispheric asymmetries, recording ERPs while volunteers performed a conjoined selection task of spatial location and spatial frequency. We reasoned that if the inhibiting function served by the left prefrontal cortex is triggered by the sources of irrelevant information within the focus of attention, as suggested by our previous studies (Zani and Proverbio, 1995; 1997a), then we should have found frontal scalp signs of this inhibition for the interfering information (i.e., the irrelevant spatial frequencies) within (i. e., the attended location) but not without (i. e., the unattended location) the focus of spatial attention.

Last but not least, since in our previous studies few electrodes were used, we investigated the topographic distribution over the scalp of visual selective processing using a whole-head 32 electrodes montage distributed over the anterior and posterior scalp.

MATERIAL AND METHODS

Participants

Nineteen young normal volunteers (10 males and 9 females; age range: 20 – 35 years; mean age = 24 years) participated in this experiment as volunteers. All participants had a normal or corrected-to-normal vision with right eye dominance. They were strictly right-handed as assessed by the Edinburgh inventory and none of them had any left-handed relatives whatsoever. Experiments were conducted with the understanding and the consent of each participant according to the declaration of Helsinki (BMJ 1991; 302: 1194) with approval from the Ethical Committee of the Italian National Research Council (CNR) and in compliance with APA ethical standards for the treatment of human volunteers (1992, American Psychological Association).

Stimuli and Procedure

Participants were seated in a dimly lit, electrically shielded cubicle and binocularly gazed on a fixation point permanently present in the centre of a visual display situated at 114 cm from them. They were instructed to avoid any kind of eye or body movement. Four sinusoidal luminance-modulated vertical gratings were used as stimuli. Gratings produced stimulation at 1, 2, 4, and 7 cycles per degree (cpd) of visual angle. Contrast was 60% and presentation duration 100 ms. The patterns were replaced for an interval randomly varying in between 850 and 1000 ms (ISI) by an isoluminant grey field (on-off). Stimulus and background had an equal average luminance to avoid flash stimulation. The mean luminance was 25 cd/m^2. The gratings were randomly presented in pattern-onset mode within the upper hemifields of a computer screen. Within each hemifield, grating stimulation began 2.5° above the horizontal meridian (HM) and 2.5° lateral to the vertical meridian (VM), and extended to 3.5° above the HM and 5° along it.

Different conjoined selective attention conditions were administered in randomised order for either 1 or 7 cpd within each hemifield to each subject. No matter the target frequency, gratings of 2 and 4 cpd always posed as potential distractors. Before the beginning of each task condition, participants were instructed to pay conjoined attention to a spatial frequency within a given hemifield (e. g., 7 cpd at the LVF) and to ignore the other combinations of frequencies and hemifields. Thus, although the physical stimuli remained unchanged, attention shifted across spatial frequency and space location.

This way, in different attention conjunction conditions a same stimulus could be:

i)   relevant both in spatial location and spatial frequency (L+F+);
ii) relevant in spatial location but irrelevant in spatial frequency (L+F-);
iii) irrelevant in spatial location but relevant in spatial frequency (L-F+); and,
iv) irrelevant in both features (L-F-).

To monitor spatial and stimulus attention selectivity, the volunteers were instructed to press a button to targets as accurately and fast as possible allowing also their reaction time

(RT) to be recorded. For each of the stimulus targets and hemifields, eight blocks of 120 trials were replicated. During a single block of trials, the 4 gratings (i. e., one target and three "distractors") were each equiprobably presented 15 times within the visual hemifields in a completely random sequence. Trial order changed randomly from block to block. In half of the blocks, participants pushed the detection-RT button with the forefinger of the left hand, whereas in the other half of the blocks they used the forefinger of the right hand. The order of the hands was counterbalanced across participants. The order with which attention tasks were administered and spatial locations attended was counterbalanced across participants and experimental sessions.

ELECTROPHYSIOLOGICAL RECORDING AND ANALYSIS

A whole-head montage was used to record EEG. Thirty scalp sites were covered using chlorized tin electrodes mounted in an elastic cap (Electro-cap, Inc.). The electrodes were located at frontal (Fp1, Fp2, FZ, F3, F4, F7, F8), central (CZ, C3, C4), temporal (T3, T4), posterior-temporal (T5, T6), parietal (PZ, P3, P4), and occipital scalp sites (O1, O2) of the International 10-20 System. Additional electrodes were placed at half the distance between C3 and T5 (CP5) and C4 and T6 (CP6), half the distance between homologous posterior-temporal and mesial occipital sites (OL, OR), half the distance between O1 and O2 sites (OZ), 10% of nasion-inion distance above OZ (POZ), 20% to the left and right of the POZ site (PO3, PO4), 10% of nasion-inion distance below OZ, INZ, and 20% to the left and right of the INZ site, IN3, IN4, respectively. Vertical eye movements were recorded by two electrodes placed below and above the right eye, while horizontal movements were recorded from electrodes placed at the outer canthi of the eyes. Balanced (i.e., two 5 kΩ resistors) yoked ears served as the reference lead. The EEG and the EOG were amplified with a half-amplitude band pass of 0.16-50 Hz and 0.01-50 Hz, respectively. Electrode impedance was kept well below 5 kΩ. Both EEG and EOG were sampled and digitized at a rate of 512 Hz.

Computerized artifact rejection was performed offline before averaging to discard epochs in which eye movements, blinks, excessive muscle potentials or amplifier blocking occurred. The criterion for defining an artifact was a peak-to-peak amplitude exceeding +/-50 µV. The rate of rejection due to artifacts was less than 5%. ERPs were averaged from 100 ms before to 600 ms after presentation of the stimuli. ERP trials associated with an incorrect behavioral response were excluded from analysis. For each subject distinct ERP averages were obtained for each frequency as a function of visual hemifield as well as of frequency and location relevance, that is L+F+, L+F-, L-F+, and L-F- conditions. Later on, ERP waveforms for these conditions were grand-averaged across the group.

Since at the earlier latency levels there were several differences in the morphology, as well as in the amplitude and latency of the ERP components elicited at occipital-temporal regions by 7 cpd and/or 1 cpd spatial frequencies (e.g., C1 greater for the former than for the latter, and vice versa for the P1), in line with the bulk of evidence since long available in the literature (e.g., Reed et al., 1984; Proverbio et al., 1996), we measured and carried out statistical analyses on ERPs separately for 7 cpd and 1 cpd.

Figure 5 displays examples of the grand-average ERPs recorded at OL and OR posterior lateral-occipital sites, as well as at dorsal frontal scalp sites in response to 7 cpd gratings as a function of attention condition. As can be seen, there were remarkable morphological differences between the ERP waveforms recorded at the posterior and anterior sites. Besides several others at an earlier post-stimulus latency, remarkable is, for instance, a late-latency positive deflection preceding the P3, much prominent in between 260-320 ms post-stimulus at anterior scalp sites for the L+F- condition only, whereas at occipital and other posterior scalp sites, in the same latency range, an N2 negativity can be clearly appreciated. Visual inspection of the figure also suggests that this L+F- condition-related positivity was largest at dorsal F3 and F4 sites.

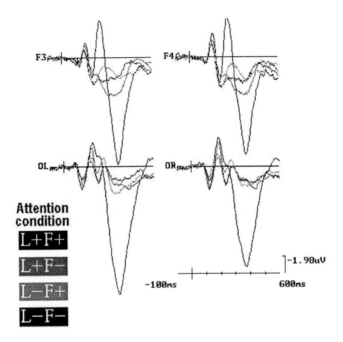

Figure 5. Grand-average ERPs collapsed across the hemifields as recorded from homologous lateral-occipital and dorsolateral prefrontal sites in response to 7 cpd as a function of attention condition. Worth of note are the morphological differences across the ERPs deriving from these distinctive brain regions as a function of attention condition.

To confirm these empirical impressions, the major ERP components were identified and measured automatically by a computer program with reference to the baseline voltage averages over the interval from -100 ms to 0 ms. ERP components were labeled according to a polarity-latency convention and quantified by measuring peak latency and baseline-to-peak, or mean area, amplitude values within a specific latency range centered approximately on the peak latency of the deflection found in the grand-average waveforms.

At the posterior scalp (O1, O2, OL, OR, IN3, IN4, T5, T6), the mean area of a small but well defined C1 component was identified in the time window between 60 and 90 ms at mesial-occipital (O1 and O2), lateral-occipital (OL, OR), lateral-ventral occipital (IN3 and IN4), and temporal (T5, T6) electrode sites (see Figure 6a). At these same sites, peak amplitude and latency were also measured of the P1 positive deflection in the time window between 80 and 140 ms (with a peak latency of about 120 ms), and of the N1 deflection, peaking at about 210 ms, in the time window between 160-230 ms.

Posterior electrode sites

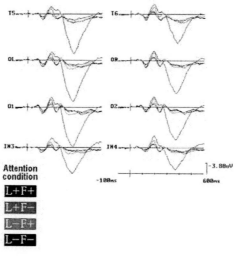

A

Anterior electrode sites

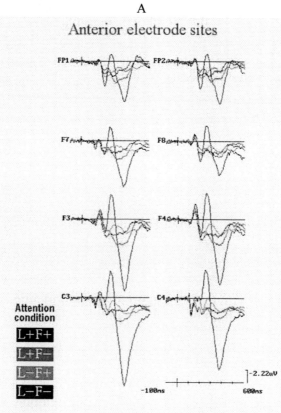

B

Figure 6. (A). Grand-average ERPs collapsed across the hemifields recorded from homologous ventral, mesial, and lateral occipital, as well as temporal sites, for 7 cpd as a function of attention condition. (B). Same as for above with the exception that ERPs were recorded from central, dorsal and inferior prefrontal, as well as fronto-polar, sites.

At anterior sites, peak amplitude and latency of an N1 deflection, peaking at an earlier 180 ms latency than at posterior sites, was measured in the time window between 140-210 ms, central (C3, C4), dorsal-frontal (F3, F4), lateral-frontal (F7, F8), and fronto-polar (Fp1, Fp2) medial scalp sites (see Figure 6b). At these same sites, the mean area was measured, as a function of attention condition, of the ERPs in the time window between 260 and 330 ms. In addition, a later P3 was also measured between 330 and 530 ms at central (C3, C4), dorsal-frontal (F3, F4), and lateral-frontal (F7, F8), scalp sites.

ERP amplitude measures were analysed with repeated measures five-way ANOVAs, separately for each ERP component and spatial frequency. Factors were 'location relevance' (L+ and L-), 'frequency relevance' (F+ and F-), 'hemifield' (LVF and RVF), 'brain hemisphere' (left and right), and 'electrode' (variable according to the component analysed). Post-hoc Tukey tests were carried out for multiple mean comparisons. Greenhouse-Geisser corrections were employed to reduce the positive bias resulting from repeated factors with more than two levels.

For each subject hit and false alarm (FAs) percentages were converted to arcsine values and subjected to a repeated measures 2-way ANOVA. Reaction times not faster than 140 msec, and not exceeding the mean value ± 2 standard deviations were subjected to a repeated-measures two-way ANOVA. Factors were 'Hemifield' (LVF and RVF), and 'spatial frequency (1 cpd and 7 cpd).

Realistic head three-dimensional topographical voltage maps of ERP components were obtained by plotting color-coded isopotential values obtained by interpolation of voltage measures between scalp electrodes at specific latencies.

RESULTS

Behavioral Data

The volunteers showed more false alarms (FAs) in response to distractors when attending the right than left hemifield. Figures 7a and b show FA percentages as a function of hemifield and spatial frequency.

As can be clearly seen, FAs were emitted on the basis of both frequency and location relevance. More in details, a congruous percentage of total amount of FAs was emitted to non-target distractors having a similar spatial frequency partially included in the same sensitivity bandwidth (that is, responses to 2 cpd gratings when targets were 1 cpd gratings, and 4 cpd, to a lesser extent, when targets were 7 cpd gratings). Interestingly, FAs occurred almost exclusively when distractors fell within the attended spatial field. Indeed, the percentage of FAs emitted to distractors irrelevant in spatial location was largely below 1%. These data suggest a space-based suppression of irrelevant visual inputs, probably mediated by PFC activity, whose failure, occurring sporadically, gave rise to erroneous responses to frequency-relevant gratings.

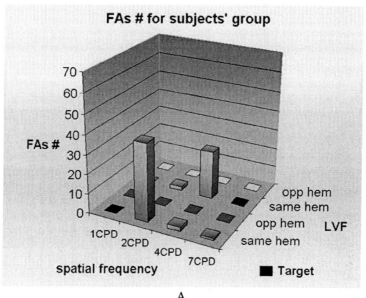

A

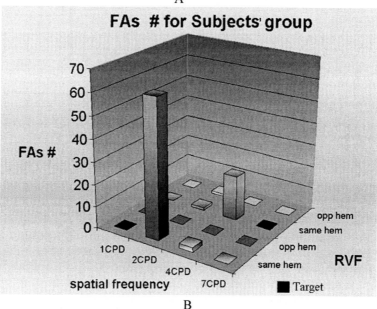

B

Figure 7. Distribution of false alarms (FAs) emitted to stimuli of varying spatial frequencies during spatial attention toward the left (A) or right (B) visual field, and to 1 cpd (first lower row) and 7 cpd (3rd row) gratings. Note that "Same hem (hemifield)." "Opp (opposite) hem" refer to visual field in relation to target location relevance.

ELECTROPHYSIOLOGICAL RESULTS

The ANOVAs provided us with manifold significant findings. Here we primarily reported those related, on the one hand, to the attention effects, both *per se* and/or in interaction with other task factors, and, on the other, to the topographic distribution over the scalp of these effects. For brevity sake, we have not reported results for the ANOVAs carried out separately on 1 cpd and 7 cpd when these attention effects showed a similar trend in both of them. For the same reason we have reported and discussed here only some of the more relevant ERP results

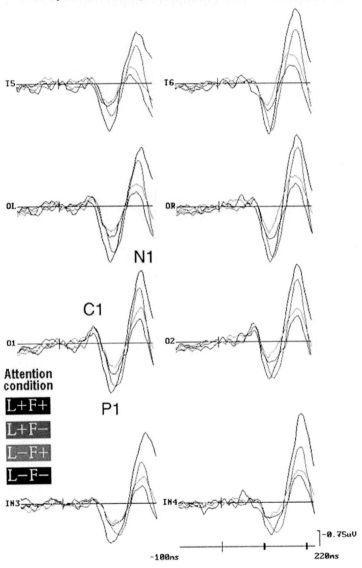

Figure 8. Grand-average ERPs collapsed across the attentional fields recorded from homologous ventral, mesial, and lateral occipital, as well as temporal sites, in response to 7 cpd as a function of attention condition. Note that the waveforms have been drawn with an expanded time scale to highlight the modulation of early sensory-evoked C1 and P1 components, as well as of N1.

POSTERIOR ELECTRODE SITES (IN3, IN4, O1, O2, OL, OR, T5, T6)

C1 Component

Mean amplitude values were measured in between 60 – 90 ms postimulus. The ANOVA on these measures yielded a significant interaction of location relevance x frequency relevance independent of the electrode site (p<0.001). Indeed, as easily discernible in the ERPs drawn with a blown-up time scale in Figure 8, unlike at the irrelevant location, at the relevant location frequency-relevant gratings elicited a greater positivity than the frequency-irrelevant gratings already starting at the earliest post-stimulus latency. This finding indicated that the visual system efficiently discriminated between the relevant and the irrelevant sources of information within the focus of attention.

Mean amplitude values for each electrode as a function of hemisphere and attention condition are reported in Table 1.

Table 1. Mean amplitude (µV) of C1 response as a function of attention condition, electrode sites and hemisphere

Occipital – temporal C1 mean amplitude (µV)									
O1					**O2**				
L+F+	L+F-	L-F+	L-F-	Pas	L+F+	L+F-	L-F+	L-F-	Pas
0.27	-0.53	-0.55	-0.59	-0.31	-0.36	-0.61	-0.58	-0.47	-025
IN3					**IN4**				
L+F+	L+F-	L-F+	L-F-	Pas	L+F+	L+F-	L-F+	L-F-	Pas
0.14	0.08	0.09	0.11	0.03	0.14	0.08	0.09	0.11	0.04
OL					**OR**				
L+F+	L+F-	L-F+	L-F-	Pas	L+F+	L+F-	L-F+	L-F-	Pas
0.07	0.26	0.21	0.28	0.06	0.03	0.24	0.23	0.17	0.01
T5					**T6**				
L+F+	L+F-	L-F+	L-F-	Pas	L+F+	L+F-	L-F+	L-F-	Pas
0.22	0.10	0.17	0.02	0.03	0.21	0.05	0.09	0.07	0.02

P1 Component

Peak amplitudes were obtained in between 80 – 140 ms post-stimulus at the same electrodes as for the C1 deflection. Statistical analyses revealed a main effect of location relevance, in that whenever within a relevant channel of attention (L+) both salient stimuli (F+) and distractors (F-) elicited a P1 of larger amplitude than when from an irrelevant channel (L-). This finding was true independent of the visual hemifield, spatial frequency, and electrode site considered. Much interestingly, the ANOVA also yielded an interaction between location relevance and frequency relevance. Post-hocs revealed that within the relevant channel (L+) frequency-relevant (F+) gratings attained a significantly larger P1 than the frequency-irrelevant (F-) ones. Conversely, within the irrelevant channel (L-) the reverse was true, as can be observed in figure 8, in that salient stimuli (F+) elicited a smaller P1 than the inconspicuous ones (F-). Although rather tiny (e.g., 0.28 μV), the difference between the P1 to the former stimuli (F+) and the latter ones (F-), proved to be overall statistically significant (see means in Table 2). These findings suggested that, at this relatively longer timing of information processing, the visual system, although overall increasing processing activation for stimuli falling within the channel of spatially-directed attention, treats the relevant and irrelevant sources of information differently. This occurs not only within the relevant channel of attention (L+), but without it (L-) too. Indeed, the present findings suggest that, while enhancing processing of frequency-relevant gratings with respect to frequency-irrelevant ones at the attended location, the system seems actively suppressing the processing of the former stimuli with respect to the latter ones at the neglected location.

Table 2. Mean amplitude (μV) of P1 response as a function of attention condition, electrode sites and hemisphere

Occipital – temporal P1 amplitude (uV)									
IN3					IN4				
L+F+	L+F-	L-F+	L-F-	Pas	L+F+	L+F-	L-F+	L-F-	Pas
1.85	1.50	0.98	1.08	0.39	1.50	1.43	0.72	0.75	1.74
O1					O2				
L+F+	L+F-	L-F+	L-F-	Pas	L+F+	L+F-	L-F+	L-F-	Pas
2.42	1.99	1.12	1.46	0.49	1.73	1.71	0.81	1.11	1.66
OL					OR				
L+F+	L+F-	L-F+	L-F-	Pas	L+F+	L+F-	L-F+	L-F-	Pas
2.59	2.12	1.46	1.78	1.31	2.63	2.32	1.17	1.54	1.84
T5					T6				
L+F+	L+F-	L-F+	L-F-	Pas	L+F+	L+F-	L-F+	L-F-	Pas
2.22	1.50	0.88	1.09	0.90	2.40	2.18	1.05	1.51	1.23

N1 Component

Peak amplitudes for the N1 component were measured at the same electrodes as for the previous components in between 150 – 210 ms post-stimulus. Interestingly, at these occipital-temporal regions N1 was overall larger for gratings from the relevant location (L+) (e. g., F+ and F-) than from the irrelevant (L-) one (see Figure 8 again). However, a significant difference was also indicated by post-hoc analyses between the frequency-relevant and frequency-irrelevant conditions as a function of the location relevance. Indeed, while at the irrelevant location no difference whatsoever was evident between the frequency-relevant and the frequency-irrelevant stimuli, at the attended location the former stimuli elicited a much larger N1 than the latter ones (see Table 3 for average N1 values). These findings further support the view that, at this relatively longer timing of information processing, the visual system, although increasing neural processing for stimuli falling within the channel of spatially-directed attention, treats the relevant and irrelevant sources of information within this channel differently. This hints at the fact that N1 reflected a discriminating function served by the posterior regions of the visual system. Additionally, our findings suggested that the system does not make any difference in responding to these same sources of information when they fall at the irrelevant location. Very probably, this occurs because processing of frequency-relevant stimuli falling at the irrelevant location had been actively suppressed at a previous level, as reflected by P1 component.

Table 3. Mean amplitude (µV) of posterior N1 as a function of attention condition, electrode sites and hemisphere

Occipital – temporal N1 amplitude (µV)									
IN3					IN4				
L+F+	L+F-	L-F+	L-F-	Pas	L+F+	L+F-	L-F+	L-F-	Pas
-3.28	-1.93	-1.22	-0.81	-0.93	-4.12	-2.57	-1.48	-1.24	-0.91
O1					O2				
L+F+	L+F-	L-F+	L-F-	Pas	L+F+	L+F-	L-F+	L-F-	Pas
-3.37	-2.55	-1.72	-1.12	-1.14	-3.57	-2.87	-1.53	-1.21	-0.96
OL					OR				
L+F+	L+F-	L-F+	L-F-	Pas	L+F+	L+F-	L-F+	L-F-	Pas
-2.73	-2.12	-1.04	-0.66	-0.68	-3.34	-2.71	-1.43	-1.06	-0.68
T5					T6				
L+F+	L+F-	L-F+	L-F-	Pas	L+F+	L+F-	L-F+	L-F-	Pas
-2.41	-1.74	-0.79	-0.44	-0.36	-3.43	-2.47	-1.39	-0.85	-0.62

Additionally, an asymmetry effect was obtained independent of any other factors. Indeed, the N1 measured over the RH was significantly larger (2.2 µV) than that recorded over the LH (1.20 µV). As for what found for the anterior electrodes, in our view the present N1 effect is functionally revealing since no lateralization resulted in the ERPs elicited by the passively gazed stimuli (see again Table 3).

ANTERIOR ELECTRODE SITES (C3, C4, F3, F4, F7, F8, FP1, FP2)

N1 Component

At the anterior scalp sites, N1 appeared within an earlier 130 – 180 ms poststimulus latency range than at the posterior sites as can be seen in Figure 9. Peak amplitudes were measured and analyzed at homologous C3 and C4, F3 and F4, F7 and F8, and FP1 and FP2 sites. Statistics showed that N1 was largest at mesial- (F3, F4) and lateral-inferior (F7 and F8) frontal sites. Table 4 reports average amplitude values as a function of homologous electrodes and attention conditions. In addition, a significant 'electrode x hemisphere' interaction indicated a right-sided lateralization for the amplitude of this response as recorded at both the frontal and prefrontal sites, but not at the central-mesial ones (C3 and C4). This effect was most interesting since no hemispheric asymmetry was found for this response in the ERPs recorded while the volunteers passively gazed the stimuli (see again Table 4 for the values relative to this condition).

Table 4. Mean amplitude (μV) of anterior N1 as a function of attention condition, electrode sites and hemisphere

Frontal-central N1 amplitude (μV)									
FP1					FP2				
L+F+	L+F-	L-F+	L-F-	Pas	L+F+	L+F-	L-F+	L-F-	Pas
-0.16	-0.33	-0.41	-0.41	-0.08	-0.49	-0.69	-0.53	-0.49	-0.04
F7					F8				
L+F+	L+F-	L-F+	L-F-	Pas	L+F+	L+F-	L-F+	L-F-	Pas
-0.16	-0.20	0.01	0.08	-0.45	-1.37	-1.02	-0.77	-0.57	-0.37
F3					F4				
L+F+	L+F-	L-F+	L-F-	Pas	L+F+	L+F-	L-F+	L-F-	Pas
-1.63	-1.30	-1.02	-0.81	-0.73	-2.66	-1.89	-1.56	-1.46	-0.73
C3					C4				
L+F+	L+F-	L-F+	L-F-	Pas	L+F+	L+F-	L-F+	L-F-	Pas
-1.02	-0.57	-0.37	-0.20	0.01	-0.24	0.28	0.45	1.02	0.01

As at posterior sites, a further result showed that N1 was larger for the L+ than for the L- conditions. Unlike at the posterior regions, however, at the anterior sites N1 responses to the targets and the distractors from the relevant location were alike. This suggests an early orienting of spatial attention function for the prefrontal regions, as reflected by this component, dissociated from the later discriminating function between frequency-relevant and frequency-irrelevant stimuli served by occipital-temporal areas. The fact that no differences were evident between the frequency-relevant (F+) and the frequency-irrelevant (F-) gratings both at the relevant (L+) and at the irrelevant locations (L-), together with the findings that the two location-relevant conditions (L+F+ and L+F-) were larger than the two location-irrelevant ones (L-F+ and L-F-), strongly advocate this assumption. The finding that N1 for F- at L+ was much larger than for F+ at L- lends further support to this proposal when bearing on mind that, although falling within the relevant channel of attention (L+), gratings eliciting such a large N1 posed as distractors because another frequency had to be attended and responded to within this channel (e.g., 7 cpd falling at the RVF when 1 cpd was relevant in this field). Conversely, the grating falling at the unattended hemifield (L-) and eliciting a smaller N1 was frequency-relevant (F+).

An additional finding lending support to the hypothesis that anterior N1 may reflect a prefrontal orienting of attention function was that hemispheres response showed to change as a function of both 'location relevance' and 'hemifield'. The post-hocs revealed that this interaction depended on a trend for which, independent of frequency relevance, stimuli elicited a larger response at the electrodes over the contralateral hemisphere with respect to the stimulation hemifield only whenever falling at the relevant location (see Figure 9).

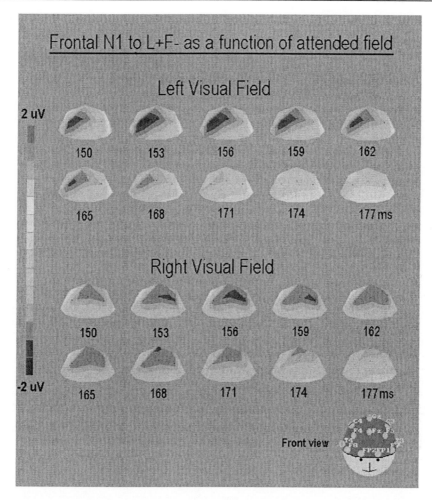

Figure 9. Isocolour voltage maps of N1 response to distractors (F-) from the attended location (L+) recorded at anterior scalp sites as a function of attended field. Note how, although N1 show a focus larger at the dorsolateral site contralateral to the attended field (i. e., F3 with the RVF, and F4 with the LVF), it was overall largest over the right-sided F4 site.

Prefrontal P290 Component

Statistical analyses on mean amplitude values of frontal P290 recorded in the latency range between 260–320 ms post-stimulus gave rise to some complex significant interactions as the location relevance x frequency relevance x hemisphere one. These factors also proved to separately interact with the electrode and the field factors, respectively. Relative post-hoc analyses indicated that the conjoined relevance of both features (L+ and F+) was associated with more negative values in the given time windows compared to all other non target stimuli (p<0.01), very probably reflecting motor preparatory processes. This effect was most evident at right central sites, but significant at all electrodes and hemispheres. The amplitude of P290 to stimuli sharing only one feature with the target was strongly affected by frequency relevance. Indeed, when the frequency was relevant, although at the unattended location (L-F+, the mean amplitude of ERPs within the given time window was still more negative (p<0.01) then when the stimulus was completely irrelevant in both features (L-F-), thus suggesting that, as for the targets, the relevance of object based dimension induced some motor preparatory processes, even if of smaller size (see Table 5 for mean values of P290).

Table 5. Mean amplitude (μV) of P290 response as a function of visual field, attention condition, electrode sites and hemisphere

Frontal P290 mean amplitude (260 –320 ms post-stimulus)							
LVF							
FP1				**FP2**			
L+F+	L+F-	L-F+	L-F-	L+F+	L+F-	L-F+	L-F-
2.15	2.99	1.70	2.71	1.67	2.77	1.52	2.60
F7				**F8**			
L+F+	L+F-	L-F+	L-F-	L+F+	L+F-	L-F+	L-F-
1.71	2.16	1.43	2.39	0.36	1.51	0.84	1.67
F3				**F4**			
L+F+	L+F-	L-F+	L-F-	L+F+	L+F-	L-F+	L-F-
0.30	3.43	1.34	3.10	-0.22	3.22	0.97	2.52
C3				**C4**			
L+F+	L+F-	L-F+	L-F-	L+F+	L+F-	L-F+	L-F-
0.11	2.86	0.98	2.39	-0.79	2.20	0.50	1.65
RVF							
FP1				**FP2**			
L+F+	L+F-	L-F+	L-F-	L+F+	L+F-	L-F+	L-F-
2.35	3.01	1.84	2.11	1.78	2.84	1.63	2.29
F7				**F8**			
L+F+	L+F-	L-F+	L-F-	L+F+	L+F-	L-F+	L-F-
1.61	2.50	0.81	1.72	0.44	2.04	0.86	1.51
F3				**F4**			
L+F+	L+F-	L-F+	L-F-	L+F+	L+F-	L-F+	L-F-
0.53	3.48	0.97	2.35	-0.84	2.86	0.88	2.40
C3				**C4**			
L+F+	L+F-	L-F+	L-F-	L+F+	L+F-	L-F+	L-F-
-0.11	2.87	0.48	1.84	-1.37	1.60	-0.18	1.37

Interestingly enough, the trend was totally different for distractors falling at the relevant location (L+F-). These stimuli elicited P290 of the largest amplitude compared to distractors irrelevant in both dimensions (L-F-) (p<0.01) and all the other conditions. The fact that both L-F- and L+F- stimuli were irrelevant, as object-feature (F-) was concerned, independent of the location-relevance, and not to be responded to, as well as the concomitant lack of contextual N2 motor negativity over the central sites, robustly suggest that DLPF areas may be strongly activated, on the bases of inputs coming from visual areas, by interfering irrelevant stimuli (F-) at the relevant channel of attention only. The increase in positivity reached its maximum at dorsolateral prefrontal (DPF) sites (F3-F4), and dropped in magnitude progressively going from the latter sites to central (C3-C4), inferior lateral (F7-F8), and fronto-polar (FP1-FP2) sites.

The change in attentional modulation of hemispheric response as a function of the field factor yielded by the ANOVA revealed to be based on changes of the RH activation for the location-relevant/frequency-irrelevant (L+F-) condition only as a function of the attended hemifield. Indeed, when the volunteers attended the RVF a clear preponderance in surface P290 positivity of the LH could be appreciated for this condition. Conversely, when the volunteers attended the LVF the preponderance of the LH relative to this condition vanished. Instead, responses of the same amplitude were obtained at the electrode sites over the LH and RH due to an increased positivity recorded at the RH (see Figure 10). As a result of this trend, at the LH the P290 resulted of similar size no matter the field attended, thus leading to a marked left-sided hemispheric asymmetry. This asymmetry found strong support in realistic 3D isocontour voltage maps of grand-average difference ERPs obtained by subtracting the L-F- condition from the L+F- one as a function of the relevant field. These maps revealed that, although larger contralateral to the side of attention, overall this positivity had a largest focus centered in between the C3-F3-F7 electrode sites over the left hemisphere, compatible with a possible activation of more inferior posterior regions of the PFC (see Figure 11).

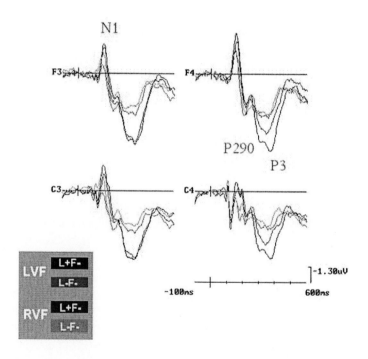

Figure 10. Grand-average ERPs to L+F- and L-F- conditions recorded at F3 and F4, as well as C3 and C4, scalp sites for 7 cpd gratings. Worth of note is the prominent positivity preceding the true P3b that changed in amplitude as a function of attended location, and as a whole largest at the left scalp sites. Remarkable is also the early N1 activation larger contralaterally to the attention direction for location-relevant stimuli, but as a whole largest over the right-sided prefrontal and frontal sites.

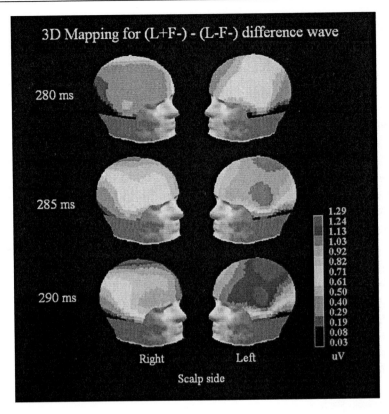

Figure 11. Time series of realistic 3D isocolour maps computed on the difference wave between the L+F-condition and the L-F- one collapsed across the attended fields. Note the remarkable left-sided asymmetry for an anterior positive focus centered at inferior-posterior dorsolateral scalp regions, as well as for a second more posterior and dorsal focus centered at central-parietal regions.

Anterior Vs. Posterior Brain Regions

Further analyses were carried out on the mean amplitude values obtained at homologous anterior F3 and F4 sites as well as posterior OL and OR sites in between 260 - 320 ms poststimulus for investigating the functional meaning of the anterior positive activation. Among other findings, the ANOVA showed that location relevance and frequency relevance separately interacted with the electrode and field factors. Post-hocs showed that whenever at frontal sites a positivity was recorded to L+F-, a rather scanty activation resulted in this same latency range at posterior scalp sites followed, later on, by a P3 as large as the one to the other two non-target conditions from the unattended location. Realistic 3D isocontour voltage maps in Figure 12 allow appreciating this trend. This pattern of results suggests that it is probable that the P290 may be an electrophysiological manifestation of an active suppressive mechanism of post-perceptual and cognitive processing of distractors falling within the attended channel (and thus implicitly oriented to via frontal N1-based spatial orienting mechanisms).

This interpretation seems to be most feasible when bearing on mind that, although these stimuli had been efficiently discriminated from targets within the relevant channel of attention at both sensory (C1) and perceptual processing levels (P1 and N1), as indicated by our results, they had anyhow demanded more attentional resources than both the distractors falling outside the focus of attention (L-F+ and L-F-). Then, it is reasonable to believe that the system has to actively suppress the demand of processing resources by these stimuli at a certain processing level. It is probable that this level might be the one reflected by our P290 activation.

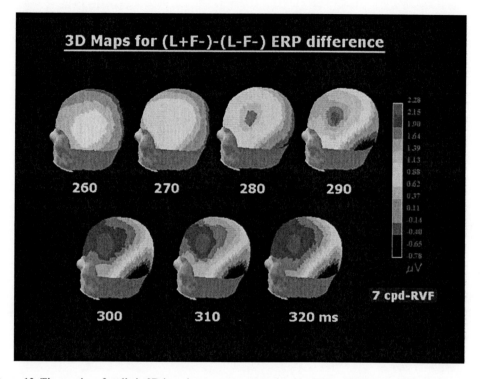

Figure 12. Time series of realistic 3D isocolour maps computed on the ERPs difference wave between the L+F- and L-F- conditions for gratings of 7 cpd presented at the attended right visual field. The maps indicate a quite opposite pattern of activation at anterior and posterior brain regions, respectively, in response to distractors occurring within the relevant channel of attention. Indeed, contralateral to the side of attention, a conspicuous positivity mounted at the inferior-posterior prefrontal regions, to which a tiny negativity corresponded at posterior occipital-temporal parietal regions.

Unlike L+F-, the targets did not show any sign of positive frontal activation at this latency (see Fig. 6B again). Conversely, they elicited prominent negativity at more dorsal and anterior sites, and a conspicuous P3 at posterior scalp sites. Figure 13 shows realistic 3D isocontour voltage time series maps of ERP grand-average difference waves obtained subtracting the L-F- condition from the L+F+ ones. These maps show that whenever a large negative dorsal focus appeared at the fronto-polar regions of the scalp, the focus of a conspicuous late-positivity progressively increased in amplitude and shifted from parietal scalp sites contralateral to the attended location toward the mesial parietal sites, very probably as a reflection of the rising of the P3 response.

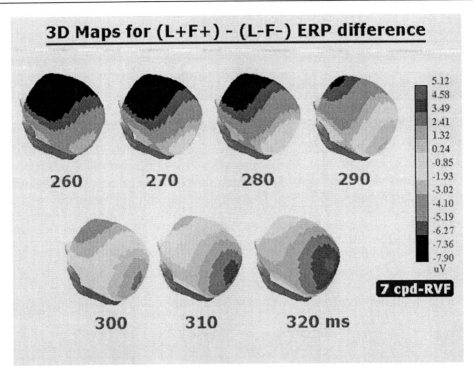

Figure 13. Time series of 3D maps obtained from the difference waves between the L+F+ and L-F-conditions for gratings of 7 cpd falling at the attended right visual field. Note that as prominent selection negativity faded at dorsal fronto-polar districts of the scalp between 260-320 ms post-stimulus, at posterior brain regions contralateral to the direction of attention a conspicuous late-positivity progressively increased in amplitude and shifted toward the mesial occipito-parietal regions.

Remarkably, in this same latency range also salient object-based stimuli (F+) from the unattended location (L-) elicited a pattern of anterior negative, as opposed to posterior positive, activation, although of smaller size, and somewhat noticeably dissimilar from the one elicited by the targets. Indeed, after the fading of a broad negative focus shifting from temporal and parietal sites toward the more dorsal fronto-polar sites, two small positive foci arose and grew in strength at contralateral occipital-temporal and ipsilateral parietal sites with respect to the stimulation side. The time series of 3D isocolour voltage maps drawn in Figure 14 depicts this intriguing trend for stimuli in the RVF. The maps were computed on the difference wave originating from the subtraction of L-F- from L-F+.

When recalling that ERPs to L-F+ were obtained while attention was oriented contralaterally to the side of stimulation, there are grounds for thinking that the two positive foci in the maps hinted at a stimulus-driven activation of occipito-temporal areas, and a concurrent parietal activation related to attention direction (for the maps in the figure, the left one), respectively.

CONCLUSION

All in all, from the general point of view the findings presented in this study are in line with the bulk of animal and human evidence in the literature indicating that attending to a location or object modulates neural processing in a distributed network of cortical areas (Kanwisher and Wojciulik, 2000; Corbetta and Shulman, 2002) including, on the one hand, the temporo-parietal cortex and inferior frontal cortex, and, on the other, the intraparietal cortex and frontal cortex (Corbetta and Shulman, 2002). This network serves different attentional functions. These functions include the facilitation of perceptual processing (Olson, 2001; Carrasco and McElree, 2001), and the tracking of an object's dynamic features and positions over time, as well as the goal-directed (top-down) selection of sensory information and responses.

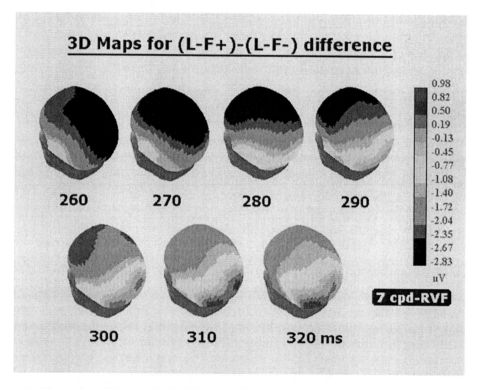

Figure 14. Time series of 3D maps obtained from the difference waves between the L-F+ and L-F- conditions for gratings of 7 cpd falling at the attended right visual field. Most interestingly, these maps show that, opposite to the distractors within the relevant channel of attention, salient stimuli falling at an unattended location elicited prominent negativity shifting from parietal to frontal districts of the scalp between 260-320 ms post-stimulus. Following the fading of this negativity, two positive foci progressively increased in amplitude over the contralateral occipito-temporal regions and the ipsilateral parietal ones, respectively.

Indeed, attention enhances neuronal response to attended stimuli at extrastriate cortex (see for instance Spitzer *et al.*, 1988, or Haenny and Schiller 1988). Generally speaking, our findings at the occipital-temporal electrode sites are pretty consistent with this view. Additionally, our discover of an enhanced C1 to stimulus targets extends this knowledge suggesting that this enhancement already starts at the earliest post-stimulus processing latency. The earliness of these effects strongly supports the hypothesis that this enhanced neural response occurs already at the lowest primary occipital cortex level of the visual system as a facilitation and/or the application of discriminative processes of the weak neural signals from attended locations. Very likely, this facilitation may serve to increase the strength of the sensory signal, as supported by our findings relative to the posterior longer-latency P1 and N1 components. Indeed, measurements of these components indicated that as processing of the stimuli from the attended location progressed in time within the visual system, the attentional facilitation or discriminative effects, already started at the earliest C1 level, progressively increase till reaching an optimal level at a late-latency level, as reflected by the P3 component.

In addition to facilitation, an additional function served by attention is the filtering of irrelevant distractors that compete for limited neural resources, especially when these appear close to a target stimulus (Desimone and Duncan, 1995). Evidence has been reported both in humans and on animals that distractors present within a neuron's receptive field produce suppression by attention of neural activity in early visual areas such as V4 (e.g., Luck et al., 1994; Kastner et al., 2001). In line with the proposal of a suppressive function reflected by the P1 component (see Luck et al., 1994), our finding of a P1 of smaller amplitude to salient stimuli (F+) than to inconspicuous stimuli (F-) from an unattended location (L-) further suggests a neural mechanism of active suppression of sensory-perceptual processing of inputs from the irrelevant channels of spatial attention by the extrastriate visual areas, where the scalp-recorded P1 reflecting spatial attention has been demonstrated by dipole modeling to have its intracortical neural sources (e.g., Clark and Hillyard, 1996; Martinez et al., 2001a).

Altogether, these results further confirm our previous findings of an enhanced early P1 response to salient, with respect to not salient, spatially attended stimuli (see Zani and Proverbio, 1997b). In addition, they extend these previous findings providing evidence for a timing of the enhancement of neural response of the visual areas as earliest as at C1 level, preceding in time the P1 effects. On the assumption that these earliest effects concern stimulus sensory processing, as reiteratively reported in the literature, it can be inferred that attention may modulate cells activation in the striate, besides in the extrastriate, visual areas. This meshes with the several reports of blood flow activation in the visual striate cortex reviewed in the Introduction section (e.g., Kastner et al., 1999; Martinez et al., 2001a), lending a reliable timing to these activations. For truth sake, it has to be said that our inference is in contrast with the assumption that attention may modulate striate cortex as the outcome of a later feedback from higher extrastriate cortices, as Martinez et al. (2001a) have recently advanced on the basis of conflicting V1-centered positive fMRI effects/negative ERP early effects.

Taken together, the findings reviewed above imply that the question about the point to which attentional modulation extends in the visual system remains still to be further investigated (see also Zani and Proverbio, 2005, for a recent critical discussion of this matter). It is exciting, however, that the most recent developments in the investigation of attentional modulation in the visual system has accounted enhanced activations in the thalamic lateral geniculate nucleus (LGN) (see Kastner et al., 2005 for such an account).

Interestingly enough, we want to outline here that the present results show to be consistent with the evidence accumulated at present that visual-spatial attention is subserved by multiple mechanisms, operating differently, able to modulate occipital-temporal neural processing just starting at the earliest cortical, if not sub-cortical, levels of the visual system.

Furthermore, we want to outline that our results seem to add to the line of research viewing spatial attention visual processing as the outcome of a dealing with space locations based on a discriminative enhanced processing of the objects or events selectively attended at the latter locations, starting from the earlier sensory levels, rather than as an undifferentiated enhanced neural processing of these objects within attended, with respect to unattended, locations of the visual space (e.g., Olson and Gettner, 1996; Olson, 2001).

Most interestingly, at the frontal regions we found effects going in the opposite direction as the functional activation and the distractors processing was concerned. Unlike at posterior brain areas, at the anterior ones a relatively early N1 activation was elicited by distractors occurring within the relevant channel of attention that matched the one elicited by target stimuli. This activation was larger contralaterally to the side where spatial attention had to be directed, thus indicating that this frontal negativity reflected an orienting of attention function of these regions, dissociated from the discriminative one reflected by the later occipital-temporal N1, to the relevant location. More in details, our data suggested that this orienting function might be mostly served by the dorso-lateral prefrontal regions, as the effects found to be largest at the F3 and F4 scalp sites induced us to believe.

It seems feasible to think that, together with our findings at posterior visual regions, the anterior N1 data hint at a parallel distributed activation in the brain during selective processing in which the frontal areas serve a relatively early voluntary orienting of attention to relevant locations so to facilitate sensory-processing and perception of information falling at the latter. The frontal-based orienting would contribute to the enhancement of the strength of the neural signal in the occipital-temporal areas while processing progresses at the P1 and N1 stages. Thus, based on this enhancement, the posterior system would allow the discrimination between the relevant and irrelevant sources of information within the relevant channel of attention.

All in all, despite their scarce localization capacity, the present N1 findings fits quite well with the findings of many hemodynamic studies investigating frontal activity related to voluntary orienting. For instance, Hopfinger and colleagues (2000) reported cue-related activations of the superior frontal gyrus and the middle frontal gyrus besides the parietal areas. Gitelman and coworkers (1999) reported consistent frontal activities during spatial precueing tasks, as did Kastner's group (1999) using fMRI.

Most importantly, they seem also to be in broad agreement with the activation in the precentral sulcus, the human homologue of the frontal eye field (FEF) in the primates, thought to be part of a more distributed "Dorsal fronto-parietal network", or *DFPN*. To this regard, Corbetta and co-workers have reiteratively reported that this area is the neural substrate of covert and overt voluntary orienting of attention (see Corbetta *et al.*, 1998; Corbetta *et al.*, 2000; Corbetta *et al.*, 2002).

A further finding deserves to be discussed here as the functional trend of N1 at both the frontal and occipito-temporal sites is concerned. In fact, during the selection tasks this component revealed to be overall larger at the right than at the left hemisphere regardless of the laterality of sensory input. These results mesh with PET findings of increased blood flow in the prefrontal and superior parietal cortex primarily in the right hemisphere during sustained attention or vigilance (Pardo *et al.*, 1991). This seems to imply that, at this stage of processing, a general arousing or vigilance function, dissociated from both the orienting and discriminative ones, is reflected by the right-sided N1 activation.

Opposite to the finding that at occipital-temporal areas interfering stimuli produced suppression of neural activity, at the frontal areas distractors that were to be ignored within the relevant channel of attention produced an enhanced late-latency processing, recorded at the scalp as a prominent positivity somehow preceding the true P3. Despite this activation was greater at the prefrontal areas contralateral to the direction of spatial attention, all in all, our topographic mappings implicated the left inferior-posterior prefrontal regions independent of the space side attended.

In our view, some lines of research support the hypothesis that this positivity may be a sign of a suppression of post-perceptual or cognitive processing of distractors present within the relevant channel of attention, so to avoid processing overload or eventually a mistaken motor response to the latter stimuli, by the ipsilateral occipital-temporal areas rather than an inhibition of motor response to such stimuli. Indeed, source analysis of the cerebral activity underlying the no-go response indicated a complex set of overlapping electrical generators in the inferior prefrontal regions, cingulate, and premotor regions (Kiefer et al., 1998). These regions do not fit well with the topographic localization of our own mapping findings. Most of all, however, whereas neuroimaging studies on inhibition of responses implicated diverse PFC foci, advances in research have now indicated the functional localization of such inhibition to right inferior frontal cortex (IFC) alone (e.g., Casey et al., 1997; Aron et al., 2004 for a review). Human lesion-mapping also supports this right-sided localization of response inhibition (see Aron et al., 2004, again).

Besides the reviewed evidence, some of our own findings too speak against this P3-preceding positivity being a sign of inhibition of motor response. Indeed, despite our volunteers inhibited their response to salient distractors (F+) presented outside the relevant channel of attention (L-), the lack of such positive activation to these stimuli contrasts the argument that these effects can be attributed solely to inhibition of motor response. In addition, such an argument is contrasted by the fact that, more or less in the same latency range, these spatially unattended distractors showed hints of a developing motor-like N2, such as the one elicited by our motorically responded targets, although much smaller than the one elicited by the latter. To this, it has to be added that inconspicuous distractors (F-) from the irrelevant location (L-) did not show any sign of frontal P290 activation, although eliciting a small and almost flatly going late positivity as processing progressed in time. Both these different electrophysiological findings recorded in the absence of motor response, we believe, suggest that it is processing suppression, not inhibition of motor response, which drives P290 activity in the left prefrontal cortex. Above all, however, the finding that lends overwhelming support to our hypothesis that this positivity might drive the suppression of processing of interfering stimuli (F-) from an attended location (L+) by the ipsilateral occipital-temporal areas is that whenever this prefrontal positivity was recorded at prefrontal regions of one hemisphere, a scant processing was observed at this stage for such stimuli, as reflected by a tiny negativity localized at the ipsilateral occipital areas in the topographic mappings. To this, it has also to be added that salient stimuli (F+) from an unattended location (L-) showed an ipsilateral posterior late P3 somewhat larger than the one elicited by distractors (F-) falling within a relevant location (L+). Overall, this implied that, despite these stimuli should have been ignored because from an unattended location, and despite they had also been actively suppressed at an early P1 processing level, they had anyhow demanded some processing resources, as our findings at both post-perceptual and cognitive processing levels strongly suggested. Very probably, this might have occurred because their processing had somehow progressed at an automatic and unconscious level. Indeed, the topographic finding that the posterior P3 to these stimuli was preceded by a parietal negativity shifting toward somewhat more anterior and dorsal frontal regions than the ones where P290 was focused meshes with this assumption. Peculiarly, topographic maps indicated that, like the salient distractors from unattended locations, target stimuli also elicited a pattern of anterior negativity and posterior positivity, although of much larger size and characterized by some topographic differences from the former. Taken together, these findings suggest that whenever occipital-temporal regions discern clues of stimulus saliency by means of sensory-perceptual processing, this evidence is pointed out to the prefrontal areas. In turn, the latter regions actively are alerted for sending a feedback to occipito-temporal-parietal regions so to enhance post-perceptual-semantic processing of such stimuli. The discover that this occurred at a greater or lesser level depending on the location relevance, also suggest that the gain of the visual signals might be modified according to stimulus relevance and distractors interfering action.

Intriguingly enough, although ERPs low spatial resolution demands cautiousness where anatomical localization is concerned, there are grounds for thinking that, altogether, these findings fit in broad terms with the attentional control model recently advanced by Corbetta and Shulman (2002). Extending earlier models (e.g., Posner and Petersen, 1990), the present one involves two partially segregated systems of brain areas that carry out different attentional functions. One system, which includes portions of the intraparietal cortex and superior frontal cortex, is preferentially involved in driving the goal-directed selection of stimuli and responses. The other system, which includes the temporo-parietal cortex and inferior frontal cortex, mainly those of the right hemisphere, would not take part in top-down attentional selection. It rather would be specialized in the detection of behaviourally relevant stimuli, particularly when they are salient or unexpected. Notwithstanding the cautiousness demanded from the anatomical viewpoint, at least from the functional viewpoint brain responses to L+F+ and L-F+ in the present study seem to be strikingly in line with the actions of the two hypothesized systems.

It is also important that, as we predicted, interfering information from the attended location only presented frontal signs of active suppression of processing by posterior brain areas. This finding is quite consistent with our previous ones of an enhanced frontal and reduced occipital processing of irrelevant stimuli as reflected by P3 component recorded during a selective attention task (Zani and Proverbio, 1995; Zani and Proverbio, 1997a).

It has to be added, however, that the finding that an electrophysiological sign functionally separated from the true P3 might reflect processing suppression in the present study hints at the possibility that there might be separate task-related selection mechanisms, as suggested by Smith and Jonides (2003) too.

The present prefrontal data fit very well with the left-sided lateralization found in our previous ERP studies (Zani and Proverbio, 1995; Zani and Proverbio, 1997a). As a matter of fact, the whole-head montage recordings from the present study extend these previous findings. Indeed, the topographic localization of our frontal P290 to the left inferior posterior regions of the scalp fits quite well with the left inferior posterior PFC localization of prefrontal damage recently found by Gerhing and Knight (2002) to be the most critical for processing selection, but not for attention switching. It also fits well with the BA45 localization of the damage shown by PET in patient R. C. who has been found to have remarkable impairments in response accuracy in the high- but not low-conflict condition of an item recognition task (Thompson-Schill et al., 2002). Interestingly, our finding also meshes with the left prefrontal activations (BA45) in normal volunteers reported by several blood-flow studies reviewed above (Thompson-Schill *et al.*, 1997; Jonides *et al.*, 1998; D'Esposito *et al.*, 1999; Milham *et al.*, 2001). In our view, we borrow a robust anatomical substrate for our suppression-related P290 finding from all these studies. In turn, however, it seems that our finding somehow lends support for the functional meaning and for the timing of the left-sided blood-flow activations and of the impairments shown by patients after damages to these structures. In fact, because of the non-verbal nature of the stimuli used in the present study, we argue that this left-lateralized activation of inferior posterior PFC reiteratively reported when selective processing is required in high-conflict conditions may reflect an hemispheric functional specialization in suppressing processing of highly interfering sources of information to guide response, and not simply the outcome of the handling of verbal stimuli as advanced in all of the scarce studies reporting hemispheric asymmetries reviewed above.

REFERENCES

Aine, C. J., Supek, S., and George, J. S. (1995). Temporal dynamics of visual-evoked neuromagnetic sources: Effects of stimulus parameters and selective attention. *International Journal of Neuroscience, 80*, 79-104.

Annlo-Vento, L, and Hillyard, S. A. (1996). Selective attention to color and the direction of moving stimuli: Electrophysiological correlates of hierarchical feature selection. *Perception & Psychophysics, 58*, 191-206.

Aron, A. R., Robbins, T. W., and Russel, A. P. (2004). Inhibition and the right inferior frontal cortex. *Trends in Cognitive Sciences, 8*, 170-177.

Aston-Jones, G. S., Desimone, R., Driver, J., Luck, S. J., and Posner, M. I. (1999). Attention. In: M. J. Zigmond, F. E. Bloom, S. C. Landis, J. L. Roberts, and L. R. Squire (Eds.), *Fundamental Neuroscience*, (pp.1385-1409). San Diego, London: Academic Press.

Barcelo, F., Suwazono, S., and Knight, R. T. (2000). Prefrontal modulation of visual processing in humans. *Nature Neuroscience, 3*, 399-403.

Brefcynski, J. A., and DeYoe, E. A. A. (1999). A physiological correlate of the 'spotlight' of visual attention. *Nature Neuroscience, 2*, 370-374.

Cabeza, R, and Nyberg, L. (2000). Imaging cognition II: An empirical review of 275 PET and fMRI studies. *Journal of Cognitive Neuroscience, 12*, 1-47.

Campbell, F. W., and Maffei, L. (1970). Electrophysiological evidence for the existence of orientation and size detectors in the human visual system. *Journal of Physiology, 207*, 635-652.

Carrasco, M., and McElree, B. (2001). Covert attention accelerates the rate of visual information processing. *Proceedings of the National Academy of Sciences USA, 98*, 5363-5367.

Carter, C. S., Braver, T. S., Barch, D. M., Botvinick, M. M., Noll, D. C., and Cohen, J. D. (1998). Anterior cingulate cortex, error detection, and the monitoring of performance. *Science, 280*, 747-749.

Casey, B. J., Trainor, R. J., Orendi, J. L., Schubert, A. B., Nystrom, L. E., Giedd, J. N., Castellanos, F. X., Haxby, J. V., Noll, D. C., Cohen, J. D., Forman, S. D., Dahl, R. E., and Rapoport, J. L. (1997). A developmental functional MRI study of prefrontal activation during performance of a go/no-go task. *Journal of Cognitive Neuroscience, 9*, 835-847.

Clark, V. P., and Hillyard, S. A. (1996). Spatial selective attention affects early extrastriate but not striate components of the visual evoked potentials. *Journal of Cognitive Neuroscience, 8*, 387-402.

Corbetta, M. (1999). Functional anatomy of visual attention in the human brain: Studies with positron emission tomography. In: R. Parasuraman, Ed., *The attentive brain* (pp. 95-122). Cambridge (Mass.): The MIT Press.

Corbetta, M., and Shulman, G. L. (1999). Human cortical mechanisms of visual attention during orienting. In: G. W. Humphreys, J. Duncan, and A. Treisman (Eds.), *Attention, Space and Action. Studies in cognitive neuroscience* (pp. 183-198). Oxford: Oxford University Press.

Corbetta, M., and Shulman, G. L. (2002). Control of goal-directed and stimulus driven attention in the brain. *Nature Reviews, 3*, 201-215.

Corbetta, M., Akbudak, E., Conturo, T. E., Snyder, A. Z., Ollinger, J. M., Drury, H. A., Lineweber, M. R., Petersen, S. E., Raichle, M. E., Van Essen, D. C., Shulman, G. L. (1998). A common network of functional areas for attention and eye movements. *Neuron, 21*, 761-773.

Corbetta, M., Kincade, J. M., Ollinger, J. M., McAvoy, M. P., and Shulman, G. L. (2000). Voluntary orienting is dissociated from target detection in human posterior parietal cortex. *Nature Neuroscience, 3*, 292-297.

Corbetta, M., Kincade, J. M., and Shulman, G. L. (2002). Neural systems for visual orienting and their relationships to spatial working memory. *Journal of Cognitive Neuroscience, 14*, 508-523.

Deouell, L. Y., and Knight, R. T. (2005). ERP measures of multiple attention deficits of multiple attention deficits following prefrontal damage. In: L. Itti, G. Rees, and J. Tsotsos (Eds.), *Neurobiology of attention* (pp. 339-344). San Diego (USA): Academic Press.

Desimone, R., and Duncan, J. (1995). Neural mechanisms of selective visual attention. *Annual Review of Neurosciences, 18*, 193-222.

D'Esposito, M., Postle, B. R., Jonides, J., and Smith, E. E. (1999). The neural substrate and temporal dynamics of interference effects in working memory as revealed by event-related functional MRI. *Proc. Natl. Acad. Sci., 96*, 7514-7519.

Donchin, E. (1981). Surprise! ... Surprise? *Psychophysiology, 9*, 493-513.

Duncan, J. (2001). Frontal lobe function and the control of visual attention. In: J. Braun, C. Koch, and J. L. Davis (Eds.), *Visual attention and cortical circuits* (pp. 69-88). Cambridge (Mass.), London (England): The MIT Press.

Dupont, P., Vogels, R., Vandenberghe, R., Rosier, A., Cornette, L., Bormans, G., Mortelmans, L., and Orban, G. A. (1998). Regions in the human brain activated by simultaneous orientation discrimination: a study with positron emission tomography. *European Journal of Neuroscience, 10*, 3689-3699.

Eimer, M. (1996). The N2pc component as an indicator of attentional selectivity. *Electroencephalography and Clinical Neurophysiology, 99*, 225-234.

Eriksen, B. A., and Eriksen, C. W. (1974). Effects of noise letters upon the identification of a target letter in a nonsearch task. *Perception and Psychophysics, 16*, 143-149.

Fabiani, M., Karis, D., and Donchin E. (1986). P300 and recall in an incidental memory paradigm. *Psychophysiology, 23*, 298-308.

Fink, G. R., Dolan, R. G., Halligan, P. W., and Marshall, J. C. (1997). Space-based and object-based visual attention: shared and specific neural domains. *Brain, 120,* 2013-2028.

FriedmaN-Hill, S. R., Robertson, L., and Treisman, A. (1995). Parietal contributions to visual feature binding: Evidence from a patient with bilateral lesions. *Science, 269,* 853-855.

Gandhi, S. P., Heeger, D. J., and Boynton, G. M. (1999). Spatial attention affects brain activity in human primary visual cortex. *Proc. Natl. Acad. Sci. USA*, *96*, 3314-3319.

Gehring, W. J., and Knight, R. T. (2000). Prefrontal-cingulate interactions in action monitoring. *Nature Neuroscience, 3*, 421-423.

Gehring, W. J., and Knight, R. T. (2002). Lateral prefrontal damage affects processing selection but not attention switching. *Brain Research: Cognitive Brain Research., 13*, 267-279.

Georgopoulos, A. P., Whang, K., Georgopoulos, M. A., Tagaris, G. A., Amirikian, B., Richter, W., Kim, S. G., and Ugurbil, K. (2001). Functional magnetic resonance imaging of visual object construction and shape discrimination: Relations among task, hemispheric lateralization, and gender. *Journal of Cognitive Neuroscience, 13*, 72-89.

Gevins, A., and Cutillo, B. (1993). Spatiotemporal dynamics of component processes in human working memory. *Electroencephalography and Clinical Neurophysiology, 87*, 128-143.

Gitelman, D. R., Nobre, A. C., Parrish, T. B., LaBar, K. S., Kim, Y. H., Meyer, J. R., and Mesulam, M. (1999). A large-scale distributed network for covert spatial attention: Further anatomical delineation based on stringent behavioural and cognitive controls. *Brain, 122*, 1093-1106.

Goldman-Rakic, P. (1987). Circuitry of primate prefrontal cortex and regulation of behavior by representational memory. In: F. Blum (Ed. by), *Handbook of Physiology. The Nervous System - Higher Functions of the Brain* (Vol. 5, Part 1, pp. 373-417). Bethesda (MD): American Physiology Association.

Gomer, F. E., Spicuzza, R. J., and O'Donnel, R. D. (1976). Evoked potentials correlates of visual item recognition during memory-scanning tasks. *Physiological Psychology, 4*, 61-65.

Grosof, D. H., Shapley, R. M., and Hawken, M. J. (1993). Macaque V1 neurones can signal "illusory" contours. *Nature, 365*, 550-552.

Haenny, P. E., and Schiller, P. H. (1988). State dependent activity in monkey visual cortex. I. Single cell activity in V1 and V4 on visual tasks. *Experimental Brain Research, 69*, 225-244.

Harter, M. R., and Aine, C. J. (1984). Brain mechanisms of visual selective attention. In: R. Parasuraman, and R. Davies (Eds.), *Varieties of attention* (pp. 293-321). San Diego, New York: Academic Press.

Harter, M. R., and Guido, W. (1980). Attention to pattern orientation: Negative cortical potentials, reaction time, and the selection process. *Electroencephalography and Clinical Neurophysiology, 49*, 461-475.

Harter, M. R., and Previc, F. H. (1978). Size-specific information channels and selective attention: Visual evoked potentials and behavioural measures. *Electroencephalography and Clinical Neurophysiology, 45*, 628-640.

Haxby, J. V., Courtney, S. M., and Clark, V. P. (1999). Functional magnetic resonance imaging and the study of attention. In: R. Parasuraman (Ed. by), *The Attentive Brain* (pp. 123-142). Cambridge (Mass.): The MIT Press.

Hazeltine, E., Poldrack, R., and Gabrieli, J. D. E. (2000). Neural activation during response competition. *Journal of Cognitive Neuroscience, 12,* 118-129.

Heinze, H. J., Mangun, G. R., Burchert, W., Hinrichs, H., Scholze, M., Münte, T. F., Gös, A., Johanne, S. S., Scherg, M., Hundeshagen, H., Gazzaniga, M. S., and Hillyard, S. A. (1994). Combined spatial and temporal imaging of spatial selective attention in humans. *Nature, 372,* 543-546.

Hermann, C. S., and Knight, R. T. (2001). Mechanisms of human attention: Event-related potentials and oscillations. *Neuroscience and Biobehavioral Reviews, 25,* 465-476.

Hess, R., and Field, D. (1999). Integration of contours: New insights. *Trends in Cognitive Sciences, 3,* 480-486.

Hillyard, S. A., Mangun, G. R, Woldorff, M. G., and Luck, S. J. (1995). Neural systems mediating selective attention. In: M. S. Gazzaniga (Ed. by), *The Cognitive Neurosciences* (pp. 665-681). Cambridge (Mass.): The MIT Press.

Hillyard, S. A., and Annlo-Vento, L. (1998). Event-related brain potentials in the study of visual selective attention. *Proceedings of the National Academy of Sciences of USA, 95,* 781-787.

Hillyard, S. A., Teder-Sälejärvi, W. A., and Münte, T. F. (1998). Temporal dynamics of early perceptual processing. *Current Opinion in Neurobiology, 8,* 202-210.

Hillyard, S. A., Vogel, E. K., and Luck, S. J. (1999). Sensory gain control (amplification) as a mechanism of selective attention: Electrophysiological and neuroimaging evidence. In: G. W. Humphreys, J. Duncan, and A. Treisman (Eds.) *Attention, Space and Action. Studies in cognitive neuroscience* (pp. 31-53). Oxford University Press, Oxford.

Hirsch, J., DeLaPaz, R., Relkin, R. N., Victor, J., Kim, K., Li, T., Borden, P., Rubin, N., and Shapley, R. (1995). Illusory contours activate specific regions in human visual cortex: Evidence from functional magnetic resonance imaging. *Proceedings of the National Academy of Sciences of USA, 92,* 6469-6473.

Hopfinger, J. B., Buonocore, M. H., and Mangun, G. R. (2000). The neural mechanisms of top-down attentional control. *Nature Neuroscience, 3,* 292-297.

Ito, M., and Gilbert, C. D. (1999). Attention modulates contextual influences in the primary visual cortex of alert monkey. *Neuron, 22,* 593-604.

Jeffreys, D. A., and Axford, J. G. (1972). Source locations of pattern specific components of human visual evoked potentials. I. Components of striate cortical origin. *Experimental Brain Research, 16,* 1-21.

Jonides, J., Smith, E. E., Marshuetz, C., Koeppe, R. A., and Reuter-Lorentz, P. A. (1998). Inhibition in verbal working memory revealed by brain activation. *Proc. Natl. Acad. Sci. 95,* 8410-8413.

Jonides, J., Badre, D., Curtis, C., Thompson-Schill, S., and Smith, E. E. (2002). Mechanisms of conflict resolution in prefrontal cortex. In: D. T. Stuss and R. T. knight (Eds.), *Principles of frontal lobe function* (pp. 233-245). Oxford: Oxford University Press.

Kanizsa, G. (1976). Subjective contours. *Scientific American, 234,* 48-52.

Kanwisher, N., and Wojciulik, E. (2000). Visual attention: Insights from brain imaging. *Nature Reviews of Neuroscience, 1,* 91-100.

Karayanidis, F., and Michie, P. T. (1997). Evidence of visual processing negativity with attention to orientation and color in central space. *Electroencephalography and Clinical Neurophysiology, 103,* 282-297.

Kastner, S., Pinsk, M. A., De Weerd, P. Desimone, R., and Ungerleider, L. G. (1999). Increased activity in human visual cortex during directed attention in the absence of visual stimulation. *Neuron, 22*, 751-761.

Kastner, S., De Weerd, P., Pinsk, M. A., Elizondo, M. I., Desimone, R., and Ungerleider, L. G. (2001). Modulation of sensory suppression: implications for receptive field sizes in the human visual cortex. *Journal of Neurophysiology, 86*, 1398-1411.

Kastner, S., Schneider, K. A., and O'Connor, D. H. (2005). Attention modulation in the human lateral geniculate nucleus and pulvinar. In: L. Itti, G. Rees, and J. Tsotsos (Eds.), *Neurobiology of attention* (pp. 435-441). San Diego (USA): Academic Press.

Kawashima, R., Satoh, K., Goto, R., Inoue, K., Itoh, M., and Fukuma, H. (1998). The role of the left inferior temporal cortex for visual pattern discrimination--a PET study. *Neuroreport, 11*, 1581-1586.

Kenemans, J. L., Kok, A., and Smulders, F. T. Y. (1993). Event-related potentials to conjunctions of spatial frequency and orientation as a function of stimulus parameters and response requirements. *Electroencephalography and Clinical Neurophysiology, 88*, 51-63.

Kiefer, M., Marzinzik, F., Weisbrod, M., Scherg, M., and Spitzer, M. (1998). The time course of brain activation during response inhibition: Evidence from event-related potentials in a go/no-go task. *NeuroReport, 9*, 765-770.

Knight, R. T. (1991). Evoked potential studies of attention capacity in human frontal lobe lesions. In: H. Levin, H. Eisenberg, and F. Benton (Eds.), *Frontal lobe function and dysfunction* (pp. 139-153). Oxford: Oxford University Press.

Knight, R. (1996). Contribution of human hippocampal region to novelty detection. *Nature, 383*, 256-259.

Knight, R. T., and Grabowecky, M. (1995). Escape from linear time: Prefrontal cortex and conscious experience. In: M. S. Gazzaniga (Ed. By), *The Cognitive Neurosciences* (pp. 1357-1371). Cambridge: The MIT Press.

Knight, R. T., Staines, W. R., Swick, D., and Chao, L. L. (1999). Prefrontal cortex regulates inhibition and excitation in distributed neural networks. *Acta Psychologica, 101*, 159-178.

Knight, R. T., and D'Esposito, M. (2003). Lateral prefrontal syndrome: A disorder of executive control. In: M. D'Esposito (Ed. by), *Neurological foundations of cognitive neuroscience* (pp. 259-279). Cambridge (Mass.), London (England): The MIT Press.

Kornblum, S., Hasbroucq, T., and Osman, A. (1990). Dimensional overlap: Cognitive basis for stimulus-response compatibility-a model and taxonomy. *Psychological Review, 97*, 253-270.

LaBerge, D. (1995). *Attentional Processing. The Brain's Art of Mindfulness*. Cambridge, Mass., London, England: Harvard University Press,.

La Berge, D., and Buchsbaum, M. S. (1990). Positron emission tomographic measurements of pulvinar activity during an attention task. *Journal of Neuroscience, 10*, 613-619.

Lamme, V. A. F., and Spekreijse, H. (2000). Modulations of primary visual cortex activity representing attentive and conscious scene perception. *Frontiers in Bioscience, 5*, 232-243.

Larsson, J., Amuntus, K., Gulys, B., Malikovic, A., Zilles, K., and Roland, P. E. (1999). Neuronal correlates of real and illusory contour perception: functional anatomy with PET. *European Journal of Neuroscience, 11*, 4024-4036.

Lee, T. S., and Nguyen, M. (2001). Dynamics of subjective contour formation in the early visual cortex. *Proceedings of the National Academy of Sciences of USA, 98*, 1907-1911.

Luck, S. J., Hillyard, S. A., Mouloua, M., Woldorff, M. G., Clark, V. P., and Hawkins, H. L. (1994). Effects of spatial cuing on luminance detectability: Psychophysical and electrophysiological evidence for early selection. *Journal of Experimental Psychology: Human Perception and Performance, 20*, 887-904.

Luck, S. J., Chelazzi, L., Hillyard, S., and Desimone, R. (1997). Neural mechanisms of spatial selective attention in areas V1, V2, and V4 of macaque visual cortex. *Journal of Neurophysiology, 77*, 24-42.

Luck, S. J., Woodman, G., and Vogel, E. K. (2000). Event-related potential studies of attention. *Trends in Cognitive Sciences, 4,* 432-440.

MacLeod, C. M. (1991). Half a century of research on the Stroop effect: an integrative review. *Psychological Bulettin, 109*, 163–203.

Mangun, G. R. (2003). Neural mechanisms of attention. In: A. Zani, and A. M. Proverbio (Eds.), *The cognitive electrophysiology of mind and brain* (pp. 247-258). Amsterdam (The Netherlands), New York (USA): Academic Press.

Mangun, G. R., Hopfinger, J. B., Kussmaul, C., Fletcher, E. M., and Heinze, H. J. (1997). Covariations in PET and ERP measures of spatial selective attention in human extrastriate visual cortex. *Human Brain Mapping, 5*, 273-279.

Mangun, G. R., Hinrichs, H., Scholz, M., Mueller-Gaertner, H. W., Herzog, H., Krause B. J., Tellman L., Kemna, L., and Heinze H. J. (2001). Integrating electrophysiology and neuroimaging of spatial selective attention to simple isolated visual stimuli. *Vision Research, 41*, 1423-35.

Martin-Loeches, M., Hinojosa, J. A., and Rubia, F. J. (1999). Insights from event-related potentials into the temporal and hierarchical organization of the ventral and dorsal streams of the visual system in selective attention. *Psychophysiology, 36*, 721-36.

Martinez, A., Anllo-Vento, L., Sereno, M. I., Frank, L. R., Buxton, R. B., Dubowitz, D. J., Wong, E. C., Hinrichs, H., Heinze, H. J., and Hillyard, S. A. (1999). Involvement of striate and extrastriate visual cortical areas in spatial attention. *Nature Neuroscience, 2*, 364-369.

Martinez, A., DiRusso, F., Annlo-Vento, L., Sereno, M. I., Buxton, R. B., and Hillyard, S. A. (2001a). Putting spatial attention on the map: timing and localization of stimulus selection processes in striate and extrastriate visual areas. *Vision Research, 41*, 1437-1547.

Martínez, A., Di Russo, F., Annlo-Vento, L., and Hillyard, S. A. (2001b). Electrophysiological analysis of cortical mechanisms of selective attention to high and low spatial frequencies. *Clinical Neurophysiology, 112*, 1980-1998.

Merigan, W. H., and Maunsell, J. H. R. (1993). How parallel are the primate visual pathways? *Annual Review of Neuroscience, 16*, 396-402.

Metha, A. D., Ulbert, D., Lindsley, R. W., and Schroeder, C. E. (1997*).* Timing and distribution of attention effects across areas in the macaque visual system. *Society of Neuroscience Abstracts, 23*, 121.1, p. 299.

Milham, M. P., Banich, M. T., Webb, A., Barad, V., Cohen, N. J., Wszalek, T., and Kramer, A. F. (2001). The relative involvement of anterior cingulate and prefrontal cortex in attentional control depends on nature of conflict. *Brain Res. Cogn. Brain Res., 12*, 467-473.

Miller, E. K., and Cohen, J. D. (2001). An integrative theory of prefrontal cortex function. *Annual Review of Neuroscience, 24,* 167-202.

Motter, B. C. (1993). Focal attention produces spatially selective processing in visual cortical areas V1, V2, and V4 in the presence of competing stimuli. *Journal of Neurophysiology, 70,* 909-919.

Mountcastle, V. B. (1998). *Perceptual Neuroscience: The cerebral cortex.* Cambridge, Mass., London, England: Harvard University Press.

Näätänen R. (1992). *Attention and Brain function.* Hillsdale (NJ): Lawrence Erlbaum Associates.

Oakley, Y. M. T., and Eason, R. G. (1990). Subcortical gating in the human visual system during spatial selective attention. *International Journal of Psychophysiology, 9,* 105-120.

Olson, C. R, and Gettner, S. N. (1996). Brain representation of object-centered space. *Current Opinion in Neurobiology, 6,* 165-170.

Olson C. R. (2001). Object-based vision and attention in primates. *Current Opinion in Neurobiology, 11,* 171-179.

Pardo, J. V., Fox, P. T., and Raichle, M. E. (1991). Localization of a human system for sustained attention by positron emission tomography. *Nature, 349,* 61-64.

Pfefferbaum, A., Ford, J. M., Weller, B. J., and Kopell, B. S. (1985). ERPs to response production and inhibition. *Electroencephalography and Clinical Neurophysiology, 60,* 423-434.

Polich, J. (1998). P300 clinical utility and control of variability. *J Clin Neurophysiol., 15,* 14-33.

Polich, J., and Herbst, K. L. (2001). P300 as a clinical assay: rationale, evaluation, and findings. *International Journal of Psychophysiology, 38,* 3-19.

Posner, M. I., and Petersen, S. E. (1990). The attention system of the human brain. *Annual Review of Neuroscience, 13,* 25-42.

Press, W. A., and Van Essen, D. C. (1997). Attentional modulation of neuronal responses in macaque area V1. *Society of Neuroscience Abstracts, 23,* 405.3, p. 1026.

Previc, F. H. (1990). Functional specialization in the lower and upper visual fields in humans: its ecological origins and neurophysiological implications. *Behavioural and Brain Sciences, 13,* 519-575.

Previc, F. H., and Harter, M. R (1982). Electrophysiological and behavioural indicants of selective attention to multifeature gratings. *Perception and Psychophysics, 32,* 465-472.

Proverbio, A. M., and Mangun, R. G. (1994). Electrophysiological and behavioral "costs" and "benefits" during sustained visual-spatial attention. *International Journal of Neuroscience, 79,* 221-233.

Proverbio, A. M., and Zani, A. (2002). Electrophysiological indexes of illusory contour perception in humans. *Neuropsychologia, 40,* 479-491.

Proverbio, A. M., and Zani, A. (2005). ERP studies of selective attention to non-spatial features, In: L. Itti, G. Rees, J. Tsotsos (Eds.), *Neurobiology of attention* (pp. 496-501). San Diego (USA): Academic Press

Proverbio, A. M., Burco, F., and Zani, A. (1999). Spatio-temporal mapping of electrocortical activity during selective processing of colour and shape. *Biomedizinische Technik, 44,* Supplement 2, 166-169.

Proverbio, A. M., Esposito, P., and Zani, A. (2002). Early involvement of temporal area in attentional selection of grating orientation: an ERP study. *Cognitive Brain Research, 13* (1), 139-151.

Proverbio, A. M., Minniti, A., and Zani, A. (1998). Electrophysiological evidence of a perceptual precedence of global vs. local visual information. *Cognitive Brain Research, 6*, 321-334.

Proverbio, A. M., Zani, A., and Avella, C. (1996). Differential activation of multiple current sources of foveal VEPs as a function of spatial frequency. *Brain Topography, 9*, 59-68.

Proverbio, A. M., Zani, A., Gazzaniga, M. S., and Mangun, R. G. (1994). ERP and RT signs of a rightward bias for spatial orienting in a split-brain patient. *Neuroreport, 5*, 2457-2461.

Proverbio A. M., Zani A., and Mangun R. G. (1993). Electrophysiological substrates of visual selective attention to spatial frequency. *Bulletin of the Psychonomic Society, 31*, 368.

Regan, D. (2000). *Multiple cues for object perception: Early visual processing of spatial form defined by luminance, color, texture, motion and binocular disparity.* Sunderland (MA): Sinauer Associates.

Reed, J. L., Marx, M. S., and May, J. G. (1984). Spatial frequency tuning in the visual evoked potential elicited by sine-wave gratings. *Vision Research, 24*, 1057-1062.

Reynolds, J. H., Gottlieb, J. P., and Kastner, S. (2003). Attention. In: L. R. Squire, F. E. Bloom, S. K., McConnell, J. L. Roberts, N. C. Spitzer, and M. J. Zigmond (Eds.), *Fundamental Neuroscience* (2nd Ed., pp. 1249-1273). Amsterdam-New York: Academic Press.

Roberts, L. E., Rau, H., Lutzenberger, W., and Birbaumer, N. (1994). Mapping P300 waves onto inhibition: Go/No-go discrimination. *Electroencephalography and Clinical Neurophysiology, 92*, 44-55.

Roelfsema, P. R., Lamme, V. A. F., and Spekreijse, H. (1997). Attentive response modulation in area V1 of the macaque during the detection of connected objects. *Society of Neuroscience Abstracts, 23*, 603.8, p. 1544.

Roelfsema, P. R., Lamme, V. A. F., and Spekreijse, H. (1998). Object-based attention in the primary visual cortex of the macaque monkey. *Nature, 395*, 376-381.

Rugg, M. D., Milner, A. D., Lines, C. R., and Phalp, R. (1987). Modulation of visual event-related potentials by spatial and non-spatial visual selective attention. *Neuropsychologia, 25*, 85-96.

Schroeder, C. E. (1995). Defining the neural bases of visual selective attention: Conceptual and empirical issues. *International Journal of Neuroscience, 80*, 65-78.

Shimamura, A. P. (2000). The role of the prefrontal cortex in dynamic filtering. *Psychobiology, 28*, 207-218.

Shimamura, A. P. (2002). Memory retrieval and executive processes. In: D. T. Stuss, and R. T. Knight (Eds.), *Principles of frontal lobe function* (pp. 210-220). Oxford (England), New York (USA): Oxford University Press.

Shulman, G. L., Corbetta, M., Fiez, J. A., Buckner, R. L., Miezin, F. M., Raichle, M. E., and Petersen, S. E. (1997). Searching for activations that generalize over tasks. *Human Brain Mapping, 5*, 317-322.

Skrandies, W. (1983). Information processing and evoked potentials: Topography of early and late components. *Advances in Biological Psychiatry, 13*, 1-12.

Smith, E. J., and Jonides, J. (2003). Executive control and thought. In: L. R. Squire, F. E. Bloom, S. K., McConnell, J, L. Roberts, N. C. Spitzer, M. J. Zigmond (Eds), *Fundamental Neuroscience* (2nd Ed., pp. 1377-1394). Amsterdam-New York: Academic Press.

Somers, D. C., Dale, A. M., Seiffert, A. E., and Tootel, R. B. (1999). Functional MRI reveals spatially specific attentional modulation in human primary visual cortex. *Proceedings of the National Academy of Sciences of USA, 96*, 1663-1668.

Spitzer, H., Desimone, R., and Moran, J. (1988). Increased attention enhances both behavioral and neuronal performance. *Science, 240*, 338-340.

Squires, N. K., Squires, K. C., and Hillyard, S. A. (1975). Two varieties of long-latency positive waves evoked by unpredictable auditory stimuli in man. *Electroencephalography and Clinical Neurophysiology, 38*, 387-401.

Stuss, D. T., Eskes, G. A., and Foster, J. K. (1994). Experimental neuropsychological studies of frontal lobe functions. In: F. Boller, and J. Grafman (Eds.), Handbook of Neuropsychology (Vol. 9, pp. 149-185). Amsterdam: Elsevier.

Sutton, S., Braren, M., Zubin, J., and John, E. R. (1965). Evoked potentials correlates of stimulus uncertainty. *Science, 26*, 1187-1188.

Swick, D., and Knight, R. T. (1999). Cortical lesions and attention. In: R. Parasuraman (Ed. by), *The attentive brain* (pp. 143-162). Cambridge (Mass.): The MIT Press.

Tanaka, K. (2000). Mechanisms of visual object recognition studied in monkeys. *Spatial Vision, 13,* 147-63.

Taylor, S. F., Kornblum, S., Lauber, E. J., Minoshima, S., and Koeppe, R. A. (1997). Isolation of specific interference processing in the Stroop task: PET activation studies. *Neuroimage, 6,* 81-92.

Thompson-Schill, S. L., D'Esposito, M., Aguirre, G. K., and Farah, M. J. (1997). Role of left inferior prefrontal cortex in retrieval of semantic knowledge: A reevaluation. *Proc. Nat. Acad. Sci. USA, 94*, 14792-14797.

Thompson-Schill, S. L., Jonides, J., Marshuetz, C., Smith, E. E., D'Esposito, M., Kan, I. P., Knight, R. T., and Swick, D. (2002). Effects of frontal lobe damage on interference effects in working memory. *Cogn. Affect. Behav. Neurosci.* 2, 109-120.

Treisman, A. (1999). Feature binding, attention and object perception. In: G. W. Humphreys, J. Duncan, and A. Treisman (Eds.), *Attention, Space and Action. Studies in cognitive neuroscience* (pp. 91-111). Oxford University Press, Oxford.

Treue, S. (2001). Neural correlates of attention in primate visual cortex. *Trends in Neuroscience, 24*, 295-300.

Ungerleider, L. G., and Mishkin, M. (1982). Two cortical visual systems. In: D. G. Ingle, M. A. Goodale, and R. J. W. Mansfield (Eds.), *Analysis of visual behaviour* (pp. 549-586). Cambridge (Mass.): The MIT Press.

Vanduffel, W., Tootell, R. B. H., and Orban, G. A. (1997). State dependent modulation of visual processing in the macaque. *Experimental Brain Research, 117*, S70.

Vandenberghe, R., Duncan, J., Arnell, K. M., Bishop, S. J., Herrod, N. J., Owen, A. M., Minhas, P. S., Dupont, P., Pickard, J. D., and Orban, G. A. (2000). Maintaining and shifting attention within left or right hemifield. *Cerebral Cortex,*10, 706-713.

Vandenberghe, R., Duncan, J., Dupont, P., Ward, R., Poline, J. B., Bormans, G., Michiels, J., Mortelmans, L., and Orban, G. A. (1997). Attention to one or two features in left or right visual field: A positron emission tomography study. *J. Neurosci. 17*, 3739-3750.

Vanduffel, W., Tootell, R., and Orban G. (2000). Attention-dependent suppression of metabolic activity in the early stages of the macaque visual system. *Cerebral Cortex, 10,* 109-126.

Verleger, R. (2003). Event-related EEG potential research in neurological patients. In: A. Zani, and A. M. Proverbio (Eds.), *The cognitive electrophysiology of mind and brain* (pp. 309-341). San Diego (USA): Academic Press.

Verleger, R., and Berg, P. (1991). The waltzing oddball. *Psychophysiology,*28, 468-477.

Vogels, R., and Orban, G. A. (1994). Activity of inferior temporal neurons during orientation discrimination with successively presented gratings. *Journal of Neurophysiology, 71,* 1428-1451.

Watanabe, T., Sasaki, Y., Miyauchi, S., Putz, B., Fujimaki, N., Nielsen, M., Takino, R., and Miyakawa, S. (1998). Attention-regulated activity in human primary visual cortex. *Rapid Communication, The American Physiological Society, 22,* 2218-2221.

Wang, J., Zhou, T. , Qiu, M., Du, A. , Cai, K., Wang, Z., Zhou, C., Meng, M., Zhuo, Y., Fan, S., and Chen, L. (1999). Relationship between ventral stream for object vision and dorsal stream for spatial vision: An fMRI+ERP study. *Human Brain Mapping, 8,* 170-181.

Webster, M. J., and Ungerleider, L. G. (1999). Neuroanatomy of visual attention. In: R. Parasuraman (Ed. by), *The attentive brain* (pp. 19-34). Cambridge (Mass.): The MIT Press.

Wijers, A. A., Mulder, G., Okita, T., and Mulder, L. J. M. (1989). An ERP study on memory search and selective attention to letter size and conjunctions of letter size and color. *Psychophysiology, 26,* 529-547.

Zani, A., and Proverbio, A. M. (1993). ERP signs of early influences of selective attention on spatial frequency channels. *Abstracts Book of the "Twenty-fifth Annual Meeting of the European Brain and Behaviour Society"* (p. 278). EBBS, Madrid.

Zani, A., and Proverbio, A. M. (1995). ERP signs of early selective attention effects to check size. *Electroencephalography and Clinical Neurophysiology, 95,* 277-292.

Zani, A., and Proverbio, A. M. (1997a). ERP indicants of frontal and occipital brain mechanisms mediating spatially directed visual processing. *Experimental Brain Research*, S68, V/18, p.117.

Zani, A., and Proverbio, A. M. (1997b). Attention modulation of short latency ERPs by selective attention to conjunction of spatial frequency and location. *Journal of Psychophysiology*, 11, 21-32.

Zani, A., and Proverbio, A. M. (1997c). Attention modulation of C1 and P1 components of visual evoked potentials. *Electroencephalography and Clinical Neurophysiology, 103,* 15-3, p. 97.

Zani, A., and Proverbio, A. M. (1997d). ERP evidence of attentional selection in the occipital primary visual areas. *Brain Topography, 10,* 49-97.

Zani, A., and Proverbio, A. M. (1997e). Selective attention modulates sensory activity of primary visual areas: Electrophysiological evidence in humans. *Soc. Neurosci. Abstr., 23(1),* 121.2, p. 299.

Zani, A., and Proverbio, A. M. (2005). The timing of attentional modulation of visual processing as indexed by ERPs. In: L. Itti, G. Rees, and J. Tsotsos (Eds.), *Neurobiology of attention* (pp. 514-519). San Diego (USA): Academic Press.

Zani, A., Avella, C., Lilli, S., and Proverbio, A. M. (1999). Scalp current density (SCD) mapping of cerebral activity during object and space selection in humans. *Biomedizinische Technik, 44,* Supplement 2, 162-165.

In: Focus on Neuropsychology Research
Editor: Joshua R. Dupri, pp. 89-101

ISBN 1-59454-779-3
© 2006 Nova Science Publishers, Inc.

Chapter 3

DIFFERENTIAL CONTRIBUTIONS OF VIEWER-CENTRED AND ENVIRONMENT-CENTRED REPRESENTATIONS IN UNILATERAL NEGLECT

*Maria Luisa Rusconi[*1], Raffaella Ricci[2] and Francesca Morganti[3]*

[1] Dipartimento di Scienza della Persona, Università di Bergamo, Italy
[2] Dipartimento di Psicologia, Università di Torino, Italy
[3] ATNP-Lab, Istituto Auxologico Italiano, Milano, Italy

ABSTRACT

Unilateral neglect refers to the failure, due to unilateral brain damage, in exploring portion of space contralateral to the side of lesion. It is a largely shared opinion that the deficit could be described with reference to specific spatial co-ordinate systems. Where neglect is referring to the mid-sagittal plane of the patient's body, it has been defined viewer–centred (or egocentric) and within it a variety of components have been distinguished, such as retinotopic-, head-, limb- and trunk-centred (Vallar, 1998). Whereas, were patients show failures in representing stimuli within the extra-personal domain, such as the surrounding 'environment' and the hand-reach visual space, disorder has been specifically defined "allocentric" neglect.

Several studies have compared the specific contribution of viewer and allocentric frames of reference on neglect (Calvanio, Petrone and Levine, 1987; Ladavas, 1987; Farah, Brunn, Wong, Wallace and Carpenter, 1990; Behrmann and Moscovitch, 1994; Chatterjee, 1994; Mennemeir, Chatterjee and Heilman, 1994). Some evidence suggests a major contribution of the environment-centred system on neglect (Mennemeir, Chatterjee and Heilman, 1994). Other data support a viewer-centred predominance when the environmental frame is derived exclusively from gravitational information without using visual cues (Karnath, Fetter and Niemeier, 1998).

---

[*] Correspondence: marialuisa.rusconi@unibg.it; Maria Luisa Rusconi, MD; Dipartimento di Scienza della Persona, Università di Bergamo, Italy; P. le S. Agostino 2 ; 24129 Bergamo ; Italy

With the current study we wished to learn how neglect allocation is affected by the differential intervention of viewer, environment and array centered spatial representations. Fifteen left-neglect patients were asked to search for visually presented targets. They performed the searching either in an upright position or lying on their right side, in a position orthogonal to the environment. This latter condition was meant to dissociate viewer-centered and environment-centered frames. The visual display, within which stimuli were presented, could be either aligned with the patient's body or rotated of 90° counterclockwise. Finally, we analyzed the effects of stimulus content on neglect severity. Numbers, letters, and drawings of objects or animals were used as stimuli. Patients' spatial neglect was found to be allocated mainly with reference to the viewer's body and, to a lesser degree, to the environment. Moreover, the amount of neglect centered on the environment was found to be enhanced by the alignment of the display with its vertical. We interpreted these data as an evidence that environment-centered neglect may be partially due to a mental rotation of viewer-based representations. This phenomenon would very likely be mediated by environmental visual cues as well as the visual display within which patients are searching for targets. Regarding stimulus material, patients manifested more severe neglect with figures, improved with letters and did even better with numbers. This pattern of results is in line with Weintraub and Mesulam's (1988) finding of a less severe neglect with 'verbal' than with 'non verbal' stimuli.

INTRODUCTION

Brain-damaged patients suffering from spatial neglect show a failure in exploring the portion of space contralateral to the lesion.

Neglect patients show generally a right parietal damage and appear to be (partially) unaware of stimuli presented on the left space. This left portion of space may be defined with respect to a variety of personal and extra-personal spatial axes (Hillis and Caramazza, 1995; Bartolomeo and Chokron, 2001; Halligan, Fink, Marshall and Vallar, 2003). In a body-centred frame of reference the representation of space is relative to the body midline axis, whereas in an environment-centred the frames of reference are independent from body orientation and the environment vertical axis is determined from features of surrounding space.

In order to dissociate the relevance of different frames of reference to spatial neglect several studies have been conducted by manipulating the location of a target in one reference frame while keeping it fixed in another (Ladavas, 1987; Calvanio, Petrone and Levine, 1987; Farah, Brunn, Wong, Wallace and Carpenter, 1990; Behrmann and Moscovitch, 1994; Beschin, Cubelli, Della Sala and Spinazzola, 1997).

According to these studies, spatial neglect has been observed with reference to multiple spatial coordinates and several specific varieties have been defined. Within an egocentric frame of references some of them have been called viewer-centred neglect. They refer to locations in space relative to the viewer's body or parts of the body. Within the viewer-centered system a variety of components have been distinguished, such as retinotopic-, head-, limb- and trunk-centred (Bisiach, 1997). Each of these frames of reference is constructed by the integration of information coming from a variety of sensory modalities, i.e. visual, proprioceptive, somato-sensory, and vestibular (Pizzamiglio, Vallar and Doricchi, 1997).

On the other hand, impairments referring to locations in space independent of the viewer's orientation have been called 'allocentric' neglect. They refers, for example, to the surrounding environment and individual objects. In particular, a deeper distinction has been proposed within neglect for object when related to the observer's viewing position. Double dissociations were found between object- based neglect, where the assignment of right/left direction is referred to patient position, versus object-centered neglect, in which the perception of right/left sides of objects is viewer independent (Vallar 1998). In an allocentric frame of references descriptions of object features will be the same regardless of the relationship of the feature to the viewer. The set of features extracted will be viewpoint invariant.

Several studies have compared the specific contribution of viewer and allocentric frames of reference on spatial neglect (Calvanio, Petrone and Levine, 1987; Ladavas, 1987; Farah, Brunn, Wong, Wallace and Carpenter, 1990; Behrmann and Moscovitch, 1994; Chatterjee, 1994; Mennemeir, Chatterjee and Heilman, 1994). Some evidence suggests a major contribution of the environment-centred system on neglect (Mennemeir, Chatterjee and Heilman, 1994). Other data support a viewer-centred predominance when the environmental frame is derived exclusively from gravitational information without using visual cues (Karnath, Fetter and Niemeier, 1998).

Generally, these studies have proposed a correspondence between patient's body-centred vertical axis and environment-centred vertical axis. In order to clarify which could be the dominant frame of reference, two studies (Calvanio, Petrone and Levine, 1987; Ladavas, 1987) have been proposed a possible experimental dissociation between viewer-centred and environment-centred frame of reference removing the alignment of the body midline with the environmental vertical axis. In Calvanio and colleagues (*ibidem*) neglect has been assessed using a set of stimuli depicted on the four visual field quadrants. Patients have been asked to name objects or real words arranged in a 5x5 matrices (constantly oriented) while sitting upright or reclining on their side. Results supports the observation that spatial neglect is bodily-centred and environment-centred. Evidences that neglect was relative to the left side of the body and also to the left side of the visual array were found. Those results have confirmed the importance of both frames of reference in the representation of space, although the results have not provided evidence in allowing a decoupling from environment to object centred frame of references. In order to explore the effect of patient's rotation on the coronal plane, Ladavas (*ibidem*) asked (Experiment 3) to five neglect patients to faster respond to visual stimuli presented on either side and above of fixation point while their head was 90° tilted either to the left or to the right body side. In the condition of left head tilt, both stimuli were presented on the ipsilesional (right) visual hemifield. Conversely in the condition of right head tilt stimuli were proposed in the contralesional (left) hemifield. Results showed how both effects, presentation and visual hemifield, were significant.

With the present study we wanted to investigate whether the viewer's body or the environment plays a dominant role in defining the distribution of space.

Fifteen left-neglect patients were asked to perform a visual search task similar to those used by Calvanio and colleagues (1987). Moreover, in defining experimental methods, we have been referred to studies proposed by Farah and colleagues (1990) and Behrmann and Moscovitch (1994). We uncoupled the two frames of reference by placing the patients in a position orthogonal to the environment. Unlike in Farah's and colleagues study (1990), the stimulus display could not be considered as representing an individual object (characterized by intrinsic left-right axis), but constituted a further 'environmental' frame.

We expect that, in the condition in which patient and environment were dissociated, left neglect could be manifested in the left side of space with respect to the viewer (i.e. the superior side of the environmentally defined space) or to the environment (relative to the mid-sagittal plane in which would be the patient's body if it were rotated from the reclined to the upright position). In case we found both viewer and environment centred neglect we could infer a possible, albeit partially, involvement of a process of "mental rotation" encoding locations in a viewer-based frame. If this hypothesis were correct, we expected to find a dominant influence on neglect by the viewer coordinates system when viewer-centred and environment-centred neglect were compared. We also expected to find a greater degree of environment-centred neglect in the condition in which the array was aligned with the environment in comparison to when it was not.

Moreover, we aimed to study the effect of stimulus content on neglect severity (Weintraub and Mesulam, 1988). According to Kinsbourne (1970 a,b), since verbal and spatial stimuli activate the left and the right hemisphere respectively, the presentation of one kind of stimulus would facilitate contralateral orientation of the activated hemisphere. This would result in a reduction of neglect in that specific hemi-field. Heilman and Watson (1978), supported Kinsbourne's theory by showing that left neglect improved when their patients had to cancel lines with respect to words. On the other hand, Caplan (1985) failed to confirm these findings, and Weintraub and Mesulam (1988) obtained the opposite result (i.e. more omissions in a cancellation task when stimuli were shapes in comparison to letters). As suggested by Weintraub and Mesulam (1988), this discordance of results might be accounted for by differences in 'non verbal' material used by the different authors. In the present study patients were presented with three different kinds of stimuli: numbers, letters, and drawings of objects or animals. Stimulus manipulation was meant to have an exploratory character more than testing a specific hypothesis.

METHOD

Subjects

Fifteen left neglect patients (5 males and 10 females), mean age 69.2 (SD= 10.27) participated in the experiment (see Table 1). Patients showed unilateral neglect on a line cancellation task (Albert, 1973) and a letters cancellation task (Diller and Weinberg, 1977). The Mini Mental State Examination (Folstein, Folstein and McHugh, 1975) was administered to exclude patients with global cognitive impairment. Ten right-handed normal subjects (5 males and 5 females), mean age 71.4 (SD= 3.85, range= 64-76) constituted the control group.

Stimuli and Procedure

Stimuli consisted of three 40x40 cm tables. On each table 25 targets were arranged in a 5x5 matrix according to a fixed random order. Targets were letters, numbers, and drawings of common objects or animals (Figure 1). Patients were asked to report what they saw without time limits. Subjects' head and eyes were aligned forward at the beginning of each trial. Each table was presented in two different orientations: either at 0° with respect to the viewer (canonical orientation), or rotated of 90° counter-clockwise with respect to the viewer. Patients were required to perform the task first sitting upright with their head and trunk aligned along the vertical mid-sagittal plane, and then lying on their right side.

Letters displays were presented first, followed by numbers and figures displays. Each subject performed 12 experimental conditions (2 subject's positions by 2 table's positions by 3 kinds of stimuli).

Table 1. Demographic and Clinical Data of Neglect Patients

Patient	Sex	Age	Education (years)	Lesion (CT scan)	Aetiology
1	F	59	5	F.T.P.	I
2	F	84	18	T.	I
3	M	66	5	T.P.O.	I
4	F	75	4	cs.	I
5	F	62	4	F.T.P.	I
6	F	72	5	cs.	I
7	F	76	4	P.	I
8	M	57	5	F.T.P.	I
9	F	80	5	T.P.O.	I
10	M	64	13	T.P.	H
11	M	68	8	Th, P.	I
12	F	73	5	F.T.P.	I
13	F	46	5	T.P.	I
14	F	79	5	bg	H
15	M	77	5	- -	- -

M= male; F= female; I= Ischemia; H= Hemorrhage; F.= Frontal; T.= Temporal; P.= Parietal ; O.= Occipital; cs = centrum semiovale; Th= Thalamus; bg= basal ganglia; - - = missing data

Analysis

Correct responses were collected. In order to analyze neglect distribution the display was divided into four quadrants: top left (1), top right (2), bottom left (3), and bottom right (4), by eliminating the 9 items on the vertical and horizontal midlines (see Figure 1). Thus, we scored 16 out of 25 items, i.e. 4 items for each quadrant.

Viewer-centred left neglect was defined as higher detection rate in the two quadrants on the right of the body midline. Environment-centred neglect was defined as higher detection rate in the two quadrants on the right of the environmental vertical. Array-centred neglect was defined as higher detection rate in the two quadrants on the right of the vertical axis of the table.

Also we analyzed the location of patients' first reports (starting points). For this purpose, the following rule was used: if the patient began in a quadrant, that quadrant received a score of 1.0; if the patient began on a midline row or column between two quadrants, each quadrant received a score of 0.5; if the patient began in the center of the array, each of the four surrounding quadrants received a score of 0.25.

A	G	K	B	F
O	S	D	R	Z
Y	N	C	T	P
V	I	M	H	E
Q	X	U	W	L

Figure 1. Example of visual search array when the stimuli were letters. The gray area indicates targets excluded from data analysis.

RESULTS

Participants assigned to the control group reported all items in all of the experimental conditions. Figure 2 shows the mean number of reports in each quadrant made by neglect patients in each experimental condition. A repeated measures ANOVA was performed on patients' data as a group, with stimulus (letters, numbers, and drawings), viewer's position (viewer upright, viewer rotated), array position (0° and 90°), and quadrant (1, 2, 3, 4) as within-subjects factors. The three main factors resulted significant. For the factor 'stimulus' [$F_{(2,28)}$= 9.27 p=0.001], an analysis post-hoc (Sheffé, p=0.05) revealed that patients performed significantly better when the stimuli were numbers (12.78) than when they were letters (12.23) and drawings (10.53). In addition, patients' performance was higher with letters than drawings. For the 'viewer's position' [$F_{(1,14)}$= 7.71 p=0.015], the number of items reported when patients performed the task in the rotated position (12.21) was higher than when they were sitting upright (11.49). Finally, for the factor 'quadrant' [$F_{(3,42)}$= 14,28 p<0.0001], an analysis post-hoc (Sheffé) revealed that reports in quadrant 1 were significantly minor than in quadrants 2 and 4. Also reports in quadrant 3 were less than those in quadrant 4. Patients had therefore the worst performance in quadrant 1, and the best in quadrant 4. Mean reports in each quadrant are presented in Figure 2.

The following interactions were also significant: stimulus x quadrant [$F_{(6, 84)}$= 5.50 p< 0.0001], array position x quadrant [$F_{(3,42)}$= 10.56 p<0.0001], and viewer's position x array position x quadrant [$F_{(3,42)}$= 2.98 p=0.042]. In order to analyze the triple interaction 'viewer's position x array position x quadrant', we performed two separate analyses of variance for each viewer's position. The interaction 'array position x quadrant' was significant for both conditions 'viewer upright' [$F_{(3,42)}$=9.47 p<0.0001], and 'viewer rotated' [$F_{(3,42)}$= 9.20 p<0.0001].

Considering the above result, we investigated how patients' performance changed, within each quadrant, by rotating the display with respect to the body midline (from 0° to minus 90°). Within each viewer's position (upright and rotated), repeated measures t-test were performed, using Bonferroni adjustment.

Patient upright (see Fig.2 conditions a and b). In this condition, we could observe the effects of removing the alignment of the array from the viewer and the environment, which were aligned.

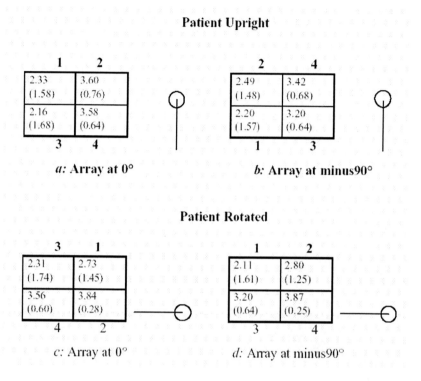

Patient Upright

a: Array at 0°   b: Array at minus90°

Patient Rotated

c: Array at 0°   d: Array at minus90°

Figure 2. Sketch of the four experimental conditions: a) viewer upright-array at 0°, b) viewer upright-array at minus 90°, c) viewer rotated-array at 0°, d) viewer rotated-array at minus 90°. Mean number of reports and standard deviations in each stimulus quadrant for each condition.

The number of targets reported to quadrant 2 significantly decreased [t(14)=3.53 p=0.003] from condition 'a' to condition 'b'. This finding together with a significant improvement [t(14)=-2.83 p=0.013] of performance within quadrant 3, from condition 'a' to condition 'b', suggests that patients' neglect was mainly allocated with reference to the viewer's and environment left space. If the array-centred frame had a critical role, performance within quadrants should not have changed when the array alignment was removed from those of the other two systems.

Patient rotated (see Fig.2 conditions c and d). In this condition, we could investigate whether patients' neglect was distributed with reference to the viewer and/or the environment. When the array was at 0°, the environment-centred frame was isolated from the other two and when the array was at minus 90°, the viewer-centred frame was isolated from the other two.

The number of reports to quadrant 2 decreased significantly [t(14)=3.41 p=0.004] from condition 'c' to condition 'd', that is when this quadrant moved from the right to the left of the viewer. Since this rotation did not change the quadrant left-right location in relation to the environment, the above result suggests a significant role of the viewer's frame of reference.

The number of reports to quadrant 1 showed a tendency to decrease from condition 'c' to condition 'd' (i.e. when this quadrant moved from the right to the left of the environment vertical). However this difference did not reach a statistically significant level when the Bonferroni correction was applied [t (14)=2.58 p=0.022>0.0125].

Neglect for the Left-Sided Quadrants

Neglect for the left-sided quadrants, within each frame of reference, was analyzed through a series of repeated measure one-tailed t-test (and Bonferroni correction).

Patient Upright

Array at 0° (Fig. 2a). Patients reported more targets on the right side (quadrants 2 and 4; mean= 7.18, SD=1.32) than on the left side (quadrants 1 and 3, mean= 4.49 SD= 3.19) of the viewer, environment and array, which in this conditions were aligned [one–tailed t(14)=-4.05 p=0.0005]. This result confirmed that patients had left neglect, when tested in a canonical position.

Array at minus 90° (Fig. 2b). The number of reports to the right (quadrants 2 and 4; mean= 5.91, SD=1.89) and to left (quadrants 1 and 3; mean=5.40 SD=2.04) of the array mid-line did not result significantly different [one-tailed t(14)= 1.89 p=0.0395>0.025, using Bonferroni's correction]. The number of reports to the right of the aligned viewer and environment frames (quadrants 3 and 4; mean= 6.62 SD=1.23) resulted to be significantly higher [one-tailed t(14)= 2.99 p=0.005] than the number of reports to the left-sided quadrants (quadrants 1 and 2, 4.69 SD= 2.97). This result suggests that overall this group of patients did not show (significant) array-centred neglect.

Patient Rotated

Array at 0° (Fig.2c). The number of reports to the right (quadrants 1 and 2; mean= 6.58 SD= 1.59) of the environment vertical was significantly higher [t(14)= 2.56 p= 0.0115] than the number of reports to its left (quadrants 3 and 4; mean= 5.87 SD= 2.20), as well as the number of reports to the right (quadrants 2 and 4, 7.40 SD=0.83) of the aligned viewer and array was higher [t(14)= 3.52 p=0.0015] than that of reports to their left (quadrants 1 and 3; mean= 5.04 SD=3.08). This result indicates the presence of significant environment-centred neglect.

Array at minus 90° (Fig. 2d). Reports to the right (quadrants 3 and 4; mean= 7.07 SD=1.00) of the viewer's mid-line were significantly more [t(14)= 3.60 p=0.0015] than reports to its left (quadrants 1 and 2, 4.91 SD=2.79) as well as reports to the right (quadrants 2 and 4; mean= 6.67 SD=1.30) of the aligned environment and array were more [t(14)= 4.80 p<0.0001] than those to the left (quadrants 1 and 3, 5.31 SD=2.24). This result indicates a significant viewer-centred neglect.

Viewer-Centred Versus Environment-Centred Neglect

The above analyses substained a significant role of the viewer's frame of reference and also the presence of environment-centred neglect. For this group of patients, the array did not appear to have a crucial role on neglect distribution.

In order to test whether the viewer's co-ordinates system had a stronger influence on neglect than the environment, the difference between right-sided reports and left-sided reports was contrasted for the condition in which the viewer (patient rotated/array minus 90°) and the environment (patient rotated/array 0°) were isolated from the other two frames. This analysis showed that left neglect was significantly greater [one-tailed $t(14)=2.66$ p=0.018 .009] within the viewer (Fig. 2d; mean difference=2.16, SD=2.32) than the environment frame of reference (Fig.2 c mean difference=0.71, SD=1.08).

Further, we wanted to test the hypothesis that environmental neglect might be partially explained by a mental rotation of spatial representations built with reference to the viewer's system, by analysing whether the alignment of the array with the environment would exacerbate environment-centred neglect. Results seem to support this hypothesis. The difference between right-sided and left-sided reports was significantly greater [$t(14)=1.98$ p=0.068, .034] within the environment co-ordinates system when the array was aligned with it (Fig. 2d; mean difference=1.36, SD=1.09) than when it was not (Fig. 2c; mean difference=0.71, SD=1.08).

To conclude, the viewer-centred space was found to have a greater influence than the environment in defining spatial neglect distribution. Our data support also the idea that environment-centred neglect might be partially accounted for by a mental rotation of viewer-centred spatial representations.

Starting Points

Patients with left neglect characteristically begin searching from the right upper side of the display (Calvanio, Petrone and Levine, 1987; Chatterjee, Mennemeir and Heilman, 1992; Mark and Heilman, 1997). In contrast, normal subjects usually start searching from the left upper side of the page.

Surprisingly, we did not find a dramatic divergence of behaviors between neglect patients and controls. All control subjects started the task in the first three conditions (a, b, c) by reporting targets located in the left upper corner with reference to the viewer's body (100%). In the last condition (d), they reported in 66% of the cases as first, targets located in the left bottom quadrant with reference to the viewer (upper left quadrant with respect to the environment). A similar, although rightwards 'biased' configuration of starting points, characterized patients' behavior (see Figure 3). They started the task from the two upper quadrants in conditions a, b, and c, and from the left bottom quadrant and the left upper quadrant, in condition d, with reference to the viewer.

Both patients and controls seemed to maintain a viewer-centred orientation in the first three conditions, in which the environment and/or the array were aligned with the body. On the other hand, in the last condition, in which the display was removed from the body orientation and aligned with the environment, patients and controls switched their orientation toward the environmental frame. Both groups manifested a behavior which is in line with the hypothesis that mental rotation of viewer-centred representations would underlie the construction of the environment-centred space representations.

STARTING POINTS

Viewer Upright

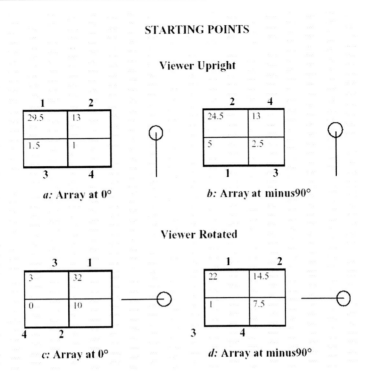

Figure 3. Starting points distribution in each stimulus quadrant (max=45) for each condition (a, b, c, d).

CONCLUSION

With the present study we investigated the influence of viewer, environment and array frames of reference on spatial neglect distribution in a group of fifteen left neglect patients. These patients' spatial disorder was found to be mainly distributed with reference to the viewer co-ordinates system. However, their spatial neglect was also affected, in a smaller degree, by environmental cues.

Our findings are apparently in contrast with those of Mennemeier and colleagues (1994) showing a main role played by the environment. This discordance of results may be due to differences in patients' lesion locations and task (line bisection). Mennemeir and colleagues' (1994) patients had bilateral lesions, while all the patients of our study showed unilateral right-hemisphere lesions.

We also tested the hypothesis that neglect centred on the environment might be (at least partially) accounted for by mental rotation of viewer-centred spatial representations. The idea that mental rotation phenomena may underlie different manifestations of unilateral neglect (Bisiach, 1997; Karnath, Fetter and Niemeier, 1998) has been invoked to explain also object-centred neglect (Buxbaum, Coslett, Montgomery and Farah, 1996). In our experiment, viewer and environment were dissociated by placing the patients in a position orthogonal to the environmental vertical. When the patients were lying on their side, both the surrounding visual cues and the display within which visual stimuli were presented were likely to mediate a mental rotation of viewer-centred representations toward the position in which they would be if standing upright. A mental rotation of the viewer's representation toward an upright position can be very likely enhanced by the alignment of the display within which patients are searching for targets, from the viewer to the environment-centred position. Our data confirmed this prediction. The amount of neglect centred on the environment was enhanced by aligning the visual display with the environment. Also starting points distribution suggested such a phenomenon in patients as well as in normal subjects.

In normal subjects the perception of the verticality of a luminous rod surrounded by a tilted frame, in a completely dark room, is dependent on the viewer's body position. When normal subjects lie at 90° to the left or to the right, gravitational information is reduced and error increases under the influence of distorted visual inputs (Zoccolotti, Antonucci, Goodenough, Pizzamiglio and Spinelli, 1992). This evidence may explain the susceptibility to external visual guidance that, in our study, patients and normal subjects (as far as starting point data) manifested when lying on their side. We based our interpretation on the analysis of the conditions in which subjects were rotated, then when the gravitational input is assumed to be weaker and the visual cueing (mediating mental rotation processes) dominant.

However, our results do not exclude the intervention of gravitational input in defining neglect patients' behavior. The fact that, overall, patients performed better in the rotated than in the upright position is in agreement with data reported by Pizzamiglio, Vallar and Doricchi (1997). They found a significant improvement of neglect when patients were in the supine position in comparison to when they were in the upright position. In the supine position the gravitational information from the otolith system is strongly reduced. In the upright position perceptual judgment would be based on the integration of visual and gravitational information, whereas in the supine position would be based predominantly on visual inputs. An improvement of patients' performance in the rotated position may be explained by a selective reduction of gravitational information (neglect referred to representations built on a gravitational input).

As far as the effects of stimulus content are concerned, overall patients had a better performance when stimuli were numbers, than letters and figures. Moreover, they did better with letters than with figures. This pattern of results seems to be in agreement with Weintraub and Mesulam's finding (1988). They showed that neglect severity increased with 'non verbal' stimuli, then with stimuli preferentially processed by the right hemisphere. Similarly, in our study, it is possible to assume that line drawings of objects and animals elicited a greater intervention of the right hemisphere than letters or number. Interestingly, stimuli associated with the worst performance (figures) seemed to be affected mostly by the left-right orientation in space as defined by the viewer's body.

ACKNOWLEDGEMENTS

We are grateful to Edoardo Bisiach , who read an early draft of this paper for his suggestions, and to Marco Franceschetti for his help in data collection.

REFERENCES

Albert, M.L. (1973). A simple test of visual neglect. *Neurology, 23*, 658-664.

Bartolomeo P., and Chokron, S. (2001). Levels of impairment in unilateral neglect. In F. Boller, M. Behrmann (Eds.) *Disorders of visual behaviour,* pp.67-98, Amsterdam: Elsevier.

Behrmann M., and Moschovitch M. (1994). Object-centered neglect in patients with unilateral neglect: Effects of left-right coordinates of objects. *Journal of Cognitive Neuroscience, 6,*1-16.

Beschin N., Cubelli R., Della Sala S., and Spinazzola L. (1997) Left of what? The role of egocentric coordinates in neglect. *Journal of Neurology Neurosurgery and Psychiatry, 63,* 483-489.

Bisiach, E. (1997). The spatial feature of unilateral neglect. In P. Thier, H.O. Karnath (Eds) *Parietal lobe contributions to orientation in 3D space,* pp.465-495, New York: Springer Verlag.

Buxbaum L.J., Coslett H.B, Montgomery M.V., and Farah M.J. (1996). Mental rotation may underlie apparent object-based neglect. *Neuropsychologia, 34(2)*, 113-126.

Calvanio R., Petrone P.N., and Levine D.N. (1987). Left visual spatial neglect is both environment-centered and body centered. *Neurology, 37,* 1179-1183

Caplan B. (1985). Stimulus effects in unilateral neglect? *Corte, 21,* 69-80

Chatterjee A. (1994) Picturing unilateral spatial neglect: viewer versus object centred reference frames. *Journal of Neurology Neurosurgery and Psychiatry, 57(10),* 1236-1240.

Chatterjee A., Mennemeir M. and Heilman K.M. (1992) Search pattern and neglect: a case study. *Neurospychologia, 30 (7),* 657-672.

Diller L., and Weinberg J.(1977). Hemi-inattention in rehabilitation: the evolution of a rational remediation program. In E.A. Weinstein and R.P. Friedland (eds) *Hemi-inattention and hemisphere specialisation: advances in neurology, 18,* New York: Raven Press.

Farah M.J., Brunn J.L., Wong A.B., Wallace M.A., and Carpenter P.A. (1990). Frames of reference for allocating attention to space: evidence from the neglect syndrome. *Neuropsychologia, 28,* 335-347.

Folstein M.F., Folstein S.E., and McHugh P.R. (1975). Mini Mental State: a practical method for grading the cognitive state of patient for the clinician. *Journal of Psychiatric Research, 12,* 189-198.

Halligan P.W., Fink G.R., Marshall J.C., and Vallar G. (2003). Spatial cognition: evidence from visual neglect. *Trends in Cognitive Sciences, 7,* 125-133.

Heilman KM, Watson RT (1978) Changes in the Symptoms of Neglect Induced by Changing Task Strategy. *Archives of Neurology, 35,* 47-49

Hillis A.E and Caramazza A. (1995) A framework for interpreting distinct patterns of hemispatial neglect. *Neurocase , 1,* 189-207.

Karnath H.O., Fetter M., and Niemeier M. (1998) Disentangling Gravitational, Environmental, and Egocentric Reference Frames in Spatial Neglect. *Journal of Cognitive Neuroscience, 10,* 680-690.

Kinsbourne M. (1970a) A model for the mechanism of unilateral neglect o space. *Trans Amer Neurol Assoc, 95,* 143-146.

Kinsbourne M. (1970b) The cerebral basis of lateral asymmetries in attention. *Acta Psychologica 33,* 193-210.

Ladavas E. (1987) Is the hemispatial deficit produced by right parietal lobe damage associated with retinal or gravitational coordinates? *Brain, 110,* 167-180.

Mark VW, Heilman KM (1997) Diagonal neglect on cancellation. *Neuropsychologia, 35 (11),* 1425-1436.

Mennemeir M, Chatterjee A, and Heilman KM (1994) A comparison of the influences of body and environment centred reference frames on neglect. *Brain, 117,* 1013-1021.

Pizzamiglio L., Vallar G., and Doricchi F. (1997) Gravitational inputs modulate visuospatial neglect. *Experimental Brain Research, 117,* 341-345.

Vallar, G. (1998). Spatial hemineglect in humans. *Trends in Cognitive Science, 2,* 87-97.

Weintraub S., and Mesulam M.M. (1988). Visual hemispatial inattention: stimulus parameters and exploratory strategies *Journal of Neurology, Neurosurgery, and Psychiatry, 51,* 1481-1488.

Zoccolotti P., Antonucci G., Goodenough D.R., Pizzamiglio L., and Spinelli D.(1992). The role of frame size on vertical and horizontal observers in the rod-and-frame illusion. *Acta Psychologica, 79,* 171-187.

In: Focus on Neuropsychology Research
Editor: Joshua R. Dupri, pp. 103-140

ISBN 1-59454-779-3
© 2006 Nova Science Publishers, Inc.

Chapter 4

NEUROPSYCHOLOGICAL PARAMETERS AFFECTING THE ACADEMIC APTITUDE TEST (AAT) ACHIEVEMENT AT THE END OF HIGH SCHOOL IN 1996 AND THEIR IMPACT ON JOB STATUS IN 2002: A MULTIFACTORIAL APPROACH IN A FOLLOW-UP STUDY

Daniza M. Ivanovic[1,], Hernán T. Pérez[1], Boris P. Leiva[1], Nora S. Díaz[1], Bárbara D. Leyton[1], Atilio Aldo F.Almagià[2], María Soledad C. Urrutia[3], Cristián G. Larraín[4], Paulina E. Olave[5], Nélida B. Inzunza[6] and Rodolfo M. Ivanovic[1]*

[1] University of Chile, Institute of Nutrition and Food Technology (INTA), Santiago, Chile.
[2] Catholic University of Valparaíso, Valparaíso, Chile.
[3] Pan American Health Organization (PAHO), Pan American Sanitary Bureau, Regional Office of the World Health Organization, Washington, D.C. USA;
[4] Department of Magnetic Resonance Imaging Service, German Clinic of Santiago. Santiago, Chile
[5] Metropolitan University of Educational Sciences. Santiago, Chile
[6] Adventist University of Chile

---

[*] Telephone (56) 2 678-1459; FAX 56 (2) 221-4030. E-mail: inta8@abello.dic.uchile.cl; daniza@inta.cl; Loma Linda University, School of Public Health, California, USA-Adventist University of Chile. Avda. Macul 5540. Casilla 138-11. Santiago. Chile.

ABSTRACT

The aim of this study was to determine the impact of neuropsychological parameters on the academic aptitude test (AAT) achievement at the end of high school in 1996 when they should be graduating from high school and on job status carried out six years later during 2002. From a representative sample of 1817 Chilean school-age children (mean age 18.0 ± 0.9 y) graduating from high school in 1996 in Chile's Metropolitan Region, 96 were selected with high (> 120 WAIS-R) and low IQ (< 100 WAIS-R) (1:1), from the high and low socio-economic strata (SES) (1:1) and of both sexes (1:1). AAT scores for university admission were obtained for 84 school-age children from University of Chile records and were divided into two groups: high AAT ($\geq$ median (Md)= score 631) and low AAT (< Md). IQ was determined by the Wechsler Intelligence Scale for Adults (WAIS-R) and the Raven Progressive Matrices Test in the school-age children and their parents. Scholastic achievement (SA) was measured applying the standard Spanish language and mathematics tests. SES was evaluated using Graffar's modified method. Nutritional status was assessed through anthropometric measurements of weight and height to establish the body mass index (BMI) according to Garrow; head circumference (HC) was compared with Tanner, Nellhaus, Roche et al. and Ivanovic et al. tables and was expressed as Z score (Z-HC); body composition parameters such as arm circumference-for-age, triceps skinfold-for-age, arm muscle area-for-age and arm fat area-for-age were calculated using data from Frisancho. Brain morphology was determined by magnetic resonance imaging (MRI). Job status was expressed as: (1) jobless, (2) workers without further schooling, (3) students at institutes and (4) students at universities. Statistical analysis included correlation and logistic regressions using the Statistical Analysis System (SAS). Results showed that students with high AAT score presented IQ, parental IQ, SA, brain volume (BV), Z-HC, maternal schooling, house-hold head occupation and quality of housing significantly higher than their peers that achieved the lowest AAT scores of whom 19% had suffered severe undernutrition in the first year of life (Fisher p< 0.0054). However, logistic regression revealed that student IQ is the best predictor of AAT score and the odds ratio value (1.252) implies that when the IQ score increases by one point, the probability to obtain a high AAT score increases in 25.2%. Students at universities presented AAT, child and maternal IQ, SA, BV, birth weight and birth height, Z-HC and socio-economic conditions significantly higher than their peers from the other three job statuses; however, AAT score at the end of high school was the best predictor of the job status six years later (odds ratio value= 1.025) which indicates that when AAT score increases by one point the probability for university admission and for university graduation increases 2.5%. In a multifactorial approach, these results point out the importance of neuropsychological parameters on children's achievement for university admission and future jobs.

INTRODUCTION

The AAT, the baccalaureate examination for university admission with national coverage in Chile, revives a permanent controversy as regards whether this instrument is the best test to select the most capable high school graduates to enroll into higher education. The question is whether AAT score is a good predictor of successful scholastic achievement at universities and later job status. As a consequence, this instrument is the object of continuous analysis in order to optimize it; however, planners have insufficient elements to consider since research carried out to assess the impact of the test on university achievement and later occupation level is scant

(Schiefelbein and Farrell, 1982). As regards to this problem, research must consider that scholastic achievement is a multifactorial process determined by multiple factors dependent on characteristics of the student, his family and the educational system that affect enrollment, attendance, school performance and desertion (Ivanovic and Ivanovic, 1988; Ivanovic, Ivanovic and Middleton, 1988).

Of all the neuropsychological parameters intelligence has been described as the most important independent variable that explains educational achievement (Ivanovic, Ivanovic, Truffello, and Buitrón, 1989a; Ivanovic et al., 2000a,b,d, 2002, 2004c). Our previous results confirm that both the child's and his parent's intellectual quotient, undernutrition in the first year of life, brain volume, birth weight and birth height significantly condition scholastic achievement; however, the child's intellectual quotient is the most important independent variable explaining approximately 90% of scholastic achievement variance in both sexes (Ivanovic el al. 2000a, 2002). Maternal intellectual quotient, brain volume and nutritional status during the first year of life have been described as the most relevant variables that contribute to explain child intelligence independently of age, sex and socio-economic strata (Ivanovic et al., 2002). Other findings reported by us in Chilean school-age children revealed that head circumference, sex, maternal and schooling of the head of the household, height, availability of sewerage at home and the quality of housing, have been also described as the most relevant independent variables associated with intellectual ability and this was independent of socio-economic strata and age (Ivanovic, Forno, and Ivanovic, 2001). These results indicate that when socio-economic, cultural, family, mass media exposure, demographic and educational variables were considered as independent variables in the statistical regression model, maternal schooling was the variable with the greatest explanatory power in the child's intellectual ability variance (Ivanovic et al., 2001). On the other hand, several authors have confirmed that variables related to family socio-economic strata and particularly maternal schooling are consistent in explaining scholastic achievement and intelligence (Ivanovic, Castro, and Ivanovic, 1995b; Özmert, et al., 2005; Sandiford, Cassel, Sanchez, and Coldham, 1997). The lack of precision concerning the relative impact of mass media exposure on scholastic achievement is evident since several authors described that for some children some television programs, has negative effects; however, for most children television is neither injurious nor beneficial and some studies even detected a positive impact of television on school performance (Gupta, Saini, Acharya, and Miglani, 1994; Hagborg, 1995; Ivanovic and Sepúlveda, 1988; Ridley-Johnson, Cooper, and Chance, 1982; Schramm, Lyle, and Parker, 1965; Strasburger, 1986). As regards to written mass media, reading ability has been described as positively and significantly associated with scholastic achievement at the onset of high school and learning disabilities are positively and significantly associated with very low birth weight (Johnson, and Breslau, 2000; Smith et al., 1996).

The nutritional status of school-age children has been reported as positively and significantly associated with scholastic achievement and intelligence. In this respect, our previous reports provide substantial evidence that this neuropsychological parameter is positively and significantly correlated with indicators of past nutrition, especially head circumference, the most important anthropometric index associated with learning and intelligence (Ivanovic, 1992; Ivanovic and Marambio, 1989; Ivanovic, Olivares, Castro, and Ivanovic, 1996; Ivanovic, Zacarías, Saitúa, and Marambio, 1988; Ivanovic et al., 1989a, 1991a, 1992, 2000a,b,c, 2002, 2004c; Toro, Almagià, and Ivanovic, 1998). Head circumference is an anthropometric indicator of both nutritional background and brain development (Rumsey and

Rapoport, 1983). Although a "normal" head circumference, mean ± 2 standard deviations, could be more related to statistical normality, this may not be the case for scholastic achievement or psychological function (Ivanovic et al., 2000c, 2004b). In this respect, although microcephaly and macrocephaly are reliable indicators of brain pathology, head circumference values below the mean but still within the normal range are associated with an increased incidence of lower intellectual quotient (Ivanovic et al., 2000c, 2004b; Menkes, 1995). This means that small differences in head size could be important in the interrelationship head circumference-intelligence-learning.

Undernutrition at an early age may have negative long-term effects on scholastic achievement; undernourished students have significantly lower birth weights, decreased head circumference, lower intellectual quotient, brain volume, school performance and maternal schooling than their peers who did not suffer from undernutrition at comparable early age (Ivanovic et al., 2000b). In Chilean school-age children graduating from high school our recent findings confirm that, independently of socio-economic condition, age and sex, high school graduates with similar intellectual quotient have similar parameters of nutritional status, brain development and scholastic achievement and that these variables are strongly and significantly interrelated (Ivanovic et al., 2002).

Undernutrition in the first year of life affects growth, especially head circumference but taking into consideration that children grow until about 18 years of age, improvements in height may be obtained through adequate nutrition. However, the brain is a notable exception since the first two years of life represent its period of maximum growth and by the end of the first year of life, 70% of it adult weight has been attained (Ivanovic, 1996; Stoch, Smythe, Moodie, and Bradshaw, 1982). In fact, head circumference has been defined by several studies as the most sensitive anthropometric index of prolonged undernutrition during infancy, associated with intellectual impairment and low scholastic achievement (Ivanovic, 1996; Ivanovic et al. 2000b; Leiva et al. 2001; Stoch et al. 1982; Winick and Rosso, 1969a). Malnutrition alters brain development and intelligence by interfering with overall health as well as with the child's activity level, rates of motor development and growth; poverty exacerbates these negative effects, especially when mothers have lower schooling levels (Brown and Pollitt, 1996; Ivanovic et al. 2000b). Independently of age, children identify their mothers as the most powerful source of nutrition information (Ivanovic, Olivares, and Ivanovic, 1991b; Ivanovic, Truffello, Buitrón, and Ivanovic, 1989b). Mothers of children who suffered from undernutrition at an early age have serious problems related to affectivity and communication with their offspring and a low degree of non-verbal expressiveness (Alvarez and Wurgaft, 1981; Alvarez, Wurgaft, and Wilder, 1982). As a result, maternal schooling may have its greatest impact on the child's health and intellectual quotient probably because mothers are the main source of intellectual stimulation and enrichment for their psycho-social environment (Smith et al., 1996). This finding could be important for the intellectual development of children since the intellectual quotient is positively influenced by adequate stimulation.

The impact of head size on intelligence and scholastic achievement increases significantly from the onset of elementary school until the end of high school, in the same way that the impact of body weight and body height decreases significantly (Ivanovic et al., 1996, 2000c). At the onset of elementary school, 59% of children had suboptimal head circumferences, a percentage that decreased significantly to 40% in high school graduates (Ivanovic et al., 1996). As a consequence, we may infer that school dropout or school delay correlates with head circumference and not with weight or height. Among high school graduates, approximately 70% of those students with the lowest scores in the scholastic achievement test had subnormal head circumference (Ivanovic et al., 1996).

Early childhood malnutrition affects head circumference, brain development and later intelligence and scholastic achievement, but this is still a matter of controversy since these variables are influenced by socio-economic and cultural factors that are co-determinants; a head circumference below -2 standard deviations of the mean may be an indicator of severe undernutrition and accurately reflects retarded brain growth during the first year of life (Winick and Rosso, 1969a). In autopsies of children who died of severe undernutrition during the first year of life, some authors have demonstrated decreased cell division rates in the brain, resulting in decreased myelination, weight, nucleic acid and protein contents, compared with normal children died of accidental causes; the decreased head circumference is proportional to the brain's weight; in fact, the magnitude of this reduction is a reliable indicator of the severity of nutritional deprivation (Winick, 1975; Winick and Rosso, 1969a,b). The long-term effects of severe undernutrition in the first year of life may result in delay of head circumference growth, of brain development and decreased intelligence and scholastic achievement, variables that are all strongly interrelated (Grantham-McGregor and Fernald, 1997; Ivanovic, 1996; Ivanovic et al., 2000b, 2002; Leiva et al., 2001; Stoch et al., 1982; Winick and Rosso, 1969a). Findings from several studies emphasize that head circumference might reflect better than body height the impact of nutritional deficiencies at an early age; this measurement is useful in the identification of the period during which malnutrition occurred (Johnston, and Lampl, 1984; Malina et al., 1975; Yarbrough, Habicht, Martorell, and Klein, 1974).

Head circumference in the first year of life may predict later intelligence as it has been described by several authors (Botting, Powls, Cooke, and Marlow, 1998; Fisch, Bilek, Horrobin, and Chang, 1976; Nelson and Deutschberger, 1970). On the other hand, the interrelationship between scholastic achievement, intelligence and nutritional background, reflected by a decreased head circumference, may be affected by birth weight and other factors (Botting et al., 1998; Grunau, Whitfield, and Fay, 2004; Ivanovic, 1996; Ivanovic et al., 1989a, 1996, 2000a,b,c, 2002, 2004a,b,c; Leiva et al., 2001; Matte, Bresnahan, Begg, and Susser, 2001; Pennington et al., 2000; Reiss, Abrams, Singer, Ross, and Denckla, 1996; Rushton, and Ankney, 1996; Sorensen et al., 1999; Stathis, O'Callaghan, Harvey, and Rogers, 1999; Stoch et al., 1982; Toro et al., 1998; Vernon, Wickett, Bazana, and Stelmack, 2000; Willerman, Schultz, Rutledge, and Bigler, 1991). However, other authors found that impaired fetal growth was not associated with poorer cognitive performance in adult life; adaptations made by the fetus in response to conditions that retard growth seem to be largely successful in maintaining brain development (Martyn, Gale, Sayer, and Fall, 1996). Recent findings support that brain growth measured indirectly by head circumference during infancy and early childhood is more important than growth during foetal life in determining cognitive function (Gale, O'Callaghan, Godfrey, Law, and Martyn, 2004).

Paul Broca (1861) and Francis Galton (1888) studied the relationships between head circumference, brain development and intelligence at the XIX century concluding that variations in brain size estimated indirectly by measuring head circumference were related with intelligence; based on these findings, many investigators tried to establish the biological basis of human intelligence (Vernon et al., 2000). Several studies have demonstrated a positive and significant correlation between head circumference, brain size and intelligence concluding that differences in human brain size are relevant in explaining differences in intelligence, although genetic and environmental factors probably affect these interrelationships (Akgun, Okuyan, Baytan, and Topbas, 2003; Botting, et al., 1998; Desch, Anderson, and Snow, 1990; Dolk, 1991; Ivanovic et al., 2000a,b,c, 2002, 2004a,b; Nelson and Deutschberger,1970; Ounsted, Moar, and Scott, 1988; Reiss et al., 1996; Rushton, and Ankney, 1996; Strauss and Dietz, 1998; Vernon et al., 2000; Willerman et al., 1991). In older people, head circumference positively and significantly correlated with intelligence and it seems to be that increased head or brain sizes may protect against intellectual impairment (Schofield, Logroscino, Andrews, Albert, and Stern, 1997; Tisserand, Bosma, Van Boxtel, and Jolles, 2001). However, some studies in monozygotic twins or in sisters, did not find any association between these variables (Schoenemann, Budinger, Sarich, and Wang, 2000; Teasdale and Pakkenberg, 1988; Yeo, Turkheimer, Raz, and Bigler, 1987) although other studies also in monozygotic and dizygotic twins, found a positive correlation between brain size and intelligence (Anderson, 1999; Pennington et al., 2000; Posthuma et al., 2003). Therefore, genetic and environmental factors could affect brain development, intelligence, head circumference and prenatal and postnatal nutritional status and scholastic achievement (Baker, Treloar, Reynolds, Heath, and Martin, 1996; Casto, DeFries, and Fulker, 1995; Luke, Keith, and Keith, 1997; McGue and Bouchard, 1998; Strauss and Dietz, 1998; Weaver and Christian, 1980). The first year of life is the most important period during brain development and whatever happens at that time will produce indelible repercussions later in life (Huttenlocher, and Dabholkar, 1997). The association between a small head circumference and impaired visuo-motor function may be the most reliable indicator of a cognitive disadvantage after undernutrition during infancy (Ivanovic et al., 2000a,b, 2002; Stoch et al., 1982).

The objective of this study was to investigate the impact of neuropsychological parameters in a multicausal context, on the AAT achievement of Chilean high school graduates in 1996 with high or low intellectual quotient and socio-economic status and on job status carried out six years later during 2002. The aim was to confirm our hypothesis that: 1) Independently of socio-economic status, AAT achievement is positively and significantly associated with child's intellectual quotient, parent's intellectual quotient, and brain size and with those indicators of past nutrition especially head circumference and 2) AAT achievement is the better predictor of later job status.

SUBJECTS AND METHODS

Subjects and Sample

This study represents an explicatively, non-experimental, cross-sectional and longitudinal research. The sample was chosen from 1817 school-age children, the total high school graduate population who attended public, private subsidized and private non-subsidized schools in the richest and poorest counties of the Santiago Metropolitan Region in Chile, according to the UNICEF classification (United Nations International Children's Fund, 1994). The final sample consisted of 96 right-handed high school graduate students (mean age 18.0 ± 0.9 y) who had no history of alcoholism, symptoms of brain damage, epilepsy, or heart disease and in whom physical growth and intellectual development processes were consolidated. IQ (WAIS-R), socio-economic strata (SES) and sex were considered for sample selection. The purpose of the main study was to compare two groups of Chilean high school graduates: Group 1, High IQ ($\geq$ 120 WAIS-R) and Group 2, Low IQ (< 100 WAIS-R). The total IQ of the school-age children from the Group 1 ($125.4a \pm 5.5$; n=47) was significantly higher than those from Group 2 ($91.4b \pm 6.8$; n=49) (t= 26.934 p< 0.0001) for both males and females (Ivanovic et al., 2002). The same proportion of school-age children according to SES (high and low) (1:1) and sexes (1:1) were included in each IQ group. This study represented a comparative investigation dividing the sample in two groups according to the scores obtained in the AAT: high AAT ($\geq$ median (Md) = score 631) and low AAT (< Md). Figure 1 shows the description of the sample that took the AAT at the end of high school (84 students) according to AAT group, SES, IQ and sex. The same proportion of school-age children from high and low SES was found in each AAT group. This study was approved by the Committee on Ethics Studies in Humans of the Institute of Nutrition and Food Technology (INTA). The subject's consent was obtained according to the norms for Human Experimentation, Code of Ethics of the World Medical Association (Declaration of Helsinki) (The World Medical Association 1964).

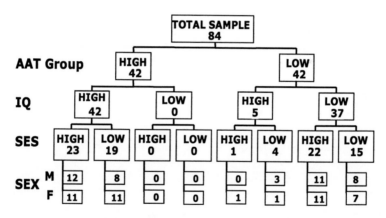

Figure 1. Description of the sample by Academic Aptitude Test (AAT) group, intellectual quotient (IQ), socio-economic strata (SES) and sex (M= males; F= females)

AAT

Results from the AAT score, both its verbal and mathematics parts, were registered for the study sample. The AAT, the baccalaureate examination for university admission with national coverage, has a maximum score of 900 for each part (verbal test with 90 items and mathematics test with 60 items) (Universidad de Chile, 1996). The data corresponding to the AAT were analyzed dividing the sample in the median (score 631) forming two groups: high AAT ($\geq$ Md) and low AAT (< Md). Table 1 describes the AAT scores expressed as mean $\pm$

SD, range and quartiles for both groups. Means of both groups were significantly different (p< 0.0001).

**Table 1. Academic Aptitude Test (AAT) score of
Chilean high school graduates by AAT groups**

AAT Groups	Score (Mean ± SD)	Range	Q1	Q2	Q3
High AAT	733.6 ± 36.9 (42)	637-790	711	737	760
Low AAT	436.8 ± 75.9 (42)	319-626	385	424	467
Student's "t" test	22.804 p< 0.0001				
Total sample	585.2 ± 160.6 (84)	319-790	424	631	737

Note. High AAT, score ≥ median (Md, = score 631); low AAT, score < Md.

Intellectual Quotient (IQ)

In this study, IQ (total, verbal and non-verbal) was assessed by means of the Wechsler Intelligence Scale for Adults-Revised (WAIS-R) adapted for Chilean population both school-age children and their parents and was carried out at the school (Wechsler, 1981; Hermosilla, 1986). WAIS-R consists of a set of six verbal and five non-verbal subtests that are individually administered requiring about 1.5 hours, and yields an age-corrected estimate of IQ. To avoid examiner bias, the WAIS-R was administered separately to each child and parent in quiet rooms by a team of educational psychologists specially trained in this type of study. Before each phase of the test, the psychologist provided a clear explanation to each child and parent, in order to clarify the problem to be solved. On the other hand, the intellectual ability (IA) was also assessed in both school-age children and their parents through the Raven Progressive Matrices Test (Raven, 1957; Ivanovic et al., 2000d, 2001) with the purpose of validating the reliability of intelligence measurement. Human intelligence exceeds all that is measured by an IQ test score, but most studies have defined "intelligence" operationally as performance on IQ or similar tests.

SES, Socio-Cultural and Family Related Variables

SES was measured applying the Graffar scale adapted for Chilean urban an rural populations which considers items such as schooling, job held by the head of the household and characteristics of the house (building materials, property status, water supply, sewerage and ownership of durable goods) (Alvarez, Muzzo, and Ivanovic, 1985). This scale allows to classify populations into six socio-economic strata: 1= High; 2= Medium-High; 3= Medium; 4= Medium-Low; 5= Low and 6= Extreme Poverty. In the present study, only High (1+2) and Low (4+5+6) SES were considered. Family variables such as the number of members and of siblings, place among siblings, crowding and promiscuity were registered. The exposure to mass media (MME), radio, cinema, TV, newspapers, magazines and books (other than school books) of the children was assessed by means of a standardized questionnaire based on open and closed questions (Ivanovic and Sepúlveda, 1988).

Scholastic Achievement (SA)

SA was evaluated through the standard Spanish language (LA) and mathematics (MA) tests. Content validity was based on the fact that, for each grade, the test was designed taking into consideration the objectives pursued by the curricular programs of the Ministry of Education (Chile. Ministerio de Educación Pública, 1996). The number of items tested were 51 for LA and 65 for MA. A pilot test was carried out in 160 school-age children during which reliability was determined applying the Spearman-Brown correlation, scores being 0.92 and 0.97 for LA and MA, respectively, when comparing paired and unpaired item (Guilford and Fruchter, 1984). Item-test consistency of each item was measured by Pearson correlation, scoring values above 0.30 in all of them (Guilford, and Fruchter, 1984). Results were expressed as percentage of achievement in overall results (SA) (mean LA + MA) as well as LA and MA.

Anthropometric Measurements

Weight (W), height (H), head circumference (HC), arm circumference (AC) and triceps skinfold (TS) were measured by the authors on both the students and their parents through standardized procedures (Gibson, 1990). Body mass index (BMI) was calculated according to Garrow, 1981. Head circumference (HC) was compared with Ivanovic, Nellhaus, Roche et al., and the tables of Tanner (Ivanovic, Olivares, Castro, and Ivanovic, 1995a; Nellhaus, 1968; Roche, Mukherjee, Guo, and Moore, 1987; Tanner, 1984) and was expressed as Z-score (Z-HC). Z-HC values are similar when applying these tables because the correlation coefficient between these patterns was 0.98 (Ivanovic et al., 1995a). HC absolute values were adjusted by body height. Percentages of adequacy to the median of arm circumference-for-age (% AC/A), triceps skinfold-for-age (% TS/A), arm muscle area-for-age (% AMA/A) and arm fat area-for-age (%AFA/A) were calculated using data from Frisancho 1981. Birth weight was used as index of prenatal nutrition, Z-HC and % AMA/A, as indicators of postnatal nutrition and BMI was used as index of current nutritional status. Nutritional diseases, especially undernutrition at an early age, were registered.

Brain Development Study

Brain development was evaluated at the German Clinic of Santiago by magnetic resonance imaging (MRI). Using the lowest margin of the cerebellum in a midsagittal view to align the first axial (horizontal) MRI slice, 18 mixed-weighted images (spin-echo pulse sequence with a TR of 2000 msec and a TE of 30 msec) were obtained from a Signa MRI General Electric unit with a field strength of 1.5 Tesla. All images were 5 mm thick and separated by 2.5 mm. Each image was 256 x 256 pixels with 256 levels of gray. The MRI tape was read into a VAS computed and the image analyzed after removing identifying information. Analyses were carried out by a trained specialist without foreknowledge of IQ or sex. For each slice, a Roberts gradient traced the boundary of the scalp by outlining large-intensity differences between adjacent pixels. All gray scale intensity values of < 96 within this boundary were converted to zero. This deleted the skull, most of the meninges, and the interhemispheric fissure; other brain membranes were deleted manually with a cursor. The computer then counted all pixels with nonzero gray scale values for brain size in each slice, and their added value serving as the index for overall brain size. Cortex thickness data, brain volume (BV), absolute and adjusted for body size (weight and height), biparietal (BD) and anteroposterior (APD) diameters are reported; corpus callosum length (CC) absolute and adjusted for brain volume (CC/BV), the thickness of the genu (CCGT), body (CCBT) and splenium (CCST), absolute and adjusted for CC (Matano, and Nakano, 1998), the presence of neuronal migration disorders, qualitative and quantitative evaluation of white matter, cortical and basal subarachnoid space and ventricular system size. Currently, there is no meaningful basis for the comparison of brain sizes within and between racial groups and sexes; the control for body size across racial groups (and sexes) is rendered difficult because bodies do not just differ only in height and weight (Peters et al., 1998). As there were practically no significant differences between absolute and adjusted values for brain parameters, only absolute values are shown in this study (Ivanovic et al., 2004a).

Job Status 2002

Student's job status 2002 was determined after six years of high school graduation and was expressed as jobless, workers without further schooling, students at technical institutes, students at universities. The procedures put in place to locate students were to send a letter to student's home, phone calls, to consult public records such as phone books and the Chilean university's registrations.

Statistical Analysis

Data were analyzed using the Statistical Analysis System (SAS) package by means of variance tests (PROC ANOVA), Scheffe's test for comparison of means, correlation, (PROC CORR) and logistic regression (PROC LOGISTIC) with the option Stepwise was used to establish the most important independent variables that affect the AAT score, dependent variable, categorized as high AAT and low AAT groups (probability modeled was high AAT=yes) and that affect job status six years later from high school graduation (probability modeled was university studies=yes). Chi-square test (X^2) and Fisher's test (PROC FREQ) were used to determine significant differences between the categorical variables (Guilford and Fruchter, 1984; SAS, 1990).

RESULTS

Table 2 shows the IQ of Chilean high school graduates and their parents by AAT groups. School-age children from the high AAT group exhibited total, verbal and non-verbal IQ significantly higher than their peers from the low AAT group ($p< 0.0001$). Total ($p< 0.01$), verbal ($p< 0.001$) and non-verbal ($p< 0.01$) paternal IQ were significantly higher in the high

AAT group compared with the low AAT group; however, differences between both groups were more significant for maternal IQ (p< 0.0001). All school-age children from the high AAT group had high IQ and in the low AAT group, 88% had low IQ (Figure 1).

Table 2. Intellectual quotient (IQ) of Chilean high school graduates and their parents by Academic Aptitude Test (AAT) groups

IQ	High AAT (42)	Low AAT (42)	Student's "t" test
Student IQ			
Total	125.6 ± 5.5	96.7 ± 11.7	14.479 ****
Verbal	125.9 ± 5.5	95.9 ± 12.2	14.609 ****
Non-verbal	121.8 ± 9.0	98.2 ± 11.6	10.414 ****
Paternal IQ			
Total	112.8 ± 12.3	99.4 ± 16.7	3.300 **
Verbal	114.7 ± 11.8	100.5 ± 17.8	3.573 ***
Non-verbal	108.7 ± 13.3	98.0 ± 14.9	2.782 **
Maternal IQ			
Total	112.3 ± 11.4	90.6 ± 14.6	7.290 ****
Verbal	113.1 ± 12.0	92.1 ± 14.6	6.786 ****
Non-verbal	107.5 ± 10.3	89.8 ± 14.4	6.014 ****

Note. Results are expressed as mean ± SD. The number of cases is indicated between parentheses.
** p< 0.01; *** p< 0.001; **** p< 0.0001

The educational variables by AAT groups are shown in Table 3. Students who obtained high AAT scores registered at the end of high school total SA, LA and MA significantly higher than the low AAT group (p< 0.0001). On the other hand, the number of repeated years was significantly higher in the low AAT group than their peers of the high AAT group (p< 0.0001). The time devoted to schoolwork at home did not differ between both groups.

Table 3. Educational variables of Chilean high school graduates by Academic Aptitude Test (AAT) groups

Educational variables	High AAT (42)	Low AAT (42)	Student's "t" Test
Scholastic achievement (SA) (percentage of achievement)			
Total SA (mean LA + MA)	78.0 ± 10.4	33.1 ± 18.0	12.852 ****
Language SA (LA)	75.6 ± 16.5	43.7 ± 17.6	7.981 ****
Mathematics SA (MA)	79.6 ± 11.6	24.1 ± 20.6	13.680 ****
Schoolwork at home (minutes/day)	123.4 ± 105.5	97.6 ± 74.8	1.288 NS
Repeated years (number)	0.02 ± 0.16	0.52 ± 0.71	4.420 ****

Note. Results are expressed as mean ± SD. The number of cases is indicated between parentheses.
**** p< 0.0001; NS = not significantly different.

The analysis of the brain development parameters by sex and AAT groups (Table 4) revealed that males with the high AAT scores exhibited BV (p< 0.01), APD (p< 0.05) and

CCST (p< 0.05) values significantly higher than those from the low AAT group and for CC length a tendency was observed. Females from the high AAT group presented BV, BD, APD and CC length values higher than their peers from the low AAT group but these differences were not significant.

Table 4. Brain development parameters of Chilean high school graduates by sex and Academic Aptitude Test (AAT) groups

Brain Development Parameters	Males (42)		Student's "t" Test	Females (42)		Student's "t" Test
	High AAT (20)	Low AAT (22)		High AAT (22)	Low AAT (20)	
BV (cm³)	1543.3 ± 85.2	1461.3 ± 102.6	2.827**	1421.0 ± 96.4	1392.7 ± 69.3	1.100 NS
BD (mm)	132.0 ± 5.6	133.3 ± 7.8	0.633 NS	129.7 ± 6.3	129.5 ± 6.6	0.139 NS
APD (mm)	167.4 ± 5.2	163.4 ± 6.4	2.245*	163.1 ± 6.6	161.1 ± 4.3	1.224 NS
CC						
CC Length (mm)	72.9 ± 4.1	70.6 ± 4.6	1.716 (t)	71.4 ± 5.8	70.4 ± 3.7	0.682 NS
CCGT (mm)	11.6 ± 1.7	11.3 ± 1.8	0.605 NS	10.5 ± 1.5	11.3 ± 1.6	1.669 NS
CCBT (mm)	6.5 ± 0.8	6.0 ± 0.8	1.569 NS	6.3 ± 0.7	6.7 ± 0.8	1.398 NS
CCST (mm)	12.0 ± 1.6	10.9 ± 1.5	2.180*	11.0 ± 1.7	11.7 ± 1.7	1.437 NS

Note. Results are expressed as mean ± SD. The number of cases is indicated between parentheses; BV= brain volume; BD= biparietal diameter; APD= anteroposterior diameter; CC= corpus callosum; CCGT= genu thickness; CCBT= body thickness; CCST= splenium thickness. * p< 0.05; ** p< 0.01; t = tendency (p> 0.05 y < 0.10); NS= not significantly different.

Table 5 illustrates the relationships between nutritional status by sex and AAT groups. As regards to prenatal nutritional parameters, birth weight and birth height values were higher in school-age children from the high AAT group both males and females, although these differences were not significant. Z-HC indicator of postnatal nutritional background and brain development was significantly higher in school-age children from the high AAT group compared with their peers from the low AAT group (p< 0.01) (Figure 2). Table 5 shows that Z-HC values were significantly higher in males from the high AAT group compared with those from the low AAT group (p< 0.01) and in females a tendency was observed. Current nutritional status and body composition parameters did no register significant differences between both groups. Figure 3 indicates the AAT score in students with and without undernutrition in the first year of life. All undernourished children and 44.7% of the non-undernourished group achieved low AAT score (Fisher= 0.00541).

The socio–economic conditions by AAT groups are shown in Table 6. No significant differences were found in the socio-economic composition of both groups, as explained in the description of the sample (Figure 1). However, maternal schooling (p< 0.01), household head occupation (p< 0.05) and the quality of housing (p< 0.02) were significantly better in the high AAT group compared with their peers with low AAT scores; both groups had access to sewerage and drinking water at home. Table 7 illustrates the socio-economic, socio-cultural, MME and demographic variables expressed as mean ± SD by AAT groups. Maternal schooling was the only socio-economic and socio-cultural variable that was significantly higher in the high AAT group compared with the low AAT group (p< 0.001). Family variables did not differ significantly between both groups. School-age children from the low AAT group had higher levels of exposure to radio, cinema and television, but radio was the only MME that presented significant differences between both groups (p< 0.05). In the high AAT group, 83% read newspapers weekly, a percentage that decreased significantly to 43% in the low AAT group (X_o^2= 23.094; 4df; p< 0.001). Books exposure were significantly different since 74% and 45% of the students belonging to the high and low AAT groups, respectively, read books (X_o^2= 7.115; 1df; p< 0.01). A high percentage of students (79.8%) read magazines without significant differences by AAT groups (X_o^2= 0.664; 1df; NS). As regards to age, students from the low AAT group were significantly older than their peers with high AAT score (p< 0.001).

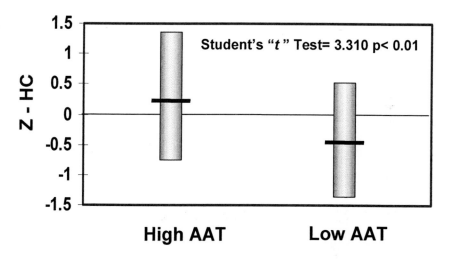

Figure 2. Head circumference-for-age Z score (Z-HC) by Academic Aptitude Test (AAT) groups of Chilean high school graduates in 1996.

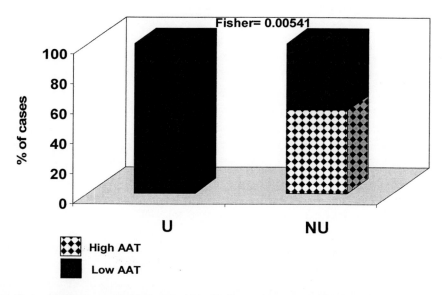

Figure 3. Academic Aptitude Test (AAT) score of Chilean high school graduates with undernutrition (U) and without severe undernutrition (NU) in the first year of life.

Table 5. Nutritional status of Chilean high school graduates by sex and Academic Aptitude Test (AAT) groups

Nutritional status parameters	Males (42)		Student's "t" Test	Females (42)		Student's "t" Test
	High AAT (20)	Low AAT (22)		High AAT (22)	Low AAT (20)	
Prenatal Nutritional Background						
Birth weight (g)	3,341.8 ± 585.9	3,083.6 ± 537.7	1.483 NS	3,127.3 ± 625.2	3,059.0 ±475.3	0.401 NS
Birth height (cm)	50.6 ± 2.6	49.2 ± 2.6	1.771 (t)	48.8 ± 2.5	48.9 ± 3.5	0.050 NS
Postnatal Nutritional Background						
Z-HC	0.56 ± 1.10	-0.38 ± 1.02	2.885 **	0.02 ± 0.88	-0.48 ± 0.85	1.846 (t)
Current Nutritional Status						
BMI	22.4 ± 2.0	22.5 ± 2.6	0.183 NS	21.6 ± 2.6	22.5 ± 2.9	1.008 NS
% W/H	104.6 ± 9.2	106.2 ± 12.8	0.449 NS	101.7 ± 12.7	104.3 ± 14.4	0.610 NS
Body Composition						
% AC/A	95.4 ± 8.2	93.6 ± 11.9	0.568 NS	95.9 ± 9.7	99.0 ± 9.3	1.046 NS
% TS/A	128.5 ± 65.8	124.8 ± 49.0	0.207 NS	97.3 ± 35.5	99.0 ± 29.6	0.174 NS
% AMA/A	87.3 ± 15.0	84.7 ± 18.0	0.516 NS	91.7 ± 18.5	99.0 ± 17.8	1.301 NS
% AFA/A	121.2 ± 63.0	119.8 ± 59.0	0.074 NS	97.5 ± 40.1	100.1 ± 33.3	0.230 NS

Note. Results are expressed as mean ± SD. The number of cases is indicated between parentheses. Z-HC = head circumference-for-age Z score; BMI= body mass index; AC/A= arm circumference-for-age; TS/A= triceps skinfold-for-age; AMA/A= arm muscle area-for-age; AFA/A= arm fat area-for-age. ** $p < 0.01$; (t) = tendency ($p > 0.05$ y < 0.10); NS= not significantly different.

Pearson correlation coefficients between AAT score and demographic, intellectual, educational, nutritional, brain development, socio-economic, socio-cultural, family and MME variables in the total sample and by sex are shown in Table 8. The high correlations observed in the total sample and in both sexes between AAT score with SA, student IQ, student IA, maternal IQ, number of repeated years, paternal IQ, maternal schooling, Z-HC and student age should be noted. In the students like in their parents, a high correlation was found between IQ and IA ($r = 0.911$ $p < 0.0001$).

The logistic regression analysis between the AAT score, dependent variable, categorized it as high AAT and low AAT (probability modeled was high AAT=yes) and most relevant parameters considering student IQ, maternal and paternal IQ, Z-HC, BV and undernutrition in the first year of life as independent variables and controlling by SES and sex, is summarized in Table 9. Only student IQ entered in the statistical model and was the best predictor of AAT achievement. The odds ratio value (1.252) implies that when the IQ score increases by one point, the probability to obtain a high AAT score increases in 25.2%.

In 2002, six years after high school graduation, 94 of these children high school graduates were located and they informed about their present job status. It found that 11.7% was jobless, 13.8% were workers without further schooling, 17% had studied at technical institutes and 57.5% had studied in universities. Table 10 describes the school-age children and parents IQ by job status 2002. Students attending universities exhibited the highest total, verbal and non-verbal IQs compared with their peers on other job categories ($p < 0.0001$). As regards parental IQ, fathers of students attending institutes or universities had the highest total ($p < 0.001$), verbal ($p < 0.001$) and non-verbal ($p < 0.05$) IQs compared with those of jobless students and with those who were workers without further schooling. However, total, verbal and non-verbal IQs of mothers of students attending universities were significantly higher than those of the other groups (p< 0.0001).

Table 6. Socio–economic conditions of Chilean high school graduates by Academic Aptitude Test (AAT) groups

Variables	High AAT (42)	Low AAT (42)	Total sample (84)	X^2 o Fisher
	% of cases			
Socio-economic status				
High	54.8	54.8	54.8	$X_o^2(1) = 0.000 <$
Low	45.2	45.2	45.2	$X_t^2(1)\ 0.05 = 3.841$
Total	100.0	100.0	100.0	
House-hold head				
Father	95.2	85.7	90.5	
Mother	2.4	14.3	8.3	Fisher = p< 0.265.
Other person	2.4	0.0	1.2	Fisher's test was
Total	100.0	100.0	100.0	calculated considering the categories father and mother + other person.
House-hold head schooling				
Illiterate	0.0	0.0	0.0	$X_o^2(1) = 0.100 <$
Incomplete elementary school	4.9	16.7	10.9	$X_t^2(1)\ 0.05 = 3.841$ Chi -square test was
Complete elementary school + Incomplete high school	39.0	23.8	31.3	calculated joined the categories (illiterate + incomplete elementary
Complete high school	4.9	14.3	9.6	school+ complete
Incomplete university education	2.4	11.9	7.2	elementary school + incomplete high
Complete university education	48.8	33.3	41.0	school) and (complete high school
Total	100.0	100.0	100.0	+incomplete university education + complete university education).
Maternal schooling				
Illiterate	0.0	0.0	0.0	
Incomplete elementary school	0.0	14.3	7.2	$X_o^2(2) = 10.600 >$ $X_t^2(2)\ 0.01 = 9.210$
Complete elementary school + Incomplete high school	16.7	28.6	22.6	Chi -square test was calculated joined the categories (illiterate +
Complete high school	45.2	45.2	45.2	incomplete elementary
Incomplete university education	4.8	0.0	2.4	school+ complete elementary school +
Complete university education	33.3	11.9	22.6	Incomplete high school) and
Total	100.0	100.0	100.0	(incomplete university education + complete university education).

Table 6. Continued

Variables	High AAT (42)	Low AAT (42)	Total sample (84)	X^2 o Fisher
House-hold head occupation				
1. Managerial positions	41.5	21.4	31.3	$X_o^2(2) = 6.710 >$
2. Mid-level employee	9.8	31.0	20.5	$X_t^2(2)\ 0.05 = 5.991$
3. Specialized worker	2.4	2.4	2.4	Chi-square test was
4. Non-specialized worker	46.3	33.3	39.8	calculated joined the
5. Jobless receiving state aid	0.0	7.2	3.6	categories (2+3) and (4+5+6).
6. Jobless without state aid	0.0	4.7	2.4	
Total	100.0	100.0	100.0	
Maternal occupation				
1. Managerial positions	7.1	4.8	6.0	
2. Mid-level employee	11.9	7.1	9.5	$X_o^2(3) = 1.500 <$
3. Specialized worker	11.9	14.2	13.1	$X_t^2(3)\ 0.05 = 7.815$
4. Non-specialized worker	11.9	19.1	15.4	Chi-square test was
5. Jobless receiving state aid	0.0	0.0	0.0	calculated joined the
6. Jobless without state aid	0.0	0.0	0.0	categories (1+2).
7. Housekeepers	57.2	54.8	56.0	
Total	100.0	100.0	100.0	
Quality of housing				
Single family unit	45.2	21.4	33.3	
Solid materials	7.2	28.6	17.9	$X_o^2(2) = 9.000 > X_t^2(2)\ 0.02 = 7.824$. Chi-
Light materials	9.5	11.9	10.7	square test was
Self-built	38.1	35.7	36.9	calculated joined the
Precarious housing ("Mejora")	0.0	2.4	1.2	categories light materials + self-built +
Total	100.0	100.0	100.0	precarious housing ("Mejora").
Property of housing				
Owner	95.2	81.0	88.1	Fisher = $p < 0.088$.
Tenant	4.8	11.9	8.3	Fisher's test was
Usufructuary	0.0	7.1	3.6	calculated joined the
Total	100.0	100.0	100.0	categories (tenant + usufructuary).

The educational variables of 1996 analyzed by job status 2002 are shown in Table 11. Students at universities presented AAT score, SA, LA and MA significantly higher ($p < 0.0001$) and their numbers of repeated years were significantly lower ($p < 0.0001$) compared with the other groups. Time devoted to schoolwork at home did not differ by job status 2002.

Table 12 summarizes the brain development parameters in 1996 as related to job status 2002. In males, jobless students registered BV ($p < 0.001$), APD ($p < 0.05$), HC ($p < 0.01$) and Z-HC ($p < 0.01$) values significantly lower than their peers from the other groups; workers without further schooling presented CCGT significantly lower than the other groups ($p < 0.05$). Among females, students at universities showed HC ($p < 0.05$) and Z-HC ($p < 0.01$) values significantly higher than the other groups; workers without further schooling presented BD values ($p < 0.05$) significantly higher than the other job status groups. Males students attending universities had a BV 179.5 cm^3 greater than the jobless group, while among the females this difference was 109 cm^3, although in these, differences were not significant. Jobless's HC was 2.1cm and 1.8 cm lower than the students at universities group in males and females, respectively.

Table 7. Socio-economic, socio-cultural, family, mass media exposure (MME) and demographic of variables of Chilean high school graduates by Academic Aptitude Test (AAT) groups

Variables	High AAT (42)	Low AAT (42)	Student's "t" Test
Socio-economic and Socio-cultural			
SES (Graffar's score)	6.7 ± 3.5	7.5 ± 3.2	1.187 NS
Paternal Schooling (y)	12.5 ± 3.1	11.5 ± 3.7	1.356 NS
Maternal Schooling (y)	12.8 ± 1.9	10.7 ± 2.8	3.958 ***
Household head's Schooling (y)	12.4 ± 3.1	11.6 ± 3.7	1.120 NS
Family			
Number of Family Members	5.7 ± 2.5	5.0 ± 1.4	1.459 NS
Number of Siblings	3.2 ± 1.5	3.0 ± 1.1	0.840 NS
Place Between Siblings	2.2 ± 1.2	2.0 ± 1.1	0.794 NS
Promiscuity (number of persons per bed)	1.1 ± 0.2	1.2 ± 0.3	1.775(t)
Crowding (number of persons by bedroom)	1.5 ± 0.8	1.5 ± 0.5	0.294 NS
MME			
Radio (minutes per day)	109.9 ± 158.7	170.1 ± 107.4	2.029 *
Cinema (times per month)	1.1 ± 1.5	1.7 ± 2.6	1.419 NS
Television (minutes per day)	138.4 ± 164.9	160.7 ± 96.7	0.755 NS
Demographic			
Age (y)	17.1 ± 0.4	17.7 ± 1.0	3.436 ***

Note. Results are expressed as mean ± SD. The number of cases is indicated between parentheses. SES= socio-economic strata. * $p < 0.05$; *** $p < 0.001$; t = tendency ($p > 0.05$ y < 0.10); NS= Not significantly different.

Table 8. Pearson correlation coefficients between Academic Aptitude Test (AAT) score and demographic, intellectual, educational, nutritional, brain development, socio-economic, socio-cultural, family and mass media exposure variables by sex

Variables	AAT		
	Total Sample (84)	Males (42)	Females (42)
Demographic			
Student age	-0.422 ****	-0.401 **	-0.471 **
Paternal age	0.023 NS	0.130 NS	0.185 NS
Maternal age	0.210 (t)	-0.058 NS	0.309 (t)
Intellectual			
Student IA	0.885 ****	0.848 ****	0.922 ****
Student total IQ	0.923 ****	0.923 ****	0.928 ****
Student verbal IQ	0.921 ****	0.934 ****	0.911 ****
Student non verbal IQ	0.830 ****	0.845 ****	0.818 ****
Total paternal IQ	0.478 ***	0.594 ***	0.248 NS

Table 8. Continued

Variables	AAT		
	Total Sample (84)	Males (42)	Females (42)
Verbal paternal IQ	0.481 ***	0.606 ***	0.229 NS
Non verbal paternal IQ	0.423 **	0.519 **	0.259 NS
Total maternal IQ	0.683 ****	0.702 ****	0.667 ****
Verbal maternal IQ	0.677 ****	0.718 ****	0.647 ****
Non verbal maternal IQ	0.599 ****	0.626 ****	0.564 ****
Educational			
Total SA (mean LA+MA)	0.925 ****	0.953 ****	0.894 ****
Spanish SA (LA)	0.804 ****	0.905 ****	0.691 ****
Mathematics SA (MA)	0.910 ****	0.930 ****	0.887 ****
Verbal AAT	0.976 ****	0.979 ****	0.974 ****
Mathematics AAT	0.977 ****	0.980 ****	0.975 ****
Repeated years	-0.511 ****	-0.430 **	-0.594 ****
Schoolwork at home	0.120 NS	0.022 NS	0.201 NS
Nutritional			
Birth weight	0.189 (t)	0.312 *	0.060 NS
Birth height	0.228 (t)	0.362 *	0.064 NS
Breastfeeding	0.207 (t)	0.142 NS	0.279 (t)
Z-HC	0.434 ****	0.475 **	0.393 **
BMI (P/T^2)	-0.060 NS	0.025 NS	-0.135 NS
% AC/A	-0.012 NS	0.143 NS	-0.177 NS
% TSA/A	0.011 NS	0.068 NS	-0.099 NS
% AMA/A	-0.022 NS	0.128 NS	-0.153 NS
% AFA/A	0.004 NS	0.057 NS	-0.091 NS
Brain development			
Brain volume	-	0.449 **	0.237 NS
Biparietal diameter	-	-0.112 NS	-0.031 NS
Anteroposterior diameter	-	0.415 **	0.314 *
Corpus callosum length	-	0.252 NS	0.198 NS
Genu thickness	-	0.103 NS	-0.104 NS
Body thickness	-	0.175 NS	-0.084 NS
Splenium thickness	-	0.228 NS	-0.076 NS
Socio-economic, socio-cultural and family			
SES (Graffar's score)	0.176 NS	0.334 *	-0.021 NS
Paternal Schooling	0.193 (t)	0.156 NS	0.235 NS
Maternal Schooling	0.435 ****	0.374 *	0.503 ***
Household head's Schooling	0.151 NS	0.150 NS	0.155 NS
Promiscuity	-0.289 **	-0.293 (t)	-0.287 (t)
Crowding	-0.098 NS	-0.348 *	0.022 NS
Number of Family Members	0.137 NS	0.044 NS	0.219 NS
Number of Siblings	0.056 NS	-0.029 NS	0.136 NS
Place Between Siblings	0.114 NS	0.128 NS	0.104 NS
Mass media exposure variables			
Radio	-0.199 (t)	-0.309 *	-0.133 NS
Cinema	-0.038 NS	0.068 NS	-0.121 NS
Television	-0.073 NS	-0.078 NS	-0.106 NS

Note. The number of cases is indicated between parentheses. IA= intellectual ability; IQ= intellectual quotient; SA= scholastic achievement; Z-HC = head circumference-for-age Z score; BMI= body mass index; AC/A= arm circumference-for-age; TS/A= triceps skinfold-for-age; AMA/A= arm muscle area-for-age; AFA/A= arm fat area-for-age; SES= socio-economic strata.

* p< 0.05; ** p< 0.01; *** p< 0.001; **** p< 0.0001; (t) = tendency (p> 0.05 y < 0.10) ; NS= not significantly different

Table 9. Logistic regression between Academic Aptitude Test (AAT) the university graduation (dependent variable), and most relevant parameters (independent variables=SES, sex, student IQ, maternal IQ, undernutrition in the first year of life, Z-HC and BV).

Parameters entered in the statistical model	DF	Parameter Estimate	Standard Error	Wald Chi-square	Standardized Estimate	Odds Ratio Estimates
INTERCEPT	1	-25.7704	7.2157	12.7552 ***	-	-
IQ	1	0.2247	0.0601	13.9843 ***	2.149866	1.252

Note: Probability modeled was High AAT (AAT ≥ Md) = yes. DF= degree of freedom; SES= socio-economic strata; IQ= intellectual quotient; Z-HC = head circumference-for-age Z score; BV= brain volume. n= 84; *** p< 0.001

Table 10. Intellectual quotient (IQ) of Chilean high school graduates in 1996 and their parents by job status 2002

IQ	Job status 2002				
	Jobless (11)	Workers without further schooling (13)	Students at technical institutes (16)	Students at universities (54)	F
Student IQ					
Total	86.5a ± 8.6	88.5a ± 5.7	94.4a ± 4.8	121.1b ± 11.6	77.33****
Verbal	85.5a ± 8.5	87.5a ± 6.9	93.8a ± 5.4	121.2b ± 11.9	77.35****
Non-Verbal	90.0a ± 9.3	91.8a ± 7.6	96.1a ± 7.4	118.3.1b ± 12.1	44.43****
Paternal IQ					
Total	95.3ab ± 22.0	88.6a ± 11.8	106.4ab ± 18.7	110.4b ± 13.2	6.40***
Verbal	94.6a ± 23.7	89.1a ± 12.6	106.8ab ± 20.0	112.5b ± 12.9	7.31***
Non-Verbal	96.1ab ± 19.3	89.3a ± 9.9	104.6ab ± 16.1	106.5b ± 13.8	4.10*
Maternal IQ					
Total	84.9a ± 16.1	79.1a ± 9.4	87.8a ± 13.2	108.5b ± 13.8	23.74****
Verbal	87.6a ± 14.4	79.7a ± 10.3	89.6a ± 12.9	109.5b ± 13.9	22.81****
Non-Verbal	84.5a ± 17.5	81.0a ± 9.9	87.4a ± 13.8	104.0b ± 13.0	15.05****

Note. Results are expressed as mean ± SD. The number of cases is indicated between parentheses. Means with the same letter are not significantly different at the 0.05 level based on Scheffe's test. F= ANOVA; * p< 0.05; *** p< 0.001; **** p< 0.0001

Figure 4 indicates that undernutrition in the first year of life had been significantly more prevalent among the jobless (54.6%) and in workers without further schooling students (61.5%) than among students attending institutes (12.5%) or universities (0%) (p< 0.00001).

**Table 11. Educational variables of Chilean high school graduates
in 1996 by job status 2002**

Educational variables	Job status 2002				F
	Jobless (11)	Workers without further schooling (13)	Students at technical institutes (16)	Students at universities (54)	
AAT (score)					
Total AAT(mean V+M)	397.8a ± 42.3	372.4a ± 45.0	428.0a ± 57.9	680.5b ± 108.8	53.32****
Verbal AAT (V)	388.0a ± 74.0	358.0a ± 56.2	424.7a ± 63.0	659.1b ± 120.9	38.38****
Mathematics AAT (M)	407.6a ± 21.2	386.9a ± 42.7	431.2a ± 74.2	702.0b ± 108.4	57.30****
Scholastic achievement (SA) (percentage of achievement)					
Total SA (mean LA+ MA)	23.6a ± 9.8	24.4a ± 5.2	24.4a ± 12.9	69.2b ± 19.8	53.15****
Language SA (LA)	28.5a ± 12.9	31.7a ± 8.4	40.6a ± 13.6	70.2b ± 19.6	32.79****
Mathematics SA (MA)	18.6a ± 10.9	19.5a ± 9.3	13.4a ± 14.5	69.1b ± 24.4	46.76****
Schoolwork at home (minutes/day)	91.4 ± 54.7	76.9 ± 43.7	97.2 ± 86.3	119.1 ± 101.0	1.03 NS
Repeated years(number)	0.90a ± 0.83	0.85a ± 0.55	0.56a ± 0.72	0.11b ± 0.37	11.99****

Note. Results are expressed as mean ± SD. The number of cases is indicated between parentheses. Means with the same letter are not significantly different at the 0.05 level based on Scheffe's test. F= ANOVA. AAT= Academic Aptitude Test; SA= scholastic achievement; **** $p < 0.0001$; NS= not significantly different.

The nutritional status 1996 and 2002 by job status 2002 is shown in Table 13. Prenatal nutritional indicators such as birth weight ($p < 0.05$) and birth height ($p < 0.001$) were significantly higher in the students attending universities and institutes compared with their peers with the other types of job status groups. As regards to postnatal nutritional parameters, in both sexes, jobless students exhibited significantly lower HC values compared with students attending universities and institutes both in 1996 and in 2002. Figure 5 shows that university students had the highest Z-HC values than the other job statuses ($p < 0.0001$). When comparing the nutritional status between both periods (Table 13), students attending technical institutes and especially university students significantly increased their %W/H and BMI values in 2002. The latter group also significantly increased their body composition parameters as %AC/A, %TS/A and %AFA/A ($p < 0.0001$).

Table 14 shows details of the socio–economic conditions of high school graduates as related to job status 2002. SES did not differ between both periods but significant differences were found by job status 2002. As a consequence, students attending technical institutes and especially university students had SES ($p < 0.001$), household head ($p < 0.001$) and maternal schooling ($p < 0.01$), household head ($p < 0.001$) and maternal occupation ($p < 0.01$) and quality of housing ($p < 0.001$) significantly higher than their peers who were workers without further schooling or jobless. Most of students had their father as household head, their parents owned housing and all of these had connections to sewerage and drinking water systems. Socio-economic, socio-cultural, family, MME and demographic variables expressed as mean ± SD by job status 2002 are shown in Table 15. Students attending technical institutes and especially university students had Graffar scores, paternal, maternal and household head schooling scores ($p < 0.0001$), significantly higher than their peers from the other job statuses. University and technical institute students showed significantly lower levels of promiscuity than the other groups ($p < 0.001$) and the former were significantly younger than their peers from the other job statuses ($p < 0.0001$).

Table 12. Brain Development Parameters of Chilean High School Graduates in 1996 by job status 2002

Brain Parameters	Job status 2002				F
	Jobless (11)	Workers without further schooling (13)	Students at technical institutes (16)	Students at universities (54)	
Males	(7)	(5)	(10)	(25)	
CC					
CC (mm)	70.0 ± 5.3	70.4 ± 5.2	70.4 ± 4.7	72.6 ± 4.6	0.90 NS
CCGT (mm)	12.1a ± 1.3	9.6b ± 1.5	10.9a ± 1.1	11.7^a ± 1.8	3.23*
CCBT (mm)	6.3 ± 1.0	5.4 ± 0.9	6.2 ± 1.0	6.3 ± 0.8	1.54 NS
CCST (mm)	11.4 ± 1.6	10.2 ± 1.5	11.3 ± 0.9	11.6 ± 1.7	1.15 NS
BV (cm^3)	1361.0a ± 125.0	1447.0ab ± 129.5	1430.0ab ± 134.4	1540.5b ± 88.5	6.31 ***
BD (mm)	130.1 ± 5.6	134.4 ± 8.6	132.0 ± 7.1	132.9 ± 6.5	0.47 NS
APD (mm)	158.3a ± 5.3	163.8ab ± 6.5	163.2ab ± 7.4	167.1b ± 5.6	4.19 *
HC (cm)	54.3a ± 1.6	54.3ab ± 1.2	55.4ab ± 1.8	56.4b ± 1.4	5.44**
Z-HC	-1.14a ± 1.23	-1.19a ± 0.95	-0.37ab ± 1.39	0.48b ± 1.06	5.66**
Females	(4)	(8)	(6)	(29)	
CC					
CC length (mm)	71.5 ± 2.4	68.6 ± 5.2	69.7 ± 2.5	71.6 ± 5.4	0.86 NS
CCGT (mm)	10.5 ± 1.7	11.6 ± 1.6	10.8 ± 1.8	10.9 ± 1.6	0.60 NS
CCBT (mm)	7.0 ± 0.8	5.9 ± 0.8	6.7 ± 0.8	6.5 ± 0.8	2.22 (t)
CCST(mm)	11.0 ± 1.4	11.0 ± 1.2	11.5 ± 0.8	11.4 ± 1.9	0.20 NS
BV (cm^3)	1309.8 ± 44.2	1383.0 ± 62.9	1374.0 ± 102.6	1418.8 ± 90.7	2.21 NS
BD (mm)	128.8ab ± 4.0	135.8a ± 5.8	126.7ab ± 5.5	128.8b ± 6.2	3.58*
APD (mm)	160.5 ± 4.4	159.6 ± 4.9	159.5 ± 2.7	163.4 ± 6.1	1.66 NS
HC (cm)	53.0a ± 0.9	53.9ab ± 1.0	54.4ab ± 1.2	54.8b ± 1.2	4.03*
Z-HC	-1.41a ± 0.68	-0.75ab ± 0.69	-0.48ab ± 1.22	0.01b ± 0.85	4.19**

Note. Results are expressed as mean ± SD. The number of cases is indicated between parentheses. F= ANOVA; CC= corpus callosum; CCGT= genu thickness; CCBT= body thickness; CCST= splenium thickness; BV= brain volume; BD= biparietal diameter; APD= anteroposterior diameter; HC= head circumference; Z-HC = head circumference-for-age Z score; * $p < 0.05$; ** $p < 0.01$; *** $p < 0.001$; NS= not significantly different; (t) = tendency ($p > 0.05$ y < 0.10).

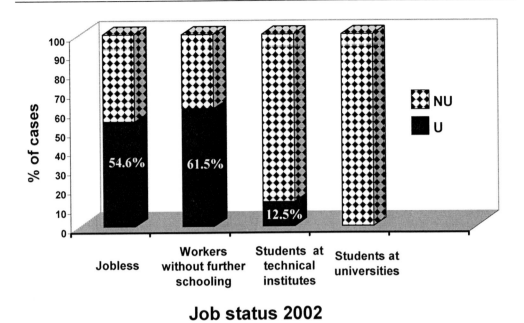

Figure 4. Undernutrition during the first year of life (U) of Chilean high school graduates in 1996 by job status 2002. NU= non-undernourished. Fisher = 0.00001.

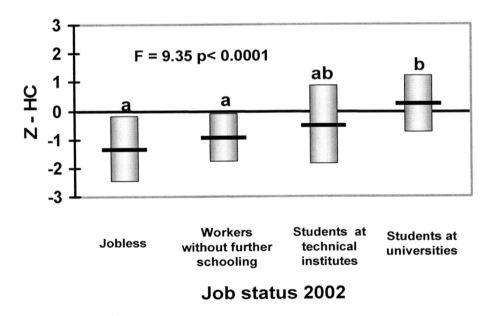

Figure 5. Head circumference-for-age Z score (Z-HC) by job status 2002 of Chilean high school graduates in 1996.

Table 13. Nutritional status 1996 and 2002 by job status 2002

Nutritional status	Job status 2002				F
	Jobless (11)	Workers without further schooling (13)	Students at technical institutes (16)	Students at universities (54)	
PPrenatal Nutritional status					
Birth weight (g)	2817.3a ± 424.7	2835.4a ± 301.3	3084.3ab ± 586.0	3214.5ab ± 594.4	2.80*
Birth height (cm)	46.6a ± 4.3	47.0a ± 3.2	49.8ab ± 1.7	49.8b ± 2.5	5.76***
Current Nutritional status					
% W/H					
1996	104.8 ± 12.4	106.1 ± 20.5	104.4 ± 17.5	104.0 ± 12.0	0.08 NS
2002	109.8 ± 19.7	118.4 ± 14.0	107.7 ± 22.0	111.4 ± 14.2	0.65 NS
Student "t" paired test	1.106 NS	0.965 NS	4.023 **	5.608****	
BMI					
1996	22.3 ± 2.5	23.0 ± 4.4	22.6 ± 3.8	22.1 ± 2.5	0.32 NS
2002	23.4 ± 3.4	24.8 ± 3.4	23.5 ± 4.7	23.8 ± 3.1	0.31 NS
Student "t" paired test	1.265 NS	1.049 NS	4.752 ***	5.810 ****	
PPostnatal Nutritional status					
HC					
Males					
1996	54.3a ± 1.6	54.3ab ± 1.2	55.4 ab ± 1.8	56.4 b ± 1.4	5.44**
2002	54.3a ± 1.7	54.6a ± 0.3	55.8 ab ± 2.2	56.4 b ± 1.5	3.01*
Student "t" paired test	1.000 NS	1.000 NS	2.792 *	1.817 NS	
Females					
1996	53.0a ± 0.9	53.9ab ± 1.0	54.4ab ± 1.2	54.8b ± 1.2	4.03*
2002	53.2a ± 1.0	53.9ab ± 1.2	54.4b ± 1.4	54.9b ± 1.2	3.13*
Student "t" paired test	1.219 NS	1.633 NS	1.000 NS	1.000 NS	
Brachial anthropometry					
%AC/A					
1996	93.8 ± 13.4	99.5 ± 19.7	96.4 ± 13.1	95.9 ± 8.8	0.47 NS
2002	92.6 ± 12.9	98.5 ± 23.4	98.0 ± 11.7	100.4 ± 9.3	1.12 NS
Student "t" paired test	0.697 NS	0.246 NS	2.677 *	4.277 ****	
%TS/A					
1996	115.1 ± 65.9	107.8 ± 51.1	121.0 ± 29.2	109.8 ± 49.6	0.26 NS
2002	110.2 ± 64.6	123.3 ± 49.7	125.3 ± 49.5	132.0 ± 44.6	0.57 NS
Student "t" paired test	0.325 NS	0.666 NS	0.766 NS	5.641****	
%AMA/A					
1996	86.7 ± 19.2	97.5 ± 30.7	89.3 ± 21.7	91.0 ± 16.6	0.65 NS
2002	85.0 ± 27.2	93.8 ± 45.1	92.0 ± 22.6	93.4 ± 13.5	0.41 NS
tudent "t" paired test	0.406 NS	0.382 NS	2.052 (t)	1.128 NS	
%AFA/A					
1996	111.1 ± 75.2	112.4 ± 71.0	117.3 ± 37.7	107.0 ± 49.5	0.16 NS
2002	102.7 ± 61.5	120.9 ± 58.1	123.9 ± 53.1	132.1 ± 50.4	0.87 NS
Student "t" paired test	0.442 NS	0.211 NS	1.242 NS	5.912 ****	

Note. Results are expressed as mean ± SD. The number of cases is indicated between parentheses. Means with the same letter are not significantly different at the 0.05 level based on Scheffe's test. F= ANOVA; W/H= % weight for height; BMI= body mass index; HC= head circumference; AC/A= arm circumference-for-age; TS/A= triceps skinfold-for-age; AMA/A= arm muscle area-for-age; AFA/A= arm fat area-for-age. * p< 0.05; ** p< 0.01; *** p< 0.001; **** p<I 0.0001; (t)= tendency (p> 0.05 y p< 0.10); NS= not significantly different

Table 14. Socio–economic conditions of Chilean high school graduates by job status 2002

Socio–economic variables	Job status 2002					X^2_o or Fisher
	Jobless (11)	Workers without further schooling (13)	Students at technical institutes (16)	Students at universities (54)	Total sample (94)	
	----------------------------- % of cases ----------------------------					
Socio-economic strata						
High	18.2	0	81.2	57.4	48.9	$X^2_o(3) = 24.858 >$
Low	81.8	100.0	18.8	42.6	51.1	$X^2_t(3)\ 0.001 = 16.268$
Total	100.0	100.0	100.0	100.0	100.0	
House-hold head						Fisher = 0.712. Fisher's
Father	90.9	84.6	81.2	92.6	89.4	test was calculated
Mother	0.0	15.4	18.8	7.4	9.6	joined the categories
Other person	9.1	0.0	0.0	0.0	1.1	(jobless + workers
Total	100.0	100.0	100.0	100.0	100.0	without further schooling), (students at institutes + students at universities) and (mother +other person)
House-hold head schooling						$X^2_o(3) = 17.920 > X^2_t(3)$
Illiterate	18.2	0.0	0.0	0.0	2.1	$0.001 = 16.268$. Chi -
Incomplete elementary school	9.0	38.5	6.2	7.4	11.7	square test was calculated joined the
Complete elementary school + Incomplete high school	36.5	53.8	12.5	33.3	33.0	categories (illiterate + incomplete elementary school+ complete
Complete high school	27.3	7.7	6.3	7.4	9.6	elementary school + incomplete high school)
Incomplete university education	9.0	0.0	25.0	3.7	7.4	and (complete high school +incomplete
Complete university education	0.0	0.0	50.0	48.2	36.2	university education + complete university
Total	100.0	100.0	100.0	100.0	100.0	education).
Maternal schooling						$X^2_o(1) = 9.270 > X^2_t(1)$
Incomplete elementary school	27.2	30.8	6.2	1.9	9.6	$0.01 = 6.635$. Chi - square test was
Complete elementary school + Incomplete high school	45.5	65.5	12.5	18.5	26.6	calculated joined the categories (incomplete elementary school
Complete high school	27.3	7.7	62.5	46.3	41.5	+complete elementary school + incomplete
Incomplete university education	0.0	0.0	0.0	3.7	2.1	high school + complete high school),
Complete university education	0.0	0.0	18.8	29.6	20.2	(incomplete university education+ complete
Total	100.0	100.0	100.0	100.0	100.0	university education), (jobless + workers without further schooling) and (students at institutes + universities).

Table 14. Continued

| Socio–economic variables | Job status 2002 | | | | | X^2_o or Fisher |
	Jobless (11)	Workers without further schooling (13)	Students at technical institutes (16)	Students at universities (54)	Total sample (94)	
House-hold head occupation						
1. Managerial positions	9.1	0.0	25.0	37.0	26.6	$X_o^2(3) = 24.860 > X_t^2(3)$ 0.001= 16.268. Chi - square test was calculated joined the categories (1+2+3) and (4+5+6).
2. Mid-level employee	9.1	0.0	56.2	16.7	20.2	
3. Specialized worker	0.0	0.0	0.0	3.7	2.1	
4. Non-specialized worker	45.4	61.5	6.2	42.6	39.4	
5. Jobless receiving state aid	27.3	30.8	6.3	0.0	8.5	
6. Jobless without state aid	9.1	7.7	6.3	0.0	3.2	
Total	100.0	100.0	100.0	100.0	100.0	
Maternal occupation						
1. Managerial positions	0.0	0.0	6.2	7.4	5.3	$X_o^2(1) = 7.190 > X_t^2(1)$ 0.01 = 6.635. Chi - square test was calculated joined the categories (1+2+3) and (4+5+6+7), (jobless + workers without further schooling) and (students at institutes + students at universities).
2. Mid-level employee	0.0	0.0	25.0	7.4	8.5	
3. Specialized worker	9.0	0.0	12.5	13.0	10.6	
4. Non-specialized worker	36.4	46.2	6.3	13.0	19.2	
5. Jobless receiving state aid	0.0	0.0	0.0	0.0	0.0	
6. Jobless without state aid	0.0	0.0	0.0	0.0	0.0	
7. Housekeepers	54.6	53.8	50.0	59.2	56.4	
Total	100.0	100.0	100.0	100.0	100.0	
Quality of housing						
Single family unit	18.2	0.0	18.8	40.7	28.7	$X_o^2(3) = 23.270 > X_t^2(3)$ 0.001 = 16.268. Chi - square test was calculated joined the categories (Single family unit + Solid materials) and (Light materials + Self-built + Precarious housing ("Mejora").
Solid materials	0.0	0.0	62.5	11.1	17.0	
Light materials	0.0	7.7	6.2	13.0	9.6	
Self-built	72.7	84.6	12.5	35.2	42.6	
Precarious housing ("Mejora")	9.1	7.7	0.0	0.0	2.1	
Total	100.0	100.0	100.0	100.0	100.0	
Property of housing						Fisher = 0.176. Fisher's test was calculated joined the categories (tenant + usufructuary), (jobless + workers without further schooling), and (students at institutes + students at universities).
Owner	72.7	84.6	75.0	94.4	87.2	
Tenant	9.1	0.0	18.8	5.6	7.4	
Usufructuary	18.2	15.4	6.3	0.0	5.3	
Total	100.0	100.0	100.0	100.0	100.0	

Table 15. Socio-economic, socio-cultural, family, mass media exposure (MME) and demographic of variables of Chilean high school graduates in 1996 by job status 2002

Variables	Job status 2002				F
	Jobless (11)	Workers without further schooling (13)	Students at technical institutes (16)	Students at universities (54)	
Socio-economic and socio-cultural variables					
SES (Graffar's score)	10.2a ± 2.6	10.8a ± 1.1	6.2b ± 2.9	6.7b ± 3.3	11.01 ****
Paternal Schooling (y)	9.2a ± 4.1	7.8a ± 3.1	13.0b ± 2.8	12.4b ± 3.3	9.86 ****
Maternal Schooling (y)	8.5a ± 2.8	8.2a ± 2.2	11.9b ± 2.4	12.5b ± 2.2	18.13 ****
Household head's Schooling (y)	8.8a ± 4.8	8.1a ± 3.0	13.3b ± 2.8	12.4b ± 3.3	9.33 ****
Family variables					
Number of Family Members	4.3 ± 1.1	5.5 ± 1.3	5.3 ± 1.3	5.5 ± 2.3	1.26 NS
Number of Siblings	2.8 ± 1.5	3.5 ± 1.1	2.6 ± 0.7	3.1 ± 1.4	1.34 NS
Place Between Siblings	1.7ab ± 1.3	2.1a ± 1.0	1.5ab ± 0.9	2.2b ± 1.1	2.31 (t)
Promiscuity (number of persons per bed)	1.2 ab± 0.2	1.4a ± 0.4	1.2ab ± 0.2	1.1b ± 0.3	5.98 ***
Crowding (number of persons by bedroom)	1.8 ± 0.7	1.8 ± 0.5	1.6 ± 0.5	1.4 ± 0.7	1.67 NS
MME variables					
Radio (minutes per day)	163.6 ± 79.7	163.8 ± 82.7	217.8 ± 134.9	124.0 ± 149.1	2.15 (t)
Cinema (times per month)	1.5 ± 3.0	1.4 ± 2.2	1.1 ± 1.2	1.3± 2.1	0.13 NS
Television (minutes per day)	159.1 ± 143.9	166.2 ± 92.2	181.9 ± 85.2	133.4 ± 146.4	0.68 NS
Demographic variables					
Age (y)	18.0a ± 1.1	18.2a ± 0.8	17.9a ± 1.1	17.2b ± 0.5	10.34****

Note. Results are expressed as mean ± SD. The number of cases is indicated between parentheses. Means with the same letter are not significantly different at the 0.05 level based on Scheffe's test. F= ANOVA; SES= socio-economic strata. *** $p < 0.001$; **** $p < 0.0001$; (t) = tendency ($p > 0.05$ y $p < 0.10$); NS = not significantly different.

Table 16. Logistic regression between the university graduation (dependent variable), and most relevant parameters (independent variables=SES, sex, student IQ, maternal IQ, AAT, SA, birth weight, birth height, undernutrition in the first year of life, Z-HC and BV).

Parameters entered in the statistical model	DF	Parameter Estimate	Standard Error	Wald Chi-square	Standardized Estimate	Odds Ratio Estimates
INTERCEPT	1	-11.3055	3.47750	10.5690 **	-	-
AAT	1	0.0244	0.00787	9.6399 **	2.232627	1.025

Note: Probability modeled was university graduation=yes. DF= degree of freedom; SES= socio-economic strata; IQ= intellectual quotient; AAT= Academic Aptitude Test; SA= scholastic achievement; Z-HC = head circumference-for-age Z score; BV= brain volume; n= 74; ** $p < 0.01$

The logistic regression analysis between the job status 2002, dependent variable, categorized them as university studies and non-university studies (probability modeled was university studies=yes) (Table 16) and most relevant parameters considering SES, sex, student IQ, maternal IQ, AAT, SA, birth weight, birth height, undernutrition in the first year of life, Z-HC and BV as independent variables, revealed that AAT score at the end of high school was the best predictor of the job status six years later. The odds ratio value (1.025) indicates that when AAT score increases by one point the probability for university admission and for university graduation increases 2.5%.

DISCUSSION

The results of this study demonstrate that AAT achievement is determined by multiple factors, such as the student IQ, maternal and paternal IQ, Z-HC, BV, undernutrition in the first year of life, maternal schooling, household head occupation, quality of housing and SA. However, after controlling by SES and sex, only student IQ entered in the logistic regression model (odds ratio value = 1.252), which means that when IQ increases by one point the probability of obtaining high AAT scores increases by 25.2%. AAT score is a good predictor of later job status and when AAT score increases by one point the probability for university admission and for university graduation increases 2.5%. This finding is interesting and probably indicates that, in fact, AAT selects the most intelligent students for admission to universities. IQ is one of the most important neuropsychological determinants of educational performance and this is in agreement with our previous findings and with those of other authors who have found that neurodevelopmental and psychological factors are major determinants of educational success (Cassidy and Lynn, 1991; Ivanovic et al., 1989a, 2000a,b, 2002, 2004c; Rostain, 1997).

We previously had reported that intelligence is the most important independent variable that explains SA at the onset of elementary school (Ivanovic et al., 1989a). However, one of our more recent reports pinpoint that this has been observed in all grades, from elementary to high school, and that its impact significantly increases from elementary to high school (Ivanovic et al., 2004c). Other recent findings in Chilean school-age children graduating from high school emphasize that SA is determined mainly by the child's IQ, that explains approximately 90% of SA variance for both males and females; this was also observed in a comparative study of Chilean undernourished and wellnourished, poor high school graduates, in whom only IQ explained SA variance (Ivanovic et al., 2000a,b, 2002). Another aspect that we should take into consideration is the heritability of intelligence, estimating that between 50-60% of the child intelligence is explained by that of the other family members (Avancini, 1982; Johnson, 1991; Lynn and Hattori, 1990). However, the degree to which genetic factors influence human intelligence remains a matter of some controversy (Reiss AL, Freund LS, Baumgardner TL, Abrams MT, and Denckla, 1995; Sternberg, Grigorenko, and Kidd, 2005).

In our study, school-age children with high AAT had significantly higher IQ, HC, BV and SA scores and had a significantly lower incidence of undernutrition in the first year of life, than their peers from the low AAT group, despite the fact that these were significantly older than the former. As a consequence, the low AAT group showed a schooling delay due to significantly more repeated years compared with their peers with high AAT scores. In addition, students from the low AAT group had significantly higher levels of exposure to radio, they attended more frequently cinemas, they watched more television and they read newspapers and books significantly less than students from the high AAT group. This could be indicative a lifestyle that does not favor learning and that might condition the quality of jobs later.

We previously described that in the sample of this study, independently of SES, high school graduates with similar IQ had similar nutritional, brain development and educational parameters and this was observed in both sexes. Maternal IQ, BV and severe undernutrition during the first year of life were the independent variables with the greatest explanatory power for child IQ variance ($r^2 = 0.707$), without interaction with age, sex or SES (Ivanovic et al. 2000a, 2002). Although paternal IQ had a significant impact on child IQ, it is important to emphasize that students from the high SES with low IQ are probably conditioned by their maternal IQ that was significantly lower from that of mothers belonging to the low SES and whose children had high IQ (Ivanovic et al., 2002). Children of the high SES with low IQ had not suffered from severe undernutrition in the first year of life but their BV, HC and SA were not different from their peers of the low SES with low IQ, of whom 64% had suffered from undernutrition in the first year of life (Ivanovic et al., 2000b, 2002). It seems that maternal IQ may be the most powerful and critical determinant of child IQ (Bacharach and Baumeister, 1998; Ivanovic et al., 2002). On the other hand, independently of SES school-age children with low IQ obtained very low SA and AAT scores (below 450) that prevented them from applying to higher education institutions (Ivanovic et al., 2002).

Parental IQ, especially maternal IQ is also an important risk factor for AAT and later job status. This could be explained by the fact that maternal IQ is the main determinant of child IQ and, as in our results, this is the only independent variable that contributes to explain AAT achievement the most important parameter explaining later job status. Our previous results pinpoint that maternal IQ is also an important risk factor for child IQ, undernutrition, decreased HC, BV and SA (Ivanovic et al., 2000a,b,c, 2002). Other investigators have reported that the greater impact of maternal IQ may be related with the quality of the stimulation received by the child; in conditions of poverty this is also conditioned by both their lower maternal schooling levels and maternal IQ (Carter, Resnick, Ariet, Shieh, and Vonesh, 1992; Crandell and Hobson, 1999; Duncan, Brooks-Gunn, and Klebanov, 1994; Melhuish, Lloyd, Martin, and Mooney, 1990; Nelson and Deutschberger, 1970; Sandiford et al. 1997; Smith et al. 1996). As regards maternal schooling this has been underlined as the most relevant socio-economic and socio-cultural variable affecting IQ and SA like in our study (Ivanovic et al., 1995b, 2000b,c,d, 2001, 2004c). In fact, in our study AAT scores were not affected by the student's SES but by maternal schooling, household head job and the quality of housing which were significantly better in the high AAT group; these findings are in agreement with previous results that demonstrated that these variables were significantly higher in students with high SA (Ivanovic et al., 1995b, 2000c,d, 2001, 2004c). Other socio-economic variables such as SES, the household head, maternal occupation, ownership of housing, connection to a sewerage system and adequate water supply were not found to be positively and significantly associated with AAT. Other findings have revealed that the presence of the father at home originates significant differences favoring learning of boys and girls (Sciara, 1975). In our study were fathers household head more frequently in the high AAT group, but differences were not significant. The considerable importance of mothers for child development has been especially emphasized by UNICEF which considers the education of girls as a high priority (United Nations International Children's Fund, 2004). Mothers from the low SES and with the lowest schooling levels also have inadequate knowledge about nutrition and health (Ivanovic, Castro, and Ivanovic, 1997) while at the same time they are the most important source of nutrition information for school-age children (Ivanovic et al. 1989b, 1991b).

Undernutrition in the first year of life is also another important risk factor for AAT and later job status since all undernourished students had low AAT scores; as regards, IQ, HC, BV and SA scores were significantly lower than their non-undernourished peers (Ivanovic et al., 2000b). For both undernourished and wellnourished poor Chilean high school graduates, the most relevant independent variable explaining IQ were, in decreasing order of importance, maternal schooling, brain volume and undernutrition in the first year of life ($r^2 = 0.714$), and only IQ explained SA variance ($r^2 = 0.860$) (Ivanovic et al., 2000b). As we previously stated, the positive and significant impact of parental schooling, especially maternal schooling, on child IQ has been described by several authors and may be related with the more intensive stimulation of the child and the same may be argued for some environmental variables such as the quality of housing in relation to SA (Agarwal et al., 1992; Carter et al., 1992; Casey, Barrett, Bradley, and Spiker, 1993; Duncan et al., 1994; Melhuish et al., 1990; Sandiford et al., 1997; Smith et al., 1996).

HC was the most important anthropometric index of postnatal nutritional status associated with AAT achievement and with later job status in the sample of this study and our previous findings revealed that its impact increased along the school years of education; thus, in high school graduates HC is the only anthropometric parameter that explains SA and IA (Ivanovic et al., 1996, 2000c). Findings from other authors have confirmed a positive and significant correlation between head size and SA (Desch et al., 1990; Ishikawa, Furuyama, Ishikawa, Ogawa, and Wada, 1988). Moreover, as we stated previously, educational selectivity correlates with HC and not with W or H (Ivanovic et al., 1996).

Considering that IQ is the most relevant independent variable explaining AAT, positive and significant correlations between intelligence, HC and SA have been reported by other authors (Botting et al., 1998; Fisch et al., 1976; Hack and Breslau, 1986; Hack et al., 1991; Ivanovic et al., 1996, 2000a,b,c, 2002, 2004a,b,c; Johnson, 1991; Nelson and Deutschberger, 1970; Ounsted et al., 1988; Rushton and Ankney, 1996; Susanne, 1979; Van Valen, 1974; Willerman et al., 1991), and in our observations. HC is a good indicator both of the quality of the nutritional background and brain development and is the most sensitive anthropometric indicator of prolonged undernutrition during infancy, which becomes associated with intellectual impairment (Stoch et al., 1982; Winick, 1975; Winick and Rosso, 1969a,b). Malnutrition and its associated conditions affect the productivity and intellectual capacity of people. This is especially significant for the quality of life in the Third World because economic development is limited by poverty of extensive social sectors that present unfavorable socio-economic, socio-cultural, intellectual and nutritional conditions; this prevents them from applying to better jobs, as seen in our study. Currently, undernutrition remains the most relevant nutritional problem in developing countries (FAO, 1996; United Nations International Children's Fund, 2005).

Several authors have shown a positive and significant association between SA and IQ, HC and BV, like in our study (Akgun et al., 2003; Botting et al.,1998; Dolk, 1991; Gale et al., 2004; Gignac, Vernon, and Wickett, 2002; Ivanovic et al., 1996, 2000a,b,c, 2002, 2004a,b,c; Nelson and Deutschberger, 1970; Ounsted et al., 1988; Reiss et al., 1996; Rushton and Ankney, 1996; Strauss and Dietz, 1998; Vernon et al., 2000; Willerman et al., 1991). In agreement with the findings of most studies, students with low AAT scores presented in our study lower IQ, HC, BV, SA and higher incidence of undernutrition in the first year of life, despite the fact that they were older than their peers with high AAT scores (Bouchard, 1998; Desch et al., 1990; Gignac et al., 2002; Ivanovic et al., 1996, 2000a,b,c, 2002, 2004a,b,c; Reynolds, Johnston, Dodge, DeKosky, and Ganguli, 1999; Vernon et al., 2000; Weinberg, Dietz, Penick, and McAlister, 1974); however, other authors did not find significant associations between the mean IQ and HC (Przytycki and Burgin, 1992; Sells, 1977).

A positive and significant correlation between intelligence, HC and BV has confirmed by several authors, suggesting that differences in human brain size are relevant in explaining differences in IQ dependent on genetic and environmental influences (Andreasen et al., 1993; Ivanovic et al., 2000a,b,c, 2002, 2004a,b,c; Reiss et al., 1996; Willerman et al., 1991). Therefore, taking into account our results we may hypothesize once more that children with low AAT scores had suboptimal HC with some degree of alteration of brain development associated with lowered IA, lowered SA and lower job status. In consequence, neuropsychological parameters are relevant to explain AAT achievement and later job status.

In summary, IQ was the best predictor of AAT achievement and this was the best predictor of later job status. This confirms that individuals with higher job status as university students have high IQ, AAT, birth weight, birth height, HC, BV, SA, better socio-economic, socio-cultural and family conditions and a lower incidence of undernutrition in the first year of life; furthermore, their parents and especially their mothers, have high IQ. This group increased significantly their %W/H, BMI, %AC/A, %TS/A and %AFA/A values from 1996 to 2002 probably because their low physical activity due to a prolonged study periods in which they remain seated.

A recent review has shown that neurocognitive assessment is frequently used as a basis for making determinations regarding a person's ability to work. Using meta-analysis to quantify objectively the association between eight neurocognitive domains and employment status revealed that performance in each domain was significantly associated with employment status, and that the associations were greatest for the following domains: intellectual functioning, executive functioning, and memory. These findings support the ecological validity of neurocognitive assessment (Kalechstein, Newton, and van Gorp, 2003). Results from a 25-year follow-up study revealed that higher IQ was also predictive of better outcome represented by a better residential placement, employment, and quality of life. (Beadle-Brown, Murphy, and Wing, 2005).

CONCLUSION

Our study confirm the hypothesis that: 1) Independently of socio-economic status, AAT achievement is positively and significantly associated with the child's intellectual quotient, his/her parent's intellectual quotient, and his/her brain size and with some indicators of past nutrition especially head circumference; and 2) AAT achievement is a good predictor of later job status. These results underline the positive impact of neuropsychological parameters on AAT achievement and later job status and may be useful for vocational guidance of school-age children in a multicausal context and in this way it may help to improve the quality of life of children through better job status.

ACKNOWLEDGEMENTS

The authors are very gratefully to the Ministry of Education of Chile for all the facilities given to carry out this research; to Dr. Oscar Brunser MD for helpful comments and suggestions. Supported in part by Grant 1961032 from the National Fund for Scientific and Technologic Development (FONDECYT), Grant 024/1997 from the University of Chile, Postgraduate Department and Grant SOC 01/13-2 from the Research Department (DI), University of Chile.

REFERENCES

Agarwal, D.K., Awasthy, A., Upadilla, S.K., Singh, P., Kumar, J., Agarwal, K.N. (1992). Growth, behavior, development and intelligence in rural children between 1-3 years of life. *Indian Pediatrics, 29*,467-480.

Akgun, A., Okuyan, O., Baytan, S.H., and Topbas, M. (2003). Relationships between nonverbal IQ and brain size in right and left-handed men and women. *International Journal of Neuroscience, 113*,893-902.

Alvarez, M.L., Muzzo, S., and Ivanovic, D. (1985). Escala para medición del nivel socioeconómico en el área de la salud. *Revista Médica de Chile,113*, 243-249.

Alvarez, M.L., and Wurgaft, F. (1981). Conducta socioafectiva de la madre con lactante desnutrido. *Revista Chilena de Nutrición,9*,101-111.

Alvarez, M.L., Wurgaft, F., and Wilder, H. (1982). Non-verbal language in mothers with malnourished infants. *Social Science and Medicine, 16*,1365-1369.

Anderson, B. (1999). Brain size, head size, and intelligence quotient in monozygotic twins. *Neurology, 53,* 239.

Andreasen, N.C., Flaum, M., Swayze, V., O'Leary, D.S., Alliger, R., Cohen, G., et al. (1993). Intelligence and brain structure in normal individuals. *American Journal of Psychiatry*,150,130-134.

Avancini, G. (1982). *El fracaso escolar*. Barcelona: Herder.

Bacharach, V.R., and Baumeister, A.A. (1998). Effects of maternal intelligence, marital status, income, and home environment on cognitive development of low birthweight infants. *Pediatric Psychology, 23*,197-205.

Baker, L.A., Treloar, S.A., Reynolds, C.A., Heath, A.C., and Martin, N.G. (1996). Genetics of scholastic achievement in Australian twins: sex differences and secular changes. *Behavior genetics,26*,89-102.

Beadle-Brown, J., Murphy, G., Wing, L. (2005). Long-term outcome for people with severe intellectual disabilities: impact of social impairment. *American Journal of Mental Retardation 110*,1-12.

Botting, N., Powls, A., Cooke, R.W., and Marlow, N. (1998). Cognitive and educational outcome of very low-birth weight children in early adolescence. *Developmental Medicine and Child Neurology, 40,* 652-660.

Bouchard, T.J. Jr. (1998). Genetic and environmental influences on adult intelligence and special mental abilities. *Human Biology,70,* 257-279.

Broca, P. (1861). Sur le volume et al forme du cerveau suivant les individus et suivant les races. *Bulletins et mémoires de la Société d'Anthropologie de Paris, 2,* 139-207, 301-321, 441-446.

Brown, L., and Pollitt, E. (1996). Malnutrition, poverty and intellectual development. *Scientific American, 274,* 38-43.

Carter, R.L., Resnick, M.B., Ariet, M., Shieh, G., and Vonesh, E.F. (1992) A random coefficient growth curve analysis of mental development in low-birth-weight infants. *Statistical in Medicine 11,* 243-256.

Casey, P.H., Barrett, K., Bradley, R.H., and Spiker, D. (1993). Pediatric clinical assessment of mother-child interaction: concurrent and predictive validity. *Journal of developmental and behavioral pediatrics,* 14,313-317.

Cassidy, T., and Lynn, R. (1991). Achievement motivation, scholastic achievement, cycles of disadvantage and social competence: some longitudinal data. *British Journal of Educational Psychology,* 61,1-12.

Casto, S.D., DeFries, J.C., and Fulker, D.W. (1995). Multivariate genetic analysis of Wechsler Intelligence Scale for Children-Revised (WISC-R) factors. *Behavior Genetics,* 25, 25-32.

Chile. Ministerio de Educación Pública. (1996). Planes y Programas de Estudio para la Educación Media. *Revista de Educación, 225.* Santiago: MINEDUC.

Crandell, L.E., and Hobson, R.P. (1999). Individual differences in young children's IQ: a social-developmental perspective. *Journal of Child Psychology and Psychiatry and Allied Disciplines,* 40,455-464.

Desch, L.W., Anderson, S.K., and Snow, J.H. (1990). Relationship of head circumference to measures of school performance. *Clinical Pediatrics, 29,* 389-392.

Dolk, H. (1991). The predictive value of microcephaly during the first year of life for mental retardation at seven years. *Developmental Medicine and Child Neurology, 33,* 974-983.

Duncan, G.J., Brooks-Gunn, J. and Klebanov, P.K. (1994) Economic deprivation and early childhood development. *Child Development 65,* 296-318.

FAO. *Sexta encuesta alimentaria mundial.* Roma: FAO. 1996.

Fisch, R.O., Bilek, M.K., Horrobin, J.M., and Chang, P.N. (1976). Children with superior intelligence at 7 years of age: a prospective study of the influence of perinatal, medical and socio-economic factors. *American Journal of Diseases of Children, 130,* 481-487.

Frisancho, A.R. (1981). New norms of upper limb fat and muscle areas for assessment of nutritional status. *American Journal of Clinical Nutrition,* 34,2540-2545.

Gale, C.R., O'Callaghan, F.J., Godfrey, K.M., Law, C.M., and Martyn, C.N. (2004). Critical periods of brain growth and cognitive function in children. *Brain,* 127,321-329.

Galton, F. (1888). Head growth in students at the University of Cambridge. *Nature, 38,* 14-15.

Garrow, J.S. (1981). *Treat Obesity Seriously: A Clinical Manual.* London: Churchill Livingstone.

Gibson, R. (1990). *Principles of Nutritional Assessment.* Oxford: Oxford University Press.

Gignac, G., Vernon, P.A., and Wickett, J.C. (2002). Factors influencing the relationship between brain size and intelligence. In: H. Nyborg (Ed.), *The Scientific Study of General Intelligence: Tribute to Arthur R. Jensen.* (pp. 93-106). Oxford, UK: Elsevier Science.

Grantham-McGregor, S.M., and Fernald, L.C. (1997). Nutritional deficiencies and subsequent effects on mental and behavioral development in children. *Southeast Asian Journal of Tropical Medicine and Public Health, 28,* 50-68.

Grunau, R.E., Whitfield, M.F., and Fay, T.B. (2004). Psychosocial and academic characteristics of extremely low birth weight (< or =800 g) adolescents who are free of major impairment compared with term-born control subjects. *Pediatrics, 114*,725-732.

Guilford, J.P., and Fruchter, B. (1984). *Estadística aplicada a la psicología y a la educación.* México: McGraw Hill.

Gupta, R.K., Saini, D.P., Acharya, U., Miglani, N. (1994). Impact of television on children. Indian Journal of *Pediatrics,61*,153-159.

Hack, M., and Breslau, N. (1986). Very low birth weight infants: effects of brain growth during infancy on intelligence quotient at 3 years of age. *Pediatrics, 77*,196-202.

Hack, M., Breslau, N., Weissman, B., Aram, D., Klein, N., and Borawski, E. (1991). Effect of very low birth weight and subnormal head size on cognitive abilities at school age. *New England Journal of Medicine, 325,* 231-237.

Hagborg, W.J. (1995). High school student television viewing time: a study of school performance and adjustment. *Child Study Journal,25,*155-167.

Hermosilla, M. (1986). *La escala de inteligencia de Wechsler para adultos (WAIS).* Santiago: Pontificia Universidad Católica de Chile, Escuela de Psicología.

Huttenlocher, P.R., and Dabholkar, A.S. (1997). Regional differences in synaptogenesis in human cerebral cortex. *Journal of Comparative Neurology, 38,*167-178.

Ishikawa, T., Furuyama, M., Ishikawa, M., Ogawa, J., and Wada, Y. (1988). Growth and achievement of large-and small-headed children in a normal population. *Brain Development,10,*295-299

Ivanovic, D. (1992). Nutrition and Education. IV. Clinical signs of malnutrition and its relationship with socio-economic, anthropometric, dietetic and educational achievement parameters. *Archivos Latinoamericanos de Nutrición, 42,*15-25.

Ivanovic, D. (1996). Does undernutrition during infancy inhibit brain growth and subsequent intellectual development?. Prospective overview. *Nutrition,12,*568-571.

Ivanovic, D., Almagià, A., Toro, T., Castro, C., Pérez, H., Urrutia, M.S., et al. (2000a). Impacto del estado nutricional en el desarrollo cerebral, inteligencia y rendimiento escolar, en el marco de un enfoque multifactorial. *La Educación (Organización de los Estados Americanos, OEA)*, 44 (134-135)I-II: 3-35.

Ivanovic, D., Castro, C., and Ivanovic, R. (1997). Conocimientos alimentarios y nutricionales de madres de escolares de Educación Básica y Media. *Archivos Latinoamericanos de Nutrición, 47,* 248-255.

Ivanovic, D., Forno, H., and Ivanovic, R. (2001). Estudio de la capacidad intelectual (Test de Matrices Progresivas de Raven) en escolares de 5 a 18 años. II. Interrelaciones con factores socioeconómicos, socioculturales, familiares, de exposición a medios de comunicación de masas, demográficos y educacionales. *Revista de Psicología General y Aplicada, 54,* 443-466.

Ivanovic, D., and Ivanovic, R. (1988). Rendimiento y deserción escolar: un enfoque multicausal. En: Ivanovic D, Ivanovic, R, Middleton S, eds. *Rendimiento escolar y estado nutricional* (pp. 3- 6) Santiago: Universidad de Chile, INTA.

Ivanovic, D., Ivanovic, R., and Middleton, S. (1988). *Rendimiento escolar y estado nutricional.* Santiago: Universidad de Chile, INTA,

Ivanovic, D., Ivanovic, R., Truffello, I., and Buitrón, C. (1989a). Nutritional status and educational achievement of elementary first grade Chilean students. *Nutrition Report International,39*, 163-175

Ivanovic, D.M., Leiva, B.P., Castro, C.G., Olivares, M.G., Jansana, J.M., Castro, V., et al. (2004a). Brain Development Parameters and Intelligence in Chilean High School Graduates. *Intelligence, 32,* 461-479

Ivanovic, D., Leiva, B., Pérez, H., Almagià, A., Toro, T., Urrutia, M.S., et al. (2002). Nutritional status, brain development and scholastic achievement of Chilean high school graduates from high and low intellectual quotient and socio-economic status. *British Journal of Nutrition, 87,* 81-92.

Ivanovic, D., Leiva, B., Pérez, H., Inzunza, N., Almagià, A., Toro, T., et al. (2000b). Long-term effects of severe undernutrition during the first year of life on brain development and learning in Chilean high school graduates. *Nutrition, 16,* 1056-1063.

Ivanovic, D.M., Leiva, B.P., Pérez, H.T., Olivares, M.G., Díaz, N.S., Urrutia, M.S.C., et al. (2004b). Head size and intelligence, learning, nutritional status and brain development. *Neuropsychologia 42,* 1118-1131

Ivanovic, D., and Marambio, M. (1989). Nutrition and Education. I. Educational achievement and anthropometric parameters of Chilean elementary and high school graduates. *Nutrition Reports International,39,*983-993

Ivanovic, D., Olivares, M., Castro, C., and Ivanovic, R. (1995a). Circunferencia craneana de escolares chilenos de 5 a 18 años. Región Metropolitana de Chile. 1986-1987, 1992. *Revista Médica de Chile, 123,* 587-599.

Ivanovic, D., Olivares, M., Castro, C., and Ivanovic, R. (1996). Nutrition and learning in Chilean school-age children. Chile's Metropolitan area. Survey 1986-1987. *Nutrition,12,*321-328.

Ivanovic, D., Pérez, H., Olivares, M., Díaz, N., Leyton, B., and Ivanovic, R. (2004c). Scholastic Achievement: A Multivariate Analysis of Nutritional, Intellectual, Socio-Economic, Socio-Cultural, Family and Demographic Variables in Chilean School-Age Children. *Nutrition, 2,* 878-889.

Ivanovic, D., Vásquez, M., Aguayo, M., Ballester, D., Marambio, M., Zacarías, I. (1992). Nutrition and Education. III. Educational achievement and food habits of Chilean elementary and high school graduates. *Archivos Latinoamericanos de Nutrición, 42,* 9-14.

Ivanovic, D., Vásquez, M., Marambio, M., Ballester, D., Zacarías, I., and Aguayo, M. (1991a). Nutrition and Education. II. Educational achievement and nutrient intake of Chilean elementary and high school graduates. *Archivos Latinoamericanos de Nutrición, 41,* 499-515.

Ivanovic, D., Zacarías, I., Saitúa, M.T., and Marambio M. (1988). Educational achievement and nutritional status of elementary and high school graduates. In: M.F. Moyal (Ed). *Dietetics in the 90s. Role of the dietitian/nutritionist* (pp. 331-334). London: John Libbey Eurotext Ltd.

Ivanovic, R., Castro, C., and Ivanovic D. (1995b). No existe una teoría sobre el rendimiento escolar. *Revista de Educación (Ministerio de Educación de Chile),224,*40-45.

Ivanovic, R., Forno, H., Castro, C.G., and Ivanovic, D. (2000c). Intellectual ability and nutritional status assessed through anthropometric measurements of Chilean school-age children from different socio-economic status. *Ecology of Food and Nutrition, 39,* 35-59.

Ivanovic, R., Forno, H., Durán, M.C., Hazbún, J., Castro, C., and Ivanovic, D. (2000d). Estudio de la capacidad intelectual (Test de Matrices Progresivas de Raven) en escolares de 5 a 18 años. I. Antecedentes generales, normas y recomendaciones. Región Metropolitana. Chile. 1986-1987. *Revista de Psicología General y Aplicada, 53,* 5-30.

Ivanovic, R., Olivares, M., and Ivanovic, D. (1991b). Sources of nutrition information of Chilean schoolers. Metropolitan Region. Chile. Survey 1986-1987. *Archivos Latinoamericanos de Nutrición, 41,*527-538.

Ivanovic R, and Sepúlveda O. (1988). Rendimiento escolar y exposición a medios de comunicación de masas en estudiantes de enseñanza media del Área Metropolitana. *Revista de Sociología,3,*73-87.

Ivanovic, R., Truffello, I., Buitrón, C., and Ivanovic, D. (1989b). Educational factors influencing the nutritional learning of elementary first grade Chilean schoolers. *Nutrition Reports International, 39,*1161-1166.

Johnson, E.O., and Breslau, N. (2000). Increased of learning disabilities in low birth weight boys at age 11 years. *Biological Psychiatry,47,*490-500.

Johnson, F.W. (1991). Biological factors and psychometric intelligence: a review. *Genetic, Social, and General Psychology Monographs, 117,* 313-357.

Johnston, F., and Lampl, M. (1984). Anthropometry in studies of malnutrition and behavior. In: J. Brožek and B. Schürch, (Eds.) *Malnutrition and Behavior: Critical Assessment of Key Issues* (pp.51-70). Lausanne: Nestlé Foundation Publication Series.

Kalechstein, A.D., Newton, T.F., and van Gorp, W.G. (2003). Neurocognitive functioning is associated with employment status: a quantitative review. *Journal of Clinical and Experimental Neuropsychology, 25,*1186-1191.

Leiva, B., Inzunza, N., Pérez, H., Castro, V., Jansana, J.M., Toro, T., et al. (2001). Algunas consideraciones sobre el impacto de la desnutrición en el desarrollo cerebral, inteligencia y rendimiento escolar. *Archivos Latinoamericanos de Nutrición, 51,* 64-71.

Luke, B., Keith, L., and Keith, D. (1997). Maternal nutrition in twin gestations: weight gain, cravings and aversions, and sources of nutrition advice. *Acta Geneticae Medicae et Gemellologiae (Roma), 46,* 157-166.

Lynn, R., and Hattori, K. (1990) The heritability of intelligence in Japan. *Behavior Genetics 20,* 545-546.

Malina, R.M., Habicht, J.P., Martorell, R., Lechtig, A., Yarbrough, C., and Klein, R.E. (1975). Head and chest circumferences in rural Guatemalan Ladino children, birth to seven years of age. *American Journal of Clinical Nutrition, 28,*1061-1070.

Martyn, C.N., Gale, C.R., Sayer, A.A., and Fall, C. (1996). Growth in utero and cognitive function in adult life: follow up study of people born between 1920 and 1943. *British Medical Journal, 312,* 1393-1396.

Matano, S., and Nakano, Y. (1998). Size comparison of the male and female human corpus callosum from autopsy samples. *Zeitschrift fur* Morphologie und Anthropologie, *82,* 67-73.

Matte, T.D., Bresnahan, M., Begg, M.D., and Susser, E. (2001). Influence of variation in birth weight within normal range and within sibships on IQ at age 7 years: cohort study. *British Medical Journal, 323,* 310-314.

McGue, M., and Bouchard, T.J. Jr. (1998). Genetic and environmental influences on human behavioral differences. *Annual Review of Neuroscience, 21,* 1-24.

Melhuish, E.C., Lloyd, E., Martin, S., and Mooney, A. (1990) Type of childcare at 18 months. II. Relations with cognitive and language development. *Journal of Child Psychology and Psychiatry and Allied Disciplines, 31,* 861-870.

Menkes, J.H. (1995). *Texbook of Child Neurology.* Baltimore: Williams and Wilkins

Nellhaus, G. (1968). Head circumference from birth to eighteen years. *Pediatrics, 41,* 106-114.

Nelson, K.B., and Deutschberger, J. (1970). Head size at one year as a predictor of four-year IQ. *Developmental Medicine and Child Neurology, 12,* 487-495.

Ounsted, M., Moar, V.A., and Scott, A. (1988). Head circumference and developmental ability at the age of seven years. *Acta Paediatrica Scanddinavica, 77,* 374-379.

Özmert, E.N., Yurdakok, K., Soysal, S., Kulak-Kayikci, M.E., Belgin, E., Ozmert, E., et al. (2005). Relationship between physical, environmental and sociodemographic factors and school erformance in primary schoolchildren. *Journal of Tropical Pediatrics, 51,*25-32

Pennington, B.F., Filipek, P.A., Lefly, D., Chhabildas, N., Kennedy, D.N., Simon, J.H., et al. (2000). A twin MRI study of size variations in human brain. *Journal of Cognitive Neuroscience, 12,* 223-232.

Peters, M., Jancke, L., Staiger, J.F., Schlaug, G., Huang, Y., and Stenmetz, H. (1998). Unsolved problems in comparing brain sizes in homo sapiens. *Brain and Cognition, 37,* 254-285.

Posthuma, D., Baare,W.F., Hulshoff Pol, H.E., Kahn, R.S., Boomsma, D.I., De Geus, E.J. (2003). Genetic correlations between brain volumes and the WAIS-III dimensions of verbal comprehension, working memory, perceptual organization, and processing speed. *Twin Research, 6,*131-9.

Przytycki, A., and Burgin, R. (1992). Microcephalic children without mental retardation. *Harefuah, 122,* 566-568.

Raven , J.C. (1957). *Test de matrices progresivas. Escala general.* Paidós, Buenos Aires.

Reiss, A.L., Abrams, M.T., Singer, H.S., Ross, J.L., and Denckla, M.B. (1996). Brain development, gender and IQ in children. A volumetric imaging study. *Brain, 119,* 1763-1774.

Reiss, A.L., Freund, L.S., Baumgardner, T.L., Abrams, M.T., and Denckla, M.B. (1995). Contribution of the FMR1 gene mutation to human intellectual dysfunction. *Nature Genetics,11,*331-334.

Reynolds, M.D., Johnston, J.M., Dodge, H.H., DeKosky, S.T., and Ganguli, M. (1999). Small head size is related to low Mini-Mental State Examination scores in a community sample of nondemented older adults. *Neurology, 53,* 228-229.

Ridley-Johnson, R., Cooper, H., and Chance, J. (1982). The relation of children's television viewing to school achievement and I.Q. *Journal of Educational Research,76,*294-297.

Roche, A.F., Mukherjee, D., Guo, S., and Moore, W. (1987). Head circumference reference data: birth to 18 years. *Pediatrics, 79,* 706-712.

Rostain, A.L. (1997). Assessing and Managing Adolescents with School Problems. *Adolescent Medicine, 8,*57-76

Rumsey, J.M., and Rapoport, J.L. (1983). Assessing behavioral and cognitive effects of diet in pediatric populations. In: R.J. Wurtman and J.J. Wurtman (Eds.), *Nutrition and the Brain* (pp. 101-161). New York, NY: Raven Press.

Rushton, J.P., and Ankney, C.D. (1996). Brain size and cognitive ability: Correlations with age, sex, social class, and race. *Psychonomic Bulletin and Review, 3,* 21-36.

SAS. (1990). *Statistical analysis system (Version 6)* [Computer software]. SAS Institute, Inc. Cary, NC: Author.

Sandiford, P., Cassel, J., Sanchez, G., and Coldham, C. (1997). Does intelligence account for the link between maternal literacy and child survival?. *Social Science and Medicine;* *45*,1231-1239.

Schiefelbein, E., and Farrel, J. (1982). *Eight years of their lives: through schooling to the labour market in Chile.* Otawa : International Development Research Centre, IDRC, 191e.

Schoenemann, P.T., Budinger, T., Sarich,V., and Wang, W. (2000). Brain size does not predict general cognitive ability within families. *Proceedings of the National Academy of Science USA, 97,* 4932-4937.

Schofield, P.W., Logroscino, G., Andrews, H.F., Albert, S., and Stern, Y. (1997). An association between head circumference and Alzheimer's disease in a population-based study of aging and dementia. *Neurology ,49,* 30-37.

Schramm, W., Lyle, J., and Parker, E. (1965). *La televisión y los niños*. Barcelona: Hispano Europea.

Sciara, F.J. (1975). Effects of father absence on the educational achievement of urban black children. *Child Study Journal,5,*45-55.

Sells, C.J. (1977). Microcephaly in a normal school population. *Pediatrics, 59,* 262-265.

Smith, K.E., Landry, S.H., Swank, P.R., Baldwin, C.D., Denson, S.E., and Wildin, S. (1996). The relation of medical risk and maternal stimulation with preterm infants' development of cognitive, language and daily living skills. *Journal of child psychology and psychiatry, and allied discipline,37,* 855-864

Sorensen, H.T., Sabroe, S., Olsen, J., Rothman, K.J., Gillman, M.W., and Fisher, P. (1999). Birth weight as a predictor of young men's intelligence. A historical cohort study. *Ugeskrift for Laeger,* 161, 791-793.

Stathis, S.L., O'Callaghan, M., Harvey, J., and Rogers, Y. (1999). Head circumference in ELBW babies is associated with learning difficulties and cognition but not ADHD in the school-aged child. *Developmental Medicine and Child Neurology, 41,* 375-380.

Sternberg, R.J., Grigorenko, E.L., and Kidd, K.K. (2005). Intelligence, race, and genetics. *The American Psychologist,60,*46-59.

Stoch, M.B., Smythe, P.M., Moodie, A.D., and Bradshaw, D. (1982). Psychosocial outcome and CT findings after gross undernourishment during infancy: a 20-year developmental study. *Developmental Medicine and Child Neurology, 24,* 419-436.

Strasburger, V.C. (1986). Does television affect learning and school performance?. *Pediatrician, 13,*141-147.

Strauss, R.S., and Dietz, W.H. (1998). Growth and development of term children born with low birth weight: effects of genetic and environmental factors. *Journal of Pediatrics, 133,* 67-72.

Susanne, C. (1979). On the relationship between psychometric and anthropometric traits. *American Journal Physical Anthropology, 51,* 421-424.

Tanner, J.M. (1984). Physical growth and development. In: J.O. Forfar and G.C. Arneil (Eds.), *Texbook of pediatrics* (pp. 278-330). Edinburgh: Churchill Livingstone.

Teasdale, T.W., and Pakkenberg, B. (1988). The association between intelligence level and brain volume measures: A negative finding. Scandinavian *Journal of Psychology, 29,* 123-125.

The World Medical Association. (1964). Human experimentation. Code of Ethics of the World Medical Association (Declaration of Helsinki). *British Medical Journal, 2,* 177.

Tisserand, D.J., Bosma, H., Van Boxtel, M.P., and Jolles, J. (2001). Head size and cognitive ability in nondemented older adults are related. *Neurology, 56,* 969-971.

Toro, T., Almagià, A., and Ivanovic, D. (1998). Evaluación antropométrica y rendimiento escolar en estudiantes de educación media de Valparaíso, Chile. *Archivos Latinoamericanos de Nutrición, 48,* 201-209.

United Nations International Children's Fund. (1994). *A proposal to classify Chilean districts by infancy situation.* Santiago: UNICEF.

United Nations International Children's Fund. (2004). *The state of the world's children 2004.* New York: UNICEF.

United Nations International Children's Fund. (2005). *The state of the world's children 2005.* New York: UNICEF.

Universidad de Chile. (1996) *Resultados de la Prueba de Aptitud Académica Proceso 1996.* Santiago: Universidad de Chile, Departamento de Evaluación, Medición y Registro Educacional (DEMRE).

Van Valen, L (1974) Brain size and intelligence in man. *American Journal of Physical Anthropology, 40,* 417-424.

Vernon, P.A., Wickett, J.C., Bazana, P.G., and Stelmack, R.M. (2000). The neuropsychology and psychophysiology of human intelligence. In: R.J. Sternberg (Ed.), *Handbook of Intelligence* (pp. 245-264). Cambridge: Cambridge University Press.

Weaver, D.D., and Christian, J.C. (1980). Familial variation of head size and adjustment for parental head circumference. *Journal of Pediatrics, 96,* 990-994.

Wechsler, D. (1981). *Manual for the Wechsler Adult Intelligence Scale—Revised.* San Antonio, TX: Psychological Corporation.

Weinberg, W.A., Dietz, S.G., Penick, E.C., and McAlister, W.H. (1974). Intelligence, reading achievement, physical size and social class. A study of St. Louis Caucasian boys aged 8-0 to 9-6 years, attending regular schools. *Journal of Pediatrics, 85,* 482-489.

Willerman, L., Schultz, R., Rutledge, J.N., and Bigler, D.E. (1991). In vivo brain size and intelligence. *Intelligence, 15,* 223-228.

Winick, M. (1975). Nutrition and brain development. In G. Serban, (Ed.), *Nutrition and Mental Functions* (pp. 65-73). New York: Plenum Press.

Winick M., and Rosso, P. (1969a). Head circumference and cellular growth of the brain in normal and marasmic children. *Journal of Pediatrics, 74,* 774-778.

Winick, M., and Rosso, P. (1969b). The effect of severe early malnutrition on cellular growth of human brain. *Pediatric Research, 3,* 181-184.

Yarbrough, C., Habicht, J.P., Martorell, R., and Klein, RE. (1974). Anthropometry as an index of nutritional status. In: A.F.Roche, & F. Falkner, (Eds.), *Nutrition and Malnutrition. Identification and measurement* (pp. 15–26). New York: Plenum press.

Yeo, R.A., Turkheimer, E., Raz, N., and Bigler, E.D. (1987). Volumetric asymmetries of the human brain: intellectual correlates. *Brain and Cognition, 6,* 15-23.

In: Focus on Neuropsychology Research
Editor: Joshua R. Dupri, pp. 141-161

ISBN 1-59454-779-3
© 2006 Nova Science Publishers, Inc.

Chapter 5

RELIABILITY AND MAGNITUDE OF LATERALITY EFFECTS IN A DICHOTIC LISTENING TASK: INFLUENCE OF THE TESTING PROCEDURE

Daniel Voyer[1], Vanessa G. Boudreau[2] and Aileen M. Russell[3]
[1]University of New Brunswick
[2]Simon Fraser University
[3]University of Windsor

ABSTRACT

Two experiments investigated the reliability of dichotic listening tasks under two conditions of administration: on tape or on a computer. Stimuli in both experiments were words (bower, dower, power, and tower) pronounced with an emotional tone of anger, happiness, neutrality, or sadness. Experiment 1 required participants to detect a target word in each dichotic pair. Accordingly, 40 right-handed participants were randomly assigned to a condition in which the dichotic word recognition task was completed twice either in a taped version or directly on a computer. Experiment 2 involved the detection of a target emotion. A different group of 40 right-handed participants completed the dichotic emotion recognition task twice either on tape or on-computer. In Experiment 1, results showed a large right ear advantage of similar magnitude and test-retest reliability on both versions of the task. In Experiment 2, the laterality effect also had a similar reliability in both versions. However, the magnitude of the observed left ear advantage (LEA) varied as a function of procedure. Specifically, on computer, the LEA was significant only in females. Implications of these findings for the use of computer tasks to measure functional lateralization in research and applied settings are discussed. Factors responsible for variability in the results obtained in Experiment 2 are also discussed.

The specialization of the cerebral hemispheres for the processing of specific task material is a phenomenon generally taken for granted in the neuropsychological literature (Iaccino, 1993). Specifically, one typically expects laterality effects to reflect the contention that verbal material is more efficiently processed by the left cerebral hemisphere, whereas non-verbal material is more efficiently processed by the right hemisphere (see Kimura, 1961a; 1961b for early findings).

It has been reported that the dichotic listening approach, in which concurrent auditory information is presented to each ear, produces some of the most robust and reliable functional laterality effects (Voyer, 1998). Specifically, a right ear advantage (REA) of large magnitude and high reliability typically emerges with verbal material, whereas a left ear advantage (LEA) is usually obtained with non-verbal material. Based on the notion that the contralateral connections in the auditory system are stronger, more numerous, and more rapidly conducting than the ipsilateral connections (see Kimura, 1967), these perceptual asymmetries for verbal and non-verbal information are interpreted as reflecting a left and right hemisphere superiority, respectively.

Several sources of evidence illustrate the high reliability and validity of dichotic listening in verbal tasks, whereas findings are more mitigated for non-verbal tasks. Voyer (1998) conducted a meta-analysis in which he examined the reliability and validity of various measures of perceptual asymmetries. He partitioned the tasks in terms of the modality of administration (visual, auditory) and their content (verbal, non-verbal). Of relevance to dichotic listening, verbal tasks presented in the auditory modality produced the most reliable findings, particularly those using digits, consonant-vowel syllables, and words. Data on the validity of the tasks were not as clear, which was likely due to the small sample size. In addition, Voyer (1998) noted that, because validity estimates are dependent on task reliability, validity assessment requires the development of reliable tasks. Unfortunately, most of the validity studies retrieved in this meta-analysis did not present reliability estimates on the tasks they used. Nevertheless, individual studies present evidence in favor of the validity of dichotic listening to assess verbal laterality. For instance, Strauss, Gaddes, and Wada (1987), Voyer, McGlone, and Savoie (1996), and Zatorre (1989) used data obtained from the intracarotid amytal technique (IAT: Wada, 1949) to determine the validity of a dichotic task using words as stimuli. Results obtained in the two procedures were quite similar in that participants who showed a left hemisphere advantage (LHA) on the IAT also generally showed a LHA (as reflected in an REA) on the dichotic listening task. Considering that the IAT is believed by some to provide the best available estimate of speech lateralization (Channon, Schugens, Daum, and Polkey, 1990; Zatorre, 1989), similar results in both tasks clearly support the validity of the dichotic listening task with verbal material.

In contrast, Voyer (1998) reported low reliability and validity estimates for non-verbal material. However, the most obvious aspect was the paucity of research on the reliability and validity of non-verbal laterality measures. Since the publication of this meta-analysis, more research conducted in our laboratory has examined the reliability of non-verbal laterality effects. Specifically, Voyer and Rodgers (2002) and Voyer, Russell, and McKenna (2002) reported relatively large reliability estimates for laterality effects in emotion recognition (.79 and .67, respectively), but only when target detection was used. In fact, Voyer et al. (2002) reported low reliability in free recall and discrimination. According to Bryden (1988) and Voyer (2003), it is likely that the target detection task produces better reliability estimates because it provides a good control of attention deployment (see below).

The importance of establishing the reliability and validity of dichotic listening lays in its potential application in clinical and experimental settings. Although the IAT arguably can be considered the best available measure of speech lateralization, it involves an invasion of a person's body through the injection of a drug (sodium amobarbytal) that anesthetizes part of the brain. Thus, this approach is an invasive measure of lateralization. Moreover, the IAT involves some degree of physical risk given the use of a drug. This technique thus requires specific medical knowledge, restricting its use in most settings. Finally, the use of an injection is often uncomfortable for the participants. For these reasons, non-invasive measures of speech lateralization are commonly used as preliminary screening procedures to ensure that speech functions are preserved in patients undergoing brain surgery (Channon et al., 1990; Zatorre, 1989). Research showing similar results with dichotic listening and IAT indicates that one can use the former task as a non-invasive alternative, thus sparing patients from further discomfort. Other, less invasive methods, such a functional magnetic resonance imaging or transcranial Doppler (see Duscheck and Schandry, 2003), require expensive equipment and thus do not provide an easy alternative to IAT.

Considering the demonstrated reliability and validity of dichotic listening as a tool for laterality assessment (at least for verbal tasks), it is often the measure of choice as screening procedure before surgery or in an experimental setting. In this context, the favored approach since the early days of dichotic listening has been to present a pre-recorded version of the task through stereophonic headphones (Broadbent, 1954; Kimura, 1961a, 1961b). Participants are typically required to report items by either repeating them or identifying them among a list (e.g., Hiscock, Cole, Benthall, Carlson, and Ricketts, 2000). Unfortunately, this method has the disadvantage that participants are relatively passive and have to wait a fixed period of time between trials. Recent advances in technology allow modifications to this classic procedure. Specifically, software packages such as the Micro-Experimental Laboratory (MEL) Version 2.0 (Schneider, 1995) and E-prime (Schneider, Eschman, and Zuccolotto, 2002a, 2002b) introduced the ability to perform dichotic listening experiments directly on a computer. Some researchers also have developed their own software to administer a dichotic listening task directly on a computer (Shtyrov et al., 2000).

The ease of administration of the task is an aspect that requires consideration. It is well-known that a greater number of trials favors internal consistency, which in turn, promotes reliability (Ghiselli, 1964). However, in applied settings, we are often dealing with individuals who have already been subjected to many tests or who are not motivated for a long task. This situation is likely to produce lapses in attention, which might result in a reduction of the observed reliability and validity estimates. Thus, there exists a tradeoff between the increased reliability and validity promoted by a lengthy task, and the decreased reliability and validity associated with extended testing periods. One way to resolve this problem is to give individuals a sense of control over task administration. On a computer version of the dichotic listening task, participants can work at their own pace, thereby reducing the influence of fatigue and boredom, which may otherwise result in poor performance over time. Specifically, in a computer task, participants can move on to the next trial immediately following their response (Shtyrov et al., 2000). In contrast, taped versions of the task force participants to wait for a fixed inter-trial interval (ITI; for examples, see Hiscock et al., 2000; Voyer and Flight, 2001).

A second advantage of the computer task is that the experimenter has the ability to randomize trials across participants, thus adding to the rigor of the experiment. In a taped task, one typically uses a limited number of versions of the recording in which a different order of trials presentation is utilized. All the participants are usually exposed to each of the randomized orders of trials. For example, Wexler and Halwes (1983) used eight randomizations of the same 15 stimulus pairings in what probably constitutes one of the most rigorous designs available. In contrast, a task completed directly on computer allows a nearly infinite number of randomizations.

A third advantage of a computer task over a taped task is the ability to provide feedback concerning accuracy on each trial. Computer tasks developed with software packages such as E-prime typically provide feedback concerning the accuracy of responses after each trial. This allows participants to be informed of their performance and is presumed to encourage them to give their full attention to the task in order to achieve optimal performance. In contrast, a task performed on the basis of a recording does not allow feedback on accuracy until the task is completed. Participants are not informed of their accuracy and they remain unaware of whether they are producing optimal performance.

A fourth advantage of computer tasks is that they produce summary statistics for individual participants or group data that are free of scorer errors. The paper-and-pencil format required in a taped task means that scoring must be performed by the experimenter. This procedure is error prone and lengthy, especially as the number of trials increases in the task.

Finally, the computer allows one to record the reaction time for response production as an additional source of information. This allows the examination of possible speed-accuracy tradeoffs and adds elements of interpretation. Previously recorded tasks typically only provide data on accuracy of responses.

The advantages listed above suggest that testing participants directly on a computer has much potential for future use. It is important to note, however, that the advantages of computer testing do not necessarily imply that it has high levels of reliability and validity. Although Voyer (1998) reported a relatively high level of reliability for laterality effects obtained with verbal dichotic listening tasks, all the estimates were obtained with taped tasks. Thus, it is currently unknown whether the reliability and validity estimates for laterality effects obtained on a computer task are comparable to those observed in the classic taped task. It was therefore the purpose of the present study to compare the magnitude and reliability of laterality effects on the same dichotic listening task administered on both computer and tape.

The present study examined the test-retest correlation for the laterality effect obtained on verbal and non-verbal tasks administered on a computer and a recording. Task validity for the verbal task was determined by means of an examination of the percentage of participants showing an REA. This approach was based on the notion that studies using invasive techniques such as the IAT have shown that about 95% of right-handers show left hemisphere dominance for language (Hiscock et al., 2000). A valid task is thus expected to show a percentage of REA close to 95%. For the non-verbal task, no such explicit criterion is available. Nevertheless, the percentage of LEA provides an approximate measure of validity, given the contention that non-verbal tasks are expected to produce a right hemisphere advantage.

The present experiments used a target detection task in which participants were presented with a dichotic pair and they were required to indicate whether a specific target stimulus was presented on each trial. In their implementation of this procedure, Bryden and MacRae (1989) presented the words bower, dower, power, or tower pronounced with an emotional tone (angry, happy, sad, neutral) and asked participants to circle "yes" on a response sheet when a specific word was presented, and "no" when it was not. For example, a participant would circle "yes" when "bower" was presented on any given trial, regardless of the ear to which it was presented. Of course, the target word used was randomized across participants. This approach produced a robust REA. One advantage of the target detection task is that participants are required to divide their attention equally between the ears in order to achieve optimal performance (Bryden, 1988). In addition, the fact that they do not directly report a stimulus, but rather they have to detect the presence of a stimulus, minimizes retrieval biases in favor of one ear or the other (Voyer, 2003).

These characteristics make the target detection task ideal for an accurate assessment of laterality effects. Voyer (2003) showed that the verbal component of this task has a high level of reliability and validity. Specifically, Voyer (2003) used the Bryden and MacRae (1989) task in three different conditions: free recall (participants reported both stimuli in a dichotic pair), focused attention (participants reported only the stimulus presented to a pre-specified ear) and target detection. Results showed that target detection produced the largest magnitude of laterality effect among the three procedures. In addition, its validity was quite high, as illustrated by the fact that as many as 95% of participants showed an REA. Finally, a test-retest reliability of .78 was observed for the laterality effect. As previously mentioned, Voyer et al. (2002) and Voyer and Rodgers (2002) showed that the non-verbal component of this task is also relatively reliable when administered under target detection. These findings make the target detection task proposed by Bryden and MacRae (1989) an ideal candidate for computer application. Although the Bryden and MacRae (1989) task was developed for the separate assessment of verbal and non-verbal laterality effects with the same material, it has been shown that these two components are independent from each other (Bulman-Fleming and Bryden, 1994). The independence of the two components integrated in this task makes it legitimate to focus on these aspects separately. Accordingly, the verbal aspect was examined in Experiment 1 and the non-verbal component was the object of Experiment 2.

The comparison of a dichotic listening task administered on tape with one administered by computer has never been performed. Thus, in view of the exploratory and descriptive nature of the present study, no predictions based on past research can be made concerning its outcome. In addition, small differences in reliability and validity can have a large impact in applied settings. This means that statistical findings that the tasks are similar (non-rejection of the null hypothesis) might be misleading. Thus, even though conventional tests of significance will be used, reliability and magnitude estimates will be interpreted as purely descriptive statistics.

EXPERIMENT 1: VERBAL TASK

Method

Participants

Forty right-handed undergraduate students (20 males, 20 females) were recruited from introductory psychology classes. Twenty participants (10 males, 10 females) completed the taped target detection condition and 20 participants (10 females, 10 males) completed the computerized procedure. Each participant performed only one of the two versions of the task (computer or taped). Participants were all native English speakers, with an age range of 18 to

32 years, and all reported normal hearing in both ears. Participation was voluntary and rewarded with course credit.

Materials

Following the approach proposed by Bryden and MacRae (1989), the words bower, dower, power, and tower were pronounced by a male speaker with an angry, happy, neutral, or sad emotional tone, and were recorded with a sampling rate of 22 kHz on a microcomputer equipped with a 16-bit soundcard. The stimuli were equated to a length of 550-msec and an intensity of 70 dB (as measured with a General Radio sound pressure level meter). All possible combinations of words and emotions in each ear resulted in 144 possibilities without dichotic pairing of the same words or emotions. For both tasks, stimuli were presented through Koss TD-60 headphones.

For the taped version of the task, the resulting combinations were recorded with an ITI of six seconds. Recording and playback were accomplished on a Fisher audiocassette recorder model CR-9005 with Dolby® noise reduction. A program written in MEL Professional Version 2.0 code (Schneider, 1995) was used to pace trial presentation during recording. A headphone amplifier (Edcor model 400 HD) was utilized to ensure that sound intensity was at the assigned level.

For the computer version of the task, a program written in MEL Professional Version 2.0 code was used to present the stimuli and to record responses. Participants were tested on microcomputers equipped with a Creative Labs Soundblaster™ 16 soundcard. Software and hardware amplification were used to ensure that sound intensity was at the assigned level.

The Waterloo Handedness Questionnaire (Steenhuis and Bryden, 1989) was used to measure hand preference. This questionnaire consists of 32 statements concerning hand preference for specific activities. It results in a score ranging from –64 (completely left-handed) to +64 (completely right-handed).

Procedure

Participants were tested in groups of at most three in a quiet room especially designed for auditory testing. Following the approach used by Bryden and MacRae (1989), a target detection task, in which participants reported the presence of a specific target word (bower, dower, power, or tower), was utilized. For the taped task, participants were seated in a small cubicle and they circled the appropriate answer (yes or no) in a response booklet. The target was written at the top of each page in the booklet and there were 36 trials per page. For the computer task, participants were seated individually in front of a computer and they responded by depressing a key on a standard computer keyboard. The response screen presented the target word (e.g., Target = BOWER) and reminded participants of the keys used in response production. Half the participants depressed the "1" key for yes responses and the "0" key for no responses. The remaining participants had the opposite key arrangement. After the response was entered, feedback concerning response accuracy was presented on the top left corner of the computer screen ("correct response" in a blue frame or "wrong response" in a red frame). Participants were then instructed to depress the spacebar for the next trial.

In both tasks, participants performed four practice trials, followed by two blocks of 72 trials, separated by a 40 seconds break. They then completed the Waterloo Handedness Questionnaire. This was followed by another run of two blocks of 72 trials, separated by a 40 seconds break. The first set of 144 trials constituted the first testing session, whereas the second set of 144 trials was the second testing session. The designation of two testing sessions allowed the calculation of a test-retest reliability estimate (i.e., the correlation of performance between two administrations of the same task). The only dependent variable available for the taped procedure was the percentage of correct responses. For the computer version, both accuracy and response time (in ms) were recorded.

From the total of 144 trials in each session for both tasks, the target was presented to the left ear on 36 trials and to the right ear on 36 trials. On 72 trials, the target was absent and a "no" response was required. These are labeled as "correct negative responses". Of course, ear of presentation is not relevant for correct negative responses as they represent cases where the target was absent. Finally, in the taped task, stimuli were presented in two different randomized orders (one order specific to each session), whereas trial order was randomized across participants in the computer task.

In both tasks, participants were instructed to switch the side of the headphones after each set of 72 trials in an ABBA fashion to avoid confounding effects due to the possibility that the sound coming out of the left and right headphones might vary in intensity. For example, when a participant started with the right headphone on the right ear for the first block, he/she would have the left headphone on the right ear for the second and third block, and would switch back to the initial arrangement for the fourth block. In both procedures, half the participants started with the right headphone on the right ear, while the other half began with the left headphone on the right ear. Headphone arrangement was therefore completely counterbalanced across testing sessions in both tasks.

In both procedures, each participant had the same specific target word for the duration of the experiment. The target was randomized across participants in such a way that each of the four words was represented equally often.

Data obtained on the Waterloo Handedness Questionnaire confirmed that all participants were right handed. Specifically, this questionnaire produced a range of scores from 2 to 64 (mean WHQ score = 37.40; SD = 13.21).

Results

In consideration of the wide range of scores obtained on the Waterloo Handedness Questionnaire, preliminary analyses were computed to ensure that the effect of the testing procedure and sex of participants variables were not confounded by variations in the degree of right-handedness. Accordingly, an analysis of variance with testing procedure (on tape or on computer) and sex as independent variables and Waterloo Handedness Questionnaire score as dependent variable was computed. This analysis showed that the Waterloo Handedness Questionnaire scores did not differ significantly between procedures ($p > .52$) and sex ($p > .37$), and that no interaction between these variables was present ($p > .59$). In addition, data obtained on accuracy in both procedures and response time in the computer task showed that Waterloo Handedness Questionnaire scores did not correlate significantly with overall performance and laterality index (as defined below) obtained in either sessions (smallest $p > .20$).

The main data analysis involved three distinct approaches. First test-retest correlations were calculated for each ear, for correct negative responses, and for the laterality effects.

Second, a mixed design analysis of variance was computed. Finally, the percentage of REA was examined in each procedure. The results are presented separately for each of these approaches.

Test-Retest Correlations

Test-retest correlations for the left and right ears, and for correct negative responses were calculated on the percentage of correct responses for both procedures and on reaction time (in ms) for the computer procedure, as presented in Table 1. The data presented in Table 1 suggest that reliability is generally satisfactory (i.e., statistically significant), except for the left ear accuracy in the computer version of the task. Comparison of the test-retest correlations obtained on the percentage of correct responses between the two procedures indicated that the correlation was significantly larger in the taped version than in the computer version for both the left, $z = 2.67$, $p < .05$, and the right ear, $z = 2.43$, $p < .05$. The two procedures did not differ in their reliability when correct negative responses were considered, $z = 1.30$, ns. It is also worth noting that the reliability for accuracy and reaction time data was statistically similar in the computer task (largest $z = 1.15$, ns).

Table 1. Test-Retest Correlations as a Function of Ear of Presentation and Procedure for the Percentage of Correct Responses and Reaction Time (ms; in parentheses) in Experiment 1

•	Procedure	•	Left Ear	•	Right Ear	•	Correct Negative	•	Laterality Effect
•	Computer	•	0.36 (0.65*)	•	0.53* (0.55*)	•	0.63* (0.76*)	•	0.66* (0.15)
•	Taped	•	0.86*	•	0.89*	•	0.83*	•	0.78*

Note: Reaction time data were collected only in the computer procedure.
* p < .05

A test-retest correlation was also calculated on the laterality effect. A simple measure of laterality consisting of performance for the right ear minus performance for the left ear was used for this purpose on both accuracy and reaction time. This laterality index is generally considered valid (Hiscock et al., 2000). The results of this analysis, also presented in Table 1, indicated that, on the accuracy measure, the test-retest correlation was significant for the both procedures. In fact, the correlation obtained in the taped procedure was statistically similar to that obtained in the computer task, $z = 0.83$, ns. For reaction time, the laterality index produced a non-significant test-retest correlation (see Table 1).

Analysis of Variance: Accuracy Data

Ear Analysis: The percentage of correct responses was subjected to a mixed design analysis of variance with ear of presentation, testing session, sex of the participants, and procedure as independent variables. This analysis revealed a significant main effect for ear of presentation, $F(1,36) = 29.16$, $p < .05$, reflecting an overall REA (see Table 2). Cohen's

(1977) d was calculated for each of the two procedures by dividing the difference between the scores of the two ears by the pooled standard deviation. These calculations revealed that the laterality effect obtained in the present study represented an effect size of 0.62 standard deviation units in the computer procedure and 1.02 in the taped procedure (overall $d = .82$).

A significant interaction between sex, session, and ear of presentation was also observed, $F(1,36) = 5.01$, $p < .05$. Simple main effect analyses of this interaction revealed that the ear effect was significant in all sex by session combinations [men, session 1: $F(1,36) = 7.65$, $p <$ .05, $\eta^2 = .18$; men, session 2: $F(1,36) = 7.81$, $p < .05$, $\eta^2 = .18$; women, session 1: $F(1,36) = 10.02$, $p < .05$, $\eta^2 = .22$; and women, session 2: $F(1,36) = 34.95$, $p < .05$, $\eta^2 = .49$]. However, examination of the percentage of variance accounted for by the ear effect through eta squared (η^2) suggests that women obtained a larger laterality effect in session 2 than in session 1. All other main effects and interactions did not achieve statistical significance at the .05 level.

Table 2. **Mean Percentage of Correct Responses with Standard Deviation (in parentheses) as a Function of Sex, Ear of Presentation, Testing Session, and Procedure in Experiment 1**

Procedure	Left Ear	Right Ear	Correct Negative
Computer			
Session 1			
Men	62.6 (14.2)	71.4 (14.3)	60.6 (15.
Women	60.4 (13.2)	70.2 (17.9)	58.2 (10.6)
Session 2			
Men	69.4 (6.5)	74.7 (14.5)	66.1 (15.5)
Women	61.2 (9.9)	75.8 (9.3)	61.0 (8.5)
Taped			
Session 1			
Men	61.9 (19.3)	74.9 (20.1)	80.4 (10.9)
Women	54.3 (17.3)	69.7 (18.7)	75.4 (11.9)
Session 2			
Men	62.4 (16.3)	74.7 (20.3)	80.9 (11.2)
Women	51.2 (14.9)	73.9 (16.5)	76.7 (23.4)
Overall	60.4 (14.1)	73.1 (15.8)	69.9 (16.2)

Correct Negative Responses: A mixed design analysis of variance with session, procedure, and sex as independent variables was computed on the percentage of correct negative responses. This analysis revealed a significant effect of procedure, $F(1,36) = 16.90$, $p < .05$. Examination of the relevant data in Table 2 indicates that the percentage of correct negatives was significantly greater on the taped task compared to the computer task. No other main effects or interactions achieved statistical significance at the .05 level.

Analysis of Variance: Reaction Time

Ear Analysis: Reaction time data obtained on the computer procedure were subjected to a mixed-design analysis of variance with ear of presentation, testing session, and sex as independent variables. Results of this analysis revealed only a significant effect of session,

$F(1,18) = 35.19, p < .05$, reflecting faster performance in session 2 ($M = 490.99$ ms; $SD = 133.02$) compared to session 1 ($M = 654.53$ ms; $SD = 213.90$).

Correct Negative Responses: A mixed design analysis of variance with session and sex as independent variables was also computed on the reaction time for correct negative responses. This analysis revealed a significant effect of session, $F(1,18) = 29.71, p < .05$, which was qualified by a significant interaction between session and sex, $F(1,18) = 6.66, p < .05$. Simple effect analyses indicated that, although the effect of session was significant in both men, $F(1,18) = 11.73, p < .05$, and women, $F(1,18) = 5.03, p < .05$, the magnitude of the F test suggests that the effect of session was more pronounced in men than in women. The means indicate that reaction time was faster in session 2 than in session 1 for men (Session 1: $M = 689.12$ ms, $SD = 220.66$; Session 2: $M = 475.67$ ms, $SD = 103.84$) and women (Session 1: $M = 642.61$ ms, $SD = 199.51$; Session 2: $M = 566.34$ ms, $SD = 160.34$). No other effects achieved statistical significance at the .05 level.

Percentage of Reas

The percentage of participants showing an REA in each testing procedure is presented in Table 3. A participant was classified as showing an REA when the percentage of correct responses for the right ear minus the percentage of correct responses for the left ear was greater than one, following the criterion used by Hiscock et al. (2000). Only one participant (5%) showed no ear advantage (right minus left between -1 and +1) in session 1 of the computer version, but showed an REA in session 2. The remaining participants showed an LEA (right minus left < -1).

Table 3. Percentage of Participants Showing a Right Ear Advantage (REA) and a Left Ear Advantage (LEA) as a Function of Testing Session and Procedure in Experiment 1

Procedure	Session 1		Session2	
	LEA	REA	LEA	REA
Computer	12.5	70.0	10.0	80.0
Taped	7.5	85.0	5.0	95.0

Note. A right ear advantage is defined as a case where accuracy for the right ear minus accuracy for the left ear is greater than 1.

Examination of Table 3 indicates that the largest percentage of participants showing an REA was 95%, in session 2 of the taped procedure. In both procedures, the percentage was relatively large, although it was larger in the taped task than in the computer version. However, the distribution of ear advantages was not statistically different in the two procedures for both sessions [session 1: $\chi^2 (2) = 1.79$, ns; session 2: $\chi^2 (2) = 2.06$, ns]. Finally, the overall percentage of REAs collapsed across procedures was 77.5% in session 1 and 87.5% in session 2.

Discussion

Experiment 1 compared the reliability and magnitude of verbal laterality effects under two testing procedures with the same task. When statistical significance was considered, the only procedure differences were found on the larger test-retest reliability for the separate ear scores, as well as the better performance on correct negative responses for the taped task. Although the taped task generally produced a percentage of REAs closer to that obtained on the IAT, both appear to be equally valid, as indicated by the absence of significant differences on the percentage of REA. Thus, it is legitimate to state that, from a statistical perspective, the taped and computer versions appear to be equally valid and reliable. However, when one considers the actual magnitude of the laterality effect and the test-retest correlation as well as the percentage of REA, the data suggest that the recorded version of the task produced larger, more reliable, and more valid laterality effects than the computer task. In fact, if one were to use such a task for applied or research purpose, the taped task would clearly provide better measurement, despite the absence of significant differences when compared to the computer task. This suggests that there are ways in which the computer task could be improved to promote better reliability and validity. However, before these possibilities are discussed, Experiment 2 will determine whether the findings obtained in Experiment 1 extend to a non-verbal task.

EXPERIMENT 2: NON-VERBAL TASK

Method

Participants

As in Experiment 1, 40 right-handed undergraduate students (19 males, 21 females) were recruited from introductory psychology classes. Twenty participants (9 males, 11 females) completed the taped target detection condition and 20 participants (10 females, 10 males) completed the computerized procedure. Each participant performed only one of the two versions of the task (computer or taped) and none of the participants were involved in Experiment 1. Participants were all native English speakers, with an age range of 18 to 32 years, and all reported normal hearing in both ears. Participation was voluntary and rewarded with course credit.

Materials and Procedure

Materials and procedure were the same as in Experiment 1 except for the following changes. Participants were tested individually in both procedures. In the taped procedure, participants listened to the stimuli by means of a Sanyo audiocassette player (model C15) through Koss TD-60 headphones. They were required to indicate whether a target emotion was presented. Other aspects of the task were the same as in Experiment 1.

Data obtained on the Waterloo Handedness Questionnaire confirmed that all participants were right handed. Specifically, this questionnaire produced a range of scores from 22 to 64 (mean WHQ score = 38.68; SD = 11.12).

Results

As in Experiment 1, preliminary analyses were computed to ensure that testing procedure and sex of participants were not confounded with variations in the degree of right-handedness. Accordingly, an analysis of variance with testing procedure (on tape or on computer) and sex as independent variables and Waterloo Handedness Questionnaire score as dependent variable was computed. This analysis showed that the Waterloo Handedness Questionnaire scores did not differ significantly between procedures ($p > .29$) and that no interaction between these variables was present ($p > .90$). However, there was a significant main effect of sex, $F(1,36) = 7.76$, $p < .01$. This reflected the findings that, on average, females ($M = 42.95$; $SD = 11.76$) scored higher than males ($M = 33.95$; $SD = 8.32$) on the Waterloo Handedness Questionnaire. In addition, data obtained on accuracy in both procedures and response time in the computer task showed that Waterloo Handedness Questionnaire scores correlated significantly with right ear accuracy in both sessions ($r = -.49$, $p < .01$ in session 1; $r = -.38$, $p < .05$ in session 2) and with the laterality index for accuracy in both sessions ($r = .32$, $p < .05$ in session 1; $r = .43$, $p < .01$ in session 2). In view of these findings, the score on the Waterloo Handedness Questionnaire was used as a covariate in the analysis of variance on accuracy data.

As in Experiment 1, the main data analysis involved the calculation of test-retest correlations for each ear, for correct negative responses, and for the laterality effects. A mixed design analysis of variance was also computed. Finally, the percentage of REA and LEA was examined in each procedure.

Test-Retest Correlations

Test-retest correlations for the left and right ears, and for correct negative responses are presented in Table 4. The data presented in Table 4 suggest that reliability is satisfactory (i.e., statistically significant) in all cases. Comparison of the test-retest correlations obtained on the percentage of correct responses for the left and right ears, and for correct negative responses indicated that the correlations were statistically similar in both procedures in all cases (largest $z = 0.38$, ns). As in Experiment 1, the reliability for accuracy and reaction time data was statistically similar in the computer task (largest $z = 1.25$, ns).

Table 4. Test-Retest Correlations as a Function of Ear of Presentation and Procedure for the Percentage of Correct Responses and Reaction Time (ms; in parentheses) for Experiment 2

Procedure	Left Ear	Right Ear	Correct Negative	Laterality Effect
Computer	.51* (0.66*)	.86* (0.83*)	.68* (0.85*)	.77* (-.37)
Taped	.60*	.86*	.75*	.73*

Note: Reaction time data were collected only in the computer procedure.
* $p < .05$

A test-retest correlation was also calculated on the laterality effect. The laterality index was calculated as in Experiment 1, but in such a way that a positive score reflected an LEA. The results of this analysis, also presented in Table 5, indicated that, on the accuracy measure, the test-retest correlation was significant for both procedures and the correlation obtained in the taped procedure was statistically similar to that obtained in the computer task, $z = 0.07$, ns. For reaction time, the laterality index produced a non-significant negative test-retest correlation (see Table 4).

Analysis of Variance: Accuracy Data

Ear Analysis: The percentage of correct responses was subjected to a mixed design analysis of variance with ear of presentation, testing session, sex of the participants, and procedure as independent variables with Waterloo Handedness Questionnaire scores as covariate. This analysis revealed a significant main effect for ear of presentation, $F(1,35) = 5.35$, $p < .05$, reflecting an overall LEA (see Table 5). Cohen's (1977) d was calculated for each of the two procedures by dividing the difference between the scores of the two ears by the pooled standard deviation. These calculations revealed that the laterality effect obtained in the present study represented an effect size of 0.37 standard deviation units in the computer procedure and 0.25 in the taped procedure (overall $d = .31$).

A significant interaction between sex, procedure, and ear of presentation was also observed, $F(1,35) = 6.62$, $p < .05$. Relevant means are found in Table 5. Simple main effect analyses of this interaction revealed that the sex by ear interaction was significant in the computer task, $F(1,35) = 5.46$, $p < .05$, but not on the taped task, $F(1,35) = 1.25$, ns. Further simple main effect analyses on the computer task revealed a significant LEA in females, $F(1,35) = 6.79$, $p < .02$, but not in males, $F(1,35) < 1$.

Table 5. Mean Percentage of Correct Responses with Standard Deviation (in parentheses) as a Function of Sex, Ear of Presentation, Testing Session, and Procedure in Experiment 2

Procedure	Left Ear	Right Ear	Correct Negatives
Computer			
Session 1			
Men	87.3 (16.4)	94.9 (7.5)	93.9 (5.8)
Women	89.4 (10.9)	74.4 (22.6)	85.9 (15.1)
Session 2			
Men	96.0 (5.3)	96.6 (6.3)	95.8 (5.6)
Women	96.5 (4.4)	86.3 (12.2)	93.9 (9.6)
Taped			
Session 1			
Men	91.5 (8.1)	84.7 (14.4)	94.4 (6.9)
Women	89.7 (16.4)	86.6 (18.4)	92.6 (13.5)
Session 2			
Men	87.0 (7.8)	87.7 (14.2)	92.1 (5.9)
Women	86.1 (15.0)	88.1 (15.2)	94.8 (10.6)
Overall	90.4 (11.7)	87.5 (15.2)	92.9 (9.7)

Correct Negative Responses: A mixed design analysis of variance with session, procedure, and sex as independent variables was computed on the percentage of correct negative responses. This analysis revealed significant main effects of procedure, $F(1,36) = 4.84$, $p < .05$, and session, $F(1,36) = 4.52$, $p < .05$. However, these main effects were qualified by a significant interaction between procedure and session, $F(1,36) = 4.26$, $p < .05$. Simple main effects analyses revealed a significant effect of session on the computer task, $F(1,36) = 8.33$, $p < .01$, but not on the taped task, $F(1,36) < 1$. Means reflect a significant increase in the percentage of correct negative responses from session 1 (M = 89.9%; SD = 11.26) to session 2 (M = 94.9%; SD = 8.36) in the computer task. Performance was statistically similar in both session for the taped task (Session 1: M = 93.5%; SD = 11.3; Session 2: M = 93.5%; SD = 8.40). No other main effects or interactions achieved statistical significance at the .05 level.

Analysis of Variance: Reaction Time

Ear Analysis: Reaction time data obtained on the computer procedure were subjected to a mixed-design analysis of variance with ear of presentation, testing session, and sex as independent variables. Results of this analysis revealed a significant effect of session, $F(1,18)$ = 36.31, $p < .01$, reflecting faster performance in session 2 (M = 632.03 ms; SD = 352.00) compared to session 1 (M = 940.23 ms; SD = 546.98).

Correct Negative Responses: A mixed design analysis of variance with session and sex as independent variables was also computed on the reaction time for correct negative responses. This analysis revealed a significant effect of session, $F(1,18) = 15.81$, $p < .01$, reflecting faster performance in session 2 (M = 661.85 ms; SD = 300.48) compared to session 1 (M = 986.55 ms; SD = 584.89). No other effects achieved statistical significance at the .05 level.

Percentage of Leas

The percentage of participants showing an LEA in each testing procedure is presented in Table 6. A participant was classified as showing an LEA when the percentage of correct responses for the left ear minus the percentage of correct responses for the right ear was greater than one, following the criterion used in Experiment 1. Remaining participants showed an REA (left minus right smaller than -1), or no ear advantage (left minus right between -1 and +1).

Table 6. Percentage of Participants Showing a Right Ear Advantage (REA) and a Left Ear Advantage (LEA) as a Function of Testing Session and Procedure in Experiment 2

Procedure	Session 1		Session 2	
	LEA	REA	LEA	REA
Computer	50.0	40.0	55.0	20.0
Taped	70.0	15.0	30.0	55.0

Examination of Table 6 indicates that the largest percentage of participants showing an LEA was 70%, in session 1 of the taped procedure. In both procedures, the percentage was relatively small, although the taped task showed more fluctuation than the computer version. In fact, there majority of participants showed an LEA in session 1 in the taped task, but this was reversed in session 2, with a slight majority (55%) showing an REA in session 2. However, the distribution of ear advantages was not statistically different in the two procedures for both sessions [session 1: χ^2 (2) = 3.14, ns; session 2: χ^2 (2) = 5.24, ns]. Finally, the overall percentage of LEAs collapsed across procedures was 60.0% in session 1 and 42.5% in session 2.

Supplemental Analysis

Results from both experiments revealed a significant main effect of procedure on correct negative response. Essentially, participants produced more correct negative responses for the taped version than for the computer task (see Table 2 and 5). This indicates that participants produced more false alarms (responding "yes" when the target was not presented) in the computer task than in the taped task. This suggests the possibility of response bias differences between the procedures. From this perspective, the elevated false alarm rate in the computer task might reflect the fact that participants possibly used a more lax criterion in that task than in the taped version. This possibility was examined by means of a nonparametric signal detection analysis (see McNicol, 1972). Correct responses to the left and right ear were used as hits, whereas one minus the rate of correct negative responses was utilized as the false alarm rate in calculating β', an index of response bias. A positive value of this index reflects a lax criterion (high propensity to say "yes"), whereas a positive value reflects a strict criterion (greater reluctance to say "yes"). A mixed design analysis of variance with material (verbal, non-verbal), procedure (taped, computer), and testing session as independent variables was computed with β' as dependent variable. Results only showed a significant main effect of procedure, $F(1, 76) = 5.58$, $p < .05$. The means relevant to this analysis indicated that the computer task produced a more lax criterion (mean $\beta' = -0.031$, $SD = 0.289$) than the taped task (mean $\beta' = 0.141$, $SD = 0.356$), regardless of material.

Discussion

Experiment 2 attempted to extend the findings of Experiment 1 to a non-verbal task. Here, when statistical significance was considered, the versions of the task appeared to be similar in terms of test-retest reliability and validity. However, the magnitude of the LEA varied as a function of procedure since it was found to be significant only in females on the computer task. This suggests that the taped task might provide a better assessment tool. However, the computer task seemed to be more stable over testing sessions in terms of percentage of LEA, although the percentages were very similar for both task when collapsed across session (52.5% LEA for the computer task; 50% LEA for the taped task). Finally, the test-retest reliability estimates were generally quite similar, with the taped task showing an advantage in two out of four values (left ear, correct negative) and the computer task showing a slight advantage for the laterality effect. In summary, the two tasks seem quite similar even when one disregards the outcomes of significance testing for the comparison of reliability and validity estimates. However, the fact that the LEA was found only in women on the computer task recommends against its use in applied and experimental settings since it does not allow generalization across the sexes.

GENERAL DISCUSSION

The purpose of the present study was to compare the reliability and validity of dichotic listening tasks administered either under the conventional pre-recorded format or directly on a computer. Two experiments were conducted with the exact same material, in which the verbal (words) and non-verbal (emotions) components were integrated in the same stimuli. Experiment 1 considered the verbal component, whereas Experiment 2 presented data obtained with the non-verbal component. Significance testing generally suggested that in both experiments, the two versions of the task are quite similar in terms of magnitude, test-retest reliability, and validity of laterality effects, although the computer task produced a significant LEA only in females in Experiment 2.

Given that the differences in reliability might be of great importance, particularly in applied settings, it is worthwhile to explore any difference between the two versions of the tasks without regard for the outcome of significance testing. From this perspective, one is compelled to conclude that the taped version is likely more appropriate than the computer version for the reliable and valid assessment of laterality effects. Specifically, the verbal task in Experiment 1 clearly produced a greater magnitude of effect, as well as larger test retest reliability, and percentage of REAs than the computer task. Although the results on the non-verbal task, in Experiment 2, were not as clear cut as on the verbal task, in Experiment 1, our findings nevertheless suggest that the taped task might be perceived as a better assessment method just based on the fact that, unlike the computer task, it did not produce a significant sex by ear of presentation interaction. In addition, since most researchers are likely to use only one testing session, the finding that 70% of participants showed an LEA in session 1 of the taped task is in its favor.

At this point, one might wonder why a repeated measures design in which participants completed both the taped task and its computer counterpart was not used in the present study. This would allow a more direct comparison of the results while minimizing the influence of differences between samples. In fact, with the current approach, it is not possible to determine whether procedural differences are due to sample effects or real procedural differences. However, the test-retest administration of the two versions of the task to the same group of participants would obviously require a longer testing period than that required with the approach used here. It is quite likely that fatigue and boredom would increasingly influence the results as testing progressed, possibly resulting in lower estimates of reliability. In fact, such repeated measures designs have been claimed to produce erratic results in laterality experiments (Russell and Voyer, 2004). From this perspective, it thus appears that, although the procedure used here could be improved, it likely minimized the influence of factors extraneous to the laterality effects, such as fatigue or participants attrition.

The results of the present study underline at least two aspects regarding the reliability and validity of the tasks considered here that require further discussion. First, the taped task appears to provide a better assessment of laterality effects. Second, the results on the verbal task are clearer than on the non-verbal task.

Considering the apparent psychometric superiority of the taped task over the computer version, it is interesting to note that many of the advantages of the computer task presented earlier constitute critical differences that might lead one to expect variations in reliability between the two procedures. Specifically, factors such as the response mode and the added participants control implied by the use of a computer could be used to explain task differences. For example, Bryden (1978) argued that leaving participants in control of aspects of a task might lead to variability in laterality effects. Even though Bryden was discussing specifically attention control, it is plausible to believe that his arguments are likely to apply to other aspects of the task. Essentially, leaving participants in control of when the next trial occurs, for example, possibly produces variation across participants in terms of task content. Essentially, this makes task administration non-standardized and might affect reliability.

The main effect of procedure on correct negative responses, reflecting an advantage for the taped procedure over the computer task (see Tables 2 and 5) is one finding that clearly suggests possible differences between the two versions of the task. This finding suggests that participants produced more false alarms (incorrectly responding "yes") in the computer task than in the taped procedure. It would be possible that this is the result of speeded responses in the computer task, since participants' ability to control when the next trial occurred in the computer task allowed them to speed their response, resulting in potential speed-accuracy tradeoffs. In contrast, participants had to wait for the ITI to elapse before presentation of the next trial in the taped task, thus reducing the possible influence of tradeoffs. However, considering that reaction time did not produce significant findings involving ear of presentation, such tradeoffs are unlikely.

The clear difference in response bias between the two procedures regardless of material provides a more plausible basis to explain the effect of procedure on correct negative responses. Specifically, results of the supplemental analysis indicated that participants used a more lax criterion in the computer task than in the taped version. Considering that feedback has been shown to affect how one makes decisions in various tasks (see, for example, Erev, 1998; Shanks, Tunney, and McCarthy, 2002), this finding most likely stemmed from the presence of feedback in the computer task. In fact, Shanks et al. (2002) showed that participants optimized their performance to reflect underlying response probability faster with than without feedback. This suggests the possibility that participants reached different conclusions concerning the distribution of responses in the two versions of the task. To help in understanding this point, the data were collapsed across ear of presentation to produce a "correct positive response" variable that can be directly compared to correct negatives. Results of this operation are presented in Table 7. An obvious observation arising from these data is that the percentage of correct negative responses for the taped task is an outlier in relation to the other means in this table. In fact, these data produced significantly more correct negative responses than correct positive responses in the taped task, $F(1,78) = 13.51, p < .01$, but not in the computer task, $F(1,78) < 1$. Thus, in signal detection terms, the findings actually reflect an inflated number of correct rejections (deflated number of false alarms) for the taped task. This suggests that, in the absence of feedback, participants possibly favored "no" responses when uncertain whether the target had been presented in the taped task, leading to an inflated number of correct rejections. In contrast, the feedback provided in the computer task allowed participants to reach correct conclusions concerning the distribution of "yes" and "no" responses, leading to a similar number of correct positive and negative responses in that task. This explanation also accounts for the somewhat lower percentage of hits in the taped task (see Table 7). Specifically, if there is a greater tendency to say "no" in the taped task than in the computer task, this bias should manifest itself as a greater number of misses (fewer hits) as well. The data in Table 7 support this point by showing fewer correct positive responses for the taped task than for the computer task, although this difference is not significant. Taken together, the results suggest that participants tried to maximize their performance for correct negative responses at the expense of correct positive responses only in the taped task. This cannot be explained as a sample specific finding as it occurred in both experiments. Nevertheless, since the presence of feedback in the computer task is the only factor that can plausibly account for this finding, it is quite likely that removal of feedback would eliminate this effect. However, this remains an empirical question.

Table 7. Percentage of Correct Positive and Negative Responses with Standard Deviation (in parentheses) as a Function of Procedure

Procedure	Correct Positive	Correct Negative
Computer	79.2 (14.1)	76.9 (18.7)
Taped	76.5 (17.7)	85.9 (14.0)

Note. Correct positive responses reflect performance collapsed across ear of presentation.

A point that requires some discussion in the present study is that the computer task was shorter in duration than the taped version in both experiments. Specifically, the taped version had a fixed duration, guided by stimulus duration (550 ms), ITI (6 seconds), the number of trials (144), and the 40 seconds break, for a total of 16 minutes 24 seconds required for the completion of one session. Although stimulus duration, duration of the break, and number of trials were the same in both tasks, the ITI varied in the computer task because it was controlled by the participants to some extent. Unfortunately, total task duration was not directly recorded for individual participants in the computer task. However, it is possible to estimate total task duration by considering the average reaction time of 682.87 ms on each trial (averaged across the two experiments), plus a conservative estimate of 3.0 seconds for feedback and to perform the spacebar press required for trial presentation. This results in an approximate average total of 9 minutes and 30 seconds for completion of the 144 trials in one session in the computer task, including the 40 seconds break. Although this difference cannot be tested for statistical significance, it is plausible to argue that, because the computer task took nearly half the time required in the taped task, some aspects relevant to boredom and fatigue might be attenuated. In fact, the experimenter observed that several participants manifested discontent at the length of the ITI in the taped task (e.g., by complaining about it upon debriefing). Thus, it is likely that the shorter length of the computer task and the added sense of control are advantageous in terms of its value as an assessment tool. However, one has to weigh these advantages against possible loss of psychometric qualities. The results suggest that the advantages of the computer task in terms of administration did not translate into advantages in terms of reliability and validity.

The above discussion makes it quite clear that that the computer version of the task could be further improved. For example, it seems plausible to believe that removal of the feedback, in addition to eliminating response bias differences between versions of the task (as previously discussed), might further improve the sense of control and affect performance positively, considering that its presence did not make participants more accurate in the computer task. In addition, the extended response period in the taped task allowed participants enough time to change their response. This should be made possible in the computer task as well. Future work should also examine whether the fact that trials order was completely randomized in the computer task affected its psychometric properties in comparison with the taped task. This could be achieved by using the same order of trials in both tasks. The influence of the ITI could also be investigated by using a fixed ITI in the computer task in order to assess the role of this factor in observed findings. In any event, despite the fact that the computer task used here requires further improvements, it appears that computer testing has much potential for future research.

The second aspect emphasized by the present experiments, concerning the greater variability of the non-verbal task used in Experiment 2 compared to the verbal task used in

Experiment 1, has relevance beyond the research questions explored here. Specifically, laterality effects obtained with non-verbal tasks are generally smaller than those observed on verbal tasks (Voyer, 1996). This finding was clearly demonstrated here. In addition, previous work suggests that the use of non-verbal tasks in laterality experiments exposes one to highly variable results, even with the same participants, as illustrated by shifts in laterality effect (from a right hemisphere advantage to a left hemisphere advantage) with practice in lateralized mental rotation (Voyer, 1995) and shape recognition (Voyer, 2005). This suggests that cerebral specialization might involve more than a simple verbal/non-verbal dichotomy. In addition, shifts in laterality effects with non-verbal tasks as a result of practice suggest that functional literalities have a greater plasticity than what is generally believed (Goldberg and Costa, 1981).

A simple explanation for smaller laterality effects in non-verbal tasks compared to verbal tasks could lie in the fact that non-verbal tasks are often easier than verbal tasks. In the present study, the verbal task produced an overall accuracy of 67.8% (SD = 15.4), whereas the non-verbal task had an overall accuracy of 90.3% (SD = 12.2), reflecting a significantly better performance in the non-verbal task, $t(78) = 7.24$, $p < .05$. It is thus plausible to conclude, as was done by Voyer et al. (2002), that the smaller laterality effects observed in the non-verbal task are the result of ceiling effects. It is worth noting that the same observation was made by Mondor and Bryden (1992), although a manipulation of task difficulty in their study failed to increase the magnitude of the LEA. In fact, it produced a significant REA in one experimental condition. Mondor and Bryden (1992) concluded from this finding that there might actually be a generalized right ear bias, regardless of the task used. This would account quite well for reduced effects with non-verbal tasks. However, these findings require replication.

To conclude, the present study suggests that, on the basis of significance testing, taped and computer administration of verbal and non-verbal dichotic listening tasks produce similar results in terms of the magnitude, reliability, and validity of laterality effects. However, descriptive evaluation of the findings favors the taped tasks. More work is required to improve the psychometric qualities of computer administration while preserving the aspects that make this type of task advantageous for use in applied and experimental settings.

ACKNOWLEDGEMENTS

This study was funded by a grant from the Natural Sciences and Engineering Research Council of Canada to D. Voyer. The authors thank Pamela Lodge and Heather-Dawn Wood for their assistance with data collection and scoring. Correspondence should be sent to Daniel Voyer, Department of Psychology, University of New Brunswick, Bag Service #45444, Fredericton, New Brunswick, Canada, E3B 6E4. Telephone: (506) 453-4974. Fax: (506) 447-3063. E-mail: voyer@unb.ca.

REFERENCES

Broadbent, D. E. (1954). The role of auditory localization in attention and memory span. *Journal of Experimental Psychology, 47,* 191-196.

Bryden, M. P. (1988). An overview of the dichotic listening procedure and its relation to cerebral organization. In K. Hugdahl (Ed.), *Handbook of dichotic listening* (pp. 1-44). Chichester, England: John Wiley.

Bryden, M. P. (1978). Strategy effects in the assessment of hemispheric asymmetry. In G. Underwood (Ed.), *Strategies of information processing* (Pp. 117-149). London: Academic Press.

Bryden, M. P., and MacRae, L. (1989). Dichotic laterality effects obtained with emotional words. *Neuropsychiatry, Neuropsychology and Behavioral Neurology, 3,* 171-176.

Bulman-Fleming, M. B., and Bryden, M. P. (1994). Simultaneous verbal and affective laterality effects. *Neuropsychologia, 32,* 787-797.

Channon, S., Schugens, M. M., Daum, I., and Polkey, C. E. (1990). Lateralisation of language functioning by the Wada procedure and divided visual field presentation of a verbal task. *Cortex, 26,* 147-151.

Cohen, J. (1977). *Statistical power analysis for the behavioral sciences* (2nd Ed.). New York: Academic Press.

Duscheck, S., and Schandry, R. (2003). Functional transcranial Doppler sonography as a tool in psychophysiological research. *Psychophysiology, 40,* 436-454.

Erev, I. (1998). Signal detection by human observers: A cutoff reinforcement learning model of categorization decisions under uncertainty. *Psychological Review, 105,* 280-298.

Ghiselli, E. E. (1964). *Theory of psychological measurement.* New York: McGraw-Hill.

Goldberg, E. and Costa, L. D. (1981). Hemisphere differences in the acquisition and use of descriptive systems. *Brain and Language, 14,* 144-173.

Hiscock, M., Cole, L. C., Benthall, J. G., Carlson, V. L., and Ricketts, J. M. (2000). Toward solving the inferential problem in laterality research: Effects of increased reliability on the validity of the dichotic listening right-ear advantage. *Journal of the International Neuropsychological Society, 6,* 539-547.

Iaccino, J. F. (1993). *Left brain-right brain differences.* Hillsdale, NJ: Lawrence Erlbaum Associates.

Kimura, D. (1967). Functional asymmetry of the brain in dichotic listening. *Cortex, 22,* 163-178.

Kimura, D. (1961a). Cerebral dominance and the perception of verbal stimuli. *Canadian Journal of Psychology, 15,* 166-171.

Kimura, D. (1961b). Some effects of temporal lobe damage on auditory perception. *Canadian Journal of Psychology, 15,* 156-165.

McNicol, D. (1972). *A primer of signal detection theory.* London: Allen and Unwin.

Mondor, T. A., and Bryden, M. P. (1992). On the relation between auditory spatial attention and auditory perceptual asymmetries. *Perception and Psychophysics, 52,* 393-402.

Russell, N. L. and Voyer, D. (2004). Reliability of laterality effects in a dichotic listening task with words and syllables. *Brain and Cognition, 54,* 266-267.

Schneider, W. (1995). *Micro-Experimental Laboratory Version 2.0 user's guide.* Pittsburgh: Psychology Software Tools.

Schneider, W., Eschman, A., and Zuccolotto, A. (2002a). *E-Prime user's guide: Version 1.0.* Pittsburgh: Psychology Software Tools, Inc.

Schneider, W., Eschman, A., and Zuccolotto, A. (2002b). *E-Prime reference guide: Version 1.0.* Pittsburgh: Psychology Software Tools, Inc.

Shanks, D. R., Tunney, R. J., and McCarthy, J. D. (2002). A re-examination of probability matching and rational choice. *Journal of Behavioral Decision Making, 15,* 233-250.

Shtyrov, Y., Kujala, T., Lyytinen, H., Kujala, J., Ilmoniemi, R. J., and Näätänen, R. (2000). Lateralization of speech processing in the brain as indicated by mismatch negativity and dichotic listening. *Brain and Cognition, 43,* 392-398.

Steenhuis, R.E. and Bryden, M. P. (1989). Different dimensions of hand preference that relate to skilled and unskilled activities. *Cortex, 25,* 289-304.

Strauss, E., Gaddes, W., and Wada, J. (1987). Performance on a free recall verbal dichotic listening task and cerebral dominance determined by the carotid amytal test. *Neuropsychologia, 25,* 747-753.

Voyer, D. (2005). Reliability of non-verbal laterality effects in the visual modality. *Laterality, 10,* 37-50.

Voyer, D. (2003). Reliability and magnitude of perceptual asymmetries in a dichotic word recognition task. *Neuropsychology, 37,* 393-401.

Voyer, D. (1998). On the reliability and validity of noninvasive laterality measures. *Brain and Cognition, 36,* 209-236.

Voyer, D. (1996). On the magnitude of laterality effects and sex differences in functional brain asymmetries. *Laterality, 1,* 51-83.

Voyer, D. (1995). Effect of practice on laterality in a mental rotation task. *Brain and Cognition, 29,* 326-335.

Voyer, D., and Flight, J. (2001). Reliability and magnitude of auditory laterality effects: The influence of attention. *Brain and Cognition, 46,* 397-413.

Voyer, D., McGlone, J., and Savoie, J. (1996). Non-invasive predictors of laterality in speech production and comprehension. *Brain and Cognition, 32,* 125-128.

Voyer, D. and Rodgers, M. A. (2002). Reliability of laterality effects in a dichotic listening task with non-verbal material. *Brain and Cognition, 48,* 602-606.

Voyer, D., Russell, A., and McKenna, J. (2002). On the reliability of laterality effects in a dichotic emotion recognition task. *Journal of Clinical and Experimental Neuropsychology, 24,* 605-614.

Wada, J. (1949). A new method for the determination of the side of cerebral dominance. A preliminary report on the intracarotid injection of sodium amytal in man. *Medical Biology, 14,* 221-222.

Wexler, B. E. and Halwes, T. (1983). Increasing the power of dichotic methods: The fused rhymed words test. *Neuropsychologia, 21,* 59-66.

Zatorre, R. J. (1989). Perceptual asymmetry on the dichotic fused words test and cerebral speech lateralization determined by the carotid sodium amytal test. *Neuropsychologia, 27,* 1207-1219.

In: Focus on Neuropsychology Research
Editor: Joshua R. Dupri, pp. 163-184

ISBN 1-59454-779-3

Chapter 6

NEUROPSYCHOLOGY AND PSEUDO-MEMORIES

Maarten J. V. Peters, Marko Jelicic and Harald Merckelbach*
Maastricht University, The Netherlands

ABSTRACT

Although the power of memory is evident in various daily life experiences (e.g., personal history, knowledge of facts and concepts, and learning of complex skills), memory also has its fallible side. Memory experiences are encoded as separate pieces of a puzzle. At retrieval, this puzzle has to be reconstructed. This reconstruction makes our memory susceptible to distortions. Inspired by ongoing discussions about recovered memories, researchers have studied personality and social factors that make people vulnerable to memory distortions, including pseudo-memories. Recent studies highlight the role of higher cognitive functions in reconstructing our memories. This chapter aims to give an overview of the current state of affairs linking executive functions to pseudo-memories. Evidence from aging, lesion, and imaging studies (Positron Emission Tomography and functional Magnetic Resonance Imaging) will be discussed. Studies conducted in our laboratory also suggest that suboptimal inhibition, monitoring and working memory functions contribute to the development of pseudo-memories. Explaining and identifying the neural basis of pseudo-memories can be regarded as a promising and new domain within neuropsychology.

INTRODUCTION

Throughout history, memory has been described in terms of different metaphors: from a wax tablet (Plato) up to the popular computer metaphor in our times (Draaisma, 2000; Merckelbach and Wessel, 1998). Although the power of memory is evident in daily life, memory is imperfect (e.g., Kopelman, 2002; Schacter, 1999). Events and experiences may be

---

* Correspondence to: Maarten Peters; Maastricht University, The Netherlands; Faculty of Psychology; Department of Experimental Psychology; PO Box 616, 6200 MD; Maastricht, The Netherlands; m.peters@psychology.unimaas.nl; Telephone: +31(0)433884026; Fax: +31(0)433884196

remembered in a distorted way. Thus, for example, an eyewitness may remember a yellow taxi, when actually the taxi's colour was blue. This is what has been termed a distortion (Gudjonsson and Clare, 1995). Sometimes events are completely fabricated, as was the case with BH (see below). But even neuropsychologically intact people may make such commission errors. An example is the eyewitness who remembers a blue taxi, when in fact there was no taxi at all. Throughout this chapter, we will refer to this type of error as pseudo-memory although we are aware of the fact that the term "false memory" is more common. Regardless of terminology, an important point about distortions and commissions is that they make plain that the idea of memory as a reproductive entity, in which events are reproduced with photographical precision, does not hold. Instead, memory is reconstructive, precisely because events are encoded in an incomplete and fragmentized way. When retrieving an experience, different fragments have to be combined to form an entity. Almost 40 years ago, Neisser used the analogy of the palaeontologist when describing memory. He wrote: "Out of the few stored bone chips we remember a dinosaur" (Neisser, 1967, p. 285).

Over the last two decades, the reconstructive nature of memory has informed scientific and popular discussions about, for example, recovered memories of childhood sexual abuse (e.g., Loftus and Ketchman, 1994; Schacter, 2001). Until recently, neuropsychological research in this domain was limited to case studies of neurological patients with peculiar memory illusions (e.g., Parkin, Bindschaedler, Harsent, and Metzler, 1996). In recent years, inspired by ongoing debates about the "accuracy" of human memory and its legal implications (Koriat, Goldsmith, and Pansky, 2000; Loftus, 2003), there has been an increased interest in neurocognitive research on pseudo-memories. The introduction of modern imaging techniques such as functional Magnetic Resonance Imaging (fMRI) and Positron Emission Tomography (PET) has also stimulated new studies in this field (e.g., Kopelman, 1999; 2002; Schacter and Slotnick, 2004). One important antecedent of pseudo-memories is a breakdown in what has been termed, *source monitoring* (Johnson, Hashtroudi and Lindsay, 1993). Source monitoring is a mechanism that serves as a screening and controlling device for memory at retrieval. It refers to cognitive processes involved in determining the source of memory information. Recent neurocognitive findings localize this function in a network encompassing the prefrontal cortex. In this chapter, we will give an overview of past, present, and future developments in neuropsychological research on pseudo-memories. A recurring theme in our review of the literature is the importance of frontal lobes for memory. The reconstructive nature of memory becomes most compelling in case studies on patients with frontal lobe damage (e.g., Parkin et al., 1996; Schacter, Curran, Gallucio, Milberg, and Bates, 1996a; Delbecq-Derousne, Beauvois, and Shallice, 1990). The patients in these case studies had a tendency to falsely recognize non-presented stimuli as being previously presented (e.g., Parkin et al., 1996), misattributed the source of their memories (e.g., Janowsky, Shimamura, and Squire, 1989), or recollected fictitious events (e.g., Dalla Barba, 1993). Following the tradition of these case studies, we will briefly describe patient BH, who underwent a neuropsychological evaluation at our memory lab. We will use this case as the starting point for a more systematic analysis of the neuropsychology of pseudo-memories.

CASE BH

On February 19th 1985, at 3 a.m., two policemen find a confused man in the red light district of Amsterdam. He is unable to respond to questions and comments. The man makes an anxious impression, is disoriented in time, place, and person and finds himself in a state of mutism. A head injury is suspected. The police believe that he might have been involved in a fight. At the hospital, a CT scan is made, but no neuroanatomical abnormalities are detected. From March 1st until June the 20th 1985, BH stays in a psychiatric hospital. He still does not talk and communicates with other patients and clinicians by writing in French. Neurological examination shows no abnormalities, but his performance on several neuropsychological tests does suggest residual signs of brain damage. His main complaint is that he cannot remember anything before February 19th 1985. Nonetheless, BH is dismissed from hospital with a diagnosis of neurotic amnesia. Since that time, BH occasionally received psychotherapeutic treatments (among which hypnotherapy), but his memory complaints did not disappear.

During spring of 2002, we saw BH, who still had no autobiographical memory for events that took place prior to February 19th 1985. We administered a neuropsychological test battery and collected psychophysiological data. We found his most recent Full Scale IQ to be 110. His score on a long term verbal memory task (Auditory Verbal Learning Test; AVLT; Deelman, Brouwer, van Zomeren, and Saan, 1980) was excellent, but he performed poorly on a working memory task (i.e., digit span subtask of the Wechsler Adult Intelligence Scale; For a Dutch translation, see Stinissen, Willems, Coetsier, and Hulsman, 1970). His performance on the Trail Making Task (Reitan, 1958; Reitan and Wolfson, 1993), which is sensitive to frontal (i.e., executive) dysfunctions, was also very poor. He scored low on memory for famous events up until 1985 (e.g., Mayes, Downes, McDonald, Rooke, Sagar, and Meudell, 1994; Sanders and Warrington, 1971). However, his memory for news facts from 1985 through 2002 was intact. His score on the SIMS (Structured Inventory of Malingered Symptomatology; Merckelbach and Smith, 2003) was above the cut off, indicating the tendency to endorse bizarre and rare symptoms. Patient BH did not show any autonomic responsivity (heart rate, skin conductance) during trials on which relevant information pertaining to his past or present state (e.g., the name of his mother) was presented. During an interview, three further features became apparent: A paresis on the left side of his body, an indifferent attitude, and a tendency to react with confabulatory responses. That is, when presented with fictitious names, BH produced bizarre confabulations that include these names.

As said, CT scans performed during the mid eighties did not reveal any abnormalities in the brain of BH. It should be noted though that a normal CT scan does not rule out the presence of prefrontal brain dysfunction. There are several examples in the literature where patients with normal CT scans had brain dysfunction that became only apparent when other neuroimaging techniques were used (e.g., Kopelman, Green, Guinan, Lewis, and Stanhope, 1994; Reed, Marsden, Lasseron, Sheldon, Lewis, Stanhope, Guinan, and Kopelman, 1999). Our patient's working memory impairments, his deficits in executive functions, and his tendency to confabulate clearly indicate right prefrontal cortex damage (see also Weinstein, 1996; Kopelman, 1999). BH's left sided paresis further support this interpretation. His autonomic hyporesponsivity is consistent with damage to the right dorsolateral prefrontal cortex (Tranel and Damasio, 1994; Caltagirone, Zoccolotti, Originale, Daniele, and Mammucari, 1989; Zocollotti, Scabini, and Violani, 1982).

The case of BH demonstrates the importance of the prefrontal cortex for accurate recall of past events. Damage to this region of the brain may lead to confabulations – one particular type of pseudo-memories. What more can neuropsychology tell us about the creation of pseudo-memories? It is to this issue that we now turn.

PAST: FROM REPRODUCTION TO RECONSTRUCTION

In line with this revival of Sir Frederic Bartlett's work (1932), cognitive psychologists have developed various experimental paradigms to elicit memory errors, some of which involve pseudo-memories (e.g., Loftus, Miller and Burns, 1978). During the nineties, research on memory errors was inspired by the debate about the accuracy of traumatic memories recovered during psychotherapy (Loftus, 1993; Loftus and Ketchman, 1994; Read and Lindsay, 1997).

Commonly used techniques in pseudo-memory research comprise the post-hoc misinformation paradigm (Ceci and Bruck, 1993; Loftus and Palmer, 1974), the imagination-inflation paradigm (Garry, Manning, Loftus, and Sherman, 1996; Horselenberg, Merckelbach, Muris, Rassin, Sijsenaar, and Spaan, 2000), and semantic relatedness paradigms (Deese, 1959; Roediger and McDermott, 1995; Peters, Jelicic, Haas, and Merckelbach, *submitted*). We will briefly discuss each technique.

Exposure to (post-hoc) misinformation can have detrimental effects on the accurate recollection of a specific event (for a review, see Loftus, Feldman and Dashiell, 1995). An example may clarify this: Suppose that person X is a witness to an accident, caused by a car that did not stop at a stop sign. During the interrogation of person X, a police officer asks person X what happened when the car did not stop at the yield sign. Research by, for example, Loftus and Palmer (1974) and Loftus, Miller, and Burns (1978), shows that there is a high probability that person X will recall the car did not stop at the yield sign. Thus, subtle suggestions provided after the event has occurred (i.e., post-hoc) may distort the way in which people come to remember the event (see also Crombag, Wagenaar, and van Koppen, 1996; Ost, Vrij, Costall, and Bull, 2002).

Encouraging people to fantasize about events that they have never experienced is the crux of the imagination-inflation paradigm. Imagining about an improbable event can lead to an increase in subjective confidence that the event did take place (Garry et al., 1996). Consider the following example: A young man is asked to imagine how he, at age 5, was a passenger in a hot air balloon. According to the man's parents, such an event never took place. After several weeks, he is asked to assign a confidence rating to the following item: "At age 5, I flew as a passenger in a hot air balloon". It is likely that he will overestimate the probability of the balloon trip compared to items that were not imagined (see also Horselenberg et al., 2000).

In semantic relatedness paradigms (Deese, 1959; Roediger and McDermott, 1995), participants are exposed to cues referring to a critical item that is never presented. For example, in the Deese/Roediger-McDermott (DRM) paradigm, initially developed by Deese (1959) and later modified by Roediger and McDermott (1995), people are asked to remember related words, such as *bed, nap, pillow,* and *snooze,* all of which are associated to a common word, in this particular example, the word *sleep.* The word *sleep,* however, is never presented in the study list and serves as a *critical lure* at test. Following each list presentation, participants are asked to recall the studied words. Once all lists have been presented and recalled, participants are given a recognition test comprising the studied words, unrelated lures, and critical lures. Roediger and McDermott (1995) reported that on average, participants falsely recognized 65-80 per cent of the non-presented critical lure words. These findings were replicated in a follow-up study by Stadler, Roediger, and McDermott (1999).

What post-hoc misinformation, imagination-inflation, and semantic-relatedness techniques have in common is that they produce source monitoring problems (e.g., Johnson, Hashtroudi, and Lindsay, 1993). That is, as a result of these techniques, participants find it difficult to differentiate between details that they really perceived and details that they only fantasized about. Obviously, the tendency to accept internally generated experiences as events that really took place is an important step in the direction of a full-blown pseudo-memory (see also, Smeets, Merckelbach, Horselenberg, and Jelicic, *in press*). Clearly, some people are more susceptible to such source monitoring problems than are others. A case in point are schizophrenic patients whose core symptoms (e.g., hallucinations) reflect serious source monitoring difficulties (e.g., Moritz, Woodward, and Ruff, 2003; Keefe, Arnold, Bayen, and Harvey, 1999). In line with this, recent studies explored whether more subtle personality traits may be related to source monitoring problems elicited by imagination-inflation techniques and so on. Thus, traits like dissociation, suggestibility, and imagery vividness have been studied to find out whether they modulate performance on these laboratory tasks (e.g., Eisen and Lynn, 2001). While research along these lines has yielded important clinical insights, its theoretical contribution is limited. This has to do with poor explanatory power of personality traits. Focussing on neuropsychological concepts may explain why certain traits are related to pseudo-memories and, therefore, this research line might be more fruitful. Indeed, recent aging and lesion studies suggest that executive functions such as monitoring and inhibition play a critical role in the creation of pseudo-memories. It is to this research domain that we now turn.

PRESENT: THE NEUROPSYCHOLOGY OF
MEMORY AND PSEUDO-MEMORY

A scholarly review on the neuropsychology of memory can be found in Greenberg and Rubin in (2003) and Squire and Schacter (2002). Briefly, these authors argue that when attention is paid to stimuli, different regions of the primary sensory and association cortex are activated (Thus, a visual stimulus activates the visual cortex, whereas auditory stimulation activates the auditory cortex). The role of the medial temporal lobe can best be regarded as a switchboard, linking up different brain regions that are simultaneously activated during the encoding of a specific event. When one wants to recollect/retrieve this specific event, certain structures in the medial temporal lobe mobilize different regions in the sensory and association cortex.

The prefrontal cortex is involved in search strategies and the evaluation of their results. Its primary role is evaluating and monitoring relevant information and inhibiting irrelevant information (retrieval). That is, the prefrontal cortex organizes, selects, and activates the correct representation from the various representations that are encoded and consolidated at different points in time (Nyberg, Cabeza, and Tulving, 1996). More specifically, the left prefrontal cortex sustains organizing the encoded information in the most efficient way for later remembering (Fletcher, Shallice, Frith, Frackowiak, and Dolan, 1998). In contrast, the right prefrontal cortex guides retrieval (Kapur, Craik, Jones, Brown, Houle, and Tulving, 1995; Wheeler, Stuss, and Tulving, 1997) and some authors (e.g., Markowitsch, 1996) believe that it is particularly involved in the retrieval of autobiographical memory.

In his review article on the neuropsychology of pseudo-memories, Parkin (1997) states that prefrontal damage may lead to different memory distortions. Patients with prefrontal damage show a decreased usage of strategic retrieval and control (e.g., monitoring, evaluation, inhibition). This often leads to an endorsement of irrelevant memory representations during the retrieval of a specific event (Shimamura, 1995). Evidence for this can be found in case studies involving patients with focal brain damage, aging research, research using functional imaging techniques, and individual difference studies.

Brain Damage and Aging

As mentioned before, initial evidence for the role of the prefrontal cortex in the creation of pseudo-memories came from several case studies (e.g., Parkin et al., 1996; Schacter et al., 1996a; Delbecq-Derousne, Beauvois, and Shallice, 1990). The patients described in these papers had the initials JB (Parkin, Leng, Stanhope, and Smith, 1988; Parkin et al., 1996), BG (Schacter et al., 1996a; Curran, Schacter, Norman, and Gallucio, 1997), and RW (Delbecq-Derousne, Beauvois, and Shallice, 1990; see also patient MR; Ward, Parkin, Powell, Squires, Townshend, and Bradley, 1999; patient JT; Young, Flude, Hay, and Ellis, 1993; Patients WJ and BH; Rapcsak, Polster, Comer, and Rubens, 1994). Patients JB and RW were both diagnosed with a ruptured aneurysm of the anterior communicating artery (ACoA), whereas patient BG was diagnosed with an infarction located in the right frontal lobe. These three patients exhibited an extremely high rate of false recognition errors in a forced-choice recognition task (indicating new unrelated words and/or critical lures as old). The data of JB further revealed a recall impairment in which intrusion rates (i.e., producing non-presented words) were abnormally high. Ward and colleagues (1999) described a patient (MR) who was able to correctly recognise famous people, but also had a strong tendency to falsely classify unfamiliar people as familiar (see also Rapcsak, Reminger, Glisky, Kaszniak, and Comer, 1999). This patient had had a lacunar infarction in the area above the left lateral ventricle adjacent to the left frontal horn.

Recent attempts to explore the separate contributions of medial temporal and prefrontal areas to memory have supported the findings from these case studies. A study by Melo, Winocur, and Moscovitch (1999) examined patients with isolated damage to the medial temporal or the prefrontal areas. The results showed that patients with medial temporal lesions made significantly less false recognition errors in comparison to those with prefrontal lesions.

Relative to younger adults, neurologically intact elderly tend to make more false recognition errors. Using the DRM paradigm, a recent study by Butler, McDaniel, Dornburg, Roediger, and Price (2004) investigated the relationship between neuropsychological measures of frontal lobe functioning and age differences in false recall. These authors found that older adults were less successful in reproducing studied items and more often falsely recalled the non-presented, critical lure words in comparison to younger adults, which is in line with other studies (Baltoa, Cortese, Duchek, Adams, et al., 1999; Intons-Peterson, Rocchi, West, McLellan, and Hackney, 1999; Norman and Schacter, 1997; Cohen and Faulkner, 1989; Dywan and Jacoby, 1990; Koutstaal and Schacter, 1997; See review by Schacter, Koutstaal, and Norman, 1997). These pseudo-memories were not related to the length or elaboration of the learning phase (Kensinger and Schacter, 1999). Most importantly, Butler and colleagues (2004) showed that these pseudo-memories were intimately linked to measures of frontal lobe functioning (i.e., executive functions). That is, only older adults characterized by poor frontal lobe functioning exhibited heightened levels of false recollections. Older adults with intact frontal lobe functioning and young adults had similar levels of accurate and false recall. In line with this, imaging studies of older adults show deviant activation patterns in the prefrontal cortex during memory tasks. This is most prominent when they have to rely on controlled retrieval strategies during these tasks (Schacter, Savage, Alpert, Rauch, and Albert, 1996b).

There are also indications that older adults are more suggestible compared to younger people. Evidence for this comes from studies using the post-hoc misinformation paradigm (e.g., Multhaup, De Leonardis, and Johnson, 1999). As stated earlier, the crux of this paradigm is that participants are exposed to an event and then later receive misleading information about this event. When older adults are asked to reproduce the original event, they typically tend to include the misinformation at higher rates relative to control conditions (see also Mitchel, Johnson, and Mather, 2002).

Recent studies have begun to explore pseudo-memories in individuals who suffer from Dementia of the Alzheimer Type (DAT; see Marsch, Baltoa, and Roediger, 2005, Waldie and Kwong See, 2003; Budson, Sullivan, Daffner, and Schacter, 2003; Watson, Baltoa, and Sergent-Marshall, 2001; Balota et al., 1999). Basically, these studies show that DAT patients are especially susceptible to pseudo-memories when pre-existing semantic information is activated. In a study with a mixed sample including various age groups and various levels of cognitive impairment (young, healthy old adults < 80 years, healthy old adults > 80 years, very mild DAT, and mild DAT), Watson and colleagues (2001) exposed their participants to a series of semantic memory tasks, including the DRM paradigm. Their results indicate that accurate recall decreased with increasing age and dementia severity. However, false recall of the non-presented critical lure words increased with age and remained fairly stable across dementia severity. In a later study by Waldie and Kwong See (2003), these findings were replicated using the DRM paradigm. These authors also gave an old-new recognition task to their participants. The recognition task comprised old (studied) words, non-presented critical lure words, and non-presented related and unrelated distracter words. The DAT group and healthy elderly showed similar rates of false recognition of non-presented critical lure words. However, in comparison to healthy elderly, patients with DAT were more likely to classify non-presented related and unrelated distracter words as old (presented) words.

An explanation for these findings is offered by an inefficient functioning of cognitive inhibitory control that occurs with aging and DAT, and is related to prefrontal (executive) dysfunction. Inhibitory control is important in limiting the spread of activation during retrieval of semantic material. Decreased inhibitory control results in increased spreading activation in the semantic network and, as a consequence, increased probability that one falsely remembers a non-presented critical lure word. Clearly, cognitive inhibition is a function of the prefrontal cortex.

Functional Imaging Data

Which functional brain areas are involved in accurate memories and pseudo-memories? To address this issue, researchers have used various neuroimaging techniques. A complete description of the different fMRI, PET, and electroencephalogram (EEG) studies is beyond the scope of this chapter (see Schacter and Slotnick, 2004, for a thorough overview of research in this area). In a prototypical PET study, Schacter, Reiman, Curran, Yun, et al. (1996c) focussed on true and false recognition in the DRM task. The authors found two trends. To begin with, an increased activation in left temporal region was found during accurate recall of presented words. Second, there appeared to be an increase in right prefrontal activity during false recognition of critical lures. Using fMRI during a follow up study, the same researchers noted a similar pattern (Schacter, Buckner, Koutstaal, Dale, and Rosen, 1997). In this study, a delayed onset of prefrontal activation during false recognition occurred, a phenomenon that the authors relate to suboptimal controlling of the prefrontal cortex during retrieval. A number of other studies have tried to disentangle the brain mechanisms involved in accurate and pseudo-memories (for reviews, see Dodson and Schacter, 2002; Gonsalves and Paller, 2002; Schacter and Slotnick, 2004). By and large, neuroimaging research demonstrates that, in addition to a (modest) involvement of the medial temporal cortex, the prefrontal cortex plays a leading role in errors that may occur during retrieval and, therefore, in pseudo-memories more specifically.

According to Dodson and Schacter (2002), delayed prefrontal activity during false recollection found in neuroimaging experiments would reflect a failure in executive functions, more specifically inhibitory functions that operate during retrieval. Inhibition can be defined in terms of accurate discrimination between target information and similar competing information in memory at retrieval (e.g., Anderson and Spellman, 1995). Accordingly, a lack of inhibitory function would lead to a less reliable retrieval, and as a consequence source monitoring difficulties.

Individual Differences

Another research line has focused on individual differences in susceptibility to pseudo-memories. As mentioned before, personality traits like dissociation, suggestibility, and imagery vividness have been studied to examine whether they predict performance on tasks that elicit pseudo-memories (e.g., Winograd, Peluso, and Glover, 1998; Horselenberg et al., 2000; Candel, Merckelbach, and Kuijpers, 2003). This research approach has found strong evidence that high scores on, for example, dissociation are linked to heightened levels of false recall (e.g., Candel, Merckelbach, and Kuijpers, 2003; Geraerts, Smeets, Jelicic, van Heerden, and Merckelbach, *in press)*. But what does this mean? Is dissociation a causal antecedent of pseudo-memories? Or is it just a manifestation of heightened susceptibility to pseudo-memories? This causal issue is extremely difficult to examine. Linking individual differences in inhibition and other executive functions to pseudo-memories is perhaps a more promising way. A fine example of this is an individual difference study by Alexander, Goodman, Schaaf, Edelstein, et al. (2002). These authors interviewed children ($\underline{n}$ = 51) between the ages of 3 and 7 years about an inoculation that they had undergone two weeks earlier. Children's memory accuracy and suggestibility were examined in relation to their stress levels during inoculation, parental attachment styles, and cognitive inhibition (i.e., suppression of irrelevant information). The authors anticipated that children with higher levels of cognitive inhibition would provide more accurate information and would be less suggestible than children with lower levels of inhibition. This was borne out by the data. That is, children with poorer cognitive inhibition exhibited more pseudo-memories on a free recall task about inoculation and more often accepted misleading information than children with adequate inhibition capacity. This difference remained, even when controlling for age. More recently, Lödvén (2003) investigated the underlying mechanisms of age effects on pseudo-memories. A total of 146 participants, aged 20 to 80 years were subjected to tasks measuring processing speed, inhibition, episodic memory performance, and pseudo-memories. Results revealed an increased level of pseudo-memories with increasing age. Using structural equation modeling, this author found that impairments in inhibitory control affected susceptibility to pseudo-memories indirectly via episodic memory performance. That is, participants scoring low on episodic memory tasks made more false recall critical lure intrusions, compared to participants scoring high on these episodic memory tasks. In explaining inhibitory control, participants with an impaired inhibition function showed limited episodic memory performance. Inhibitory control influenced pseudo-memories only indirectly, via an influence on episodic memory.

Empirical Intermezzo

Although the neuropsychology of pseudo-memories has mostly been studied in neurological patients (Melo, Winocur, and Moscovitch, 1999), older people (Lödvén, 2003), and children (Alexander et al., 2002), it is not unreasonable to assume that even in healthy samples, there is individual variation in the efficacy of executive functions. This variation, in turn, might be the origin of individual differences in susceptibility to pseudo-memories. To address this issue, we explored whether executive function in undergraduate students is linked to false recall and recognition as measured with the DRM paradigm (Peters et al., submitted). Because monitoring of memory retrieval does involve inhibition of competing schemata, we expected that individual differences in the ability to inhibit cognitive schemata were related to false recollections in the DRM paradigm. The Random Number Generation (RNG) task was used to assess individual differences in the ability to inhibit cognitive schemata (as measured by the seriation subscale of the RNG task; Ginsburg and Karpiuk, 1994; Williams, Moss, Bradshaw, and Rinehart, 2002). In this task, participants have to generate digits in a random sequence. Participants are asked to produce long sequences of the numbers 1-10 in a random fashion. Successful performance on the RNG requires efficient control of response generation and suppression, as people have to suppress (i.e., inhibit) their natural preference for counting in series. The RNG has been effective in detecting loss of cognitive flexibility in a number of neurological diseases like, for example Parkinson's disease (Brown, Soliveri, and Jahanshahi, 1998) and autism (Williams et al., 2002). Several RNG parameters have been proposed to measure the various departures from randomness and, thus, lack of inhibitory control

(Ginsburg and Karpiuk, 1995). A factor analysis on RNG data revealed three types of parameters. The first type involves repetition, which is related to output inhibition. The second is cycling and relates to successful monitoring of previous output, while the third and most important type is seriation, which contain inhibition of cognitive schemata (Williams et al., 2002). High seriation scores indicate a lack of inhibition of cognitive schemata (i.e., less efficient executive functioning), with low seriation indicating efficient executive functioning (i.e., one can inhibit the cognitive schema of counting in series).

Seventy-two undergraduate students took part in our study. They were subjected to both the DRM and the RNG. The DRM paradigm (Deese, 1959; Roediger and McDermott, 1995) involves 10 selected lists, each consisting of 15 words semantically related to a non-presented critical lure. After each list presentation, participants were given 2 min to write down all the words they could remember. After the final recall test, participants were given an old-new recognition task consisting of 10 critical lures of the studied lists completely intermixed with 30 study words (the 1st, 8th and 10th word of each studied list) and 20 unrelated lures. Mean DRM recall and recognition scores together with RNG task scores can be found in table 1. We found a significant link between recognition of critical lures of the DRM and the seriation scores (r = 0.36) of the RNG. Similarly, there was a borderline significant correlation between recall of critical lures and seriation (r = 0.23). When extreme groups were formed on the basis of participants' RNG seriation subscale performance (i.e., performance below the 25th or above the 75th percentile), no differences between these groups emerged in terms of accurate recall or recognition. However, those scoring high on seriation (reflecting a lack of inhibition of cognitive schemata) also had high false recognition rates of critical lures compared to those scoring low on seriation, mean proportion recognition rates being 0.63 (SD = 0.24) and 0.37 (SD = 0.3), respectively. Likewise, participants scoring high on seriation had higher false recall rates of critical lures relative to those scoring low on seriation, means being 0.28 (SD = 0.17) and 0.19 (SD = 0.16), respectively (see figure1).

Table 1. Mean scores of an undergraduate sample ($\underline{n}$ = 70) on DRM recall and recognition of studied words (overall mean and proportion) and critical lure words (overall mean for the 16 studied lists and proportion), and seriation subscale of Random Number Generation (RNG)

DRM		Mean (proportion)	SD(proportion)	Range(proportion)
	Subtests			
	Recall studied words	9.64 (0.64)	1.09 (0.07)	7.20-11.63 (0.48-0.77)
	Recognition studied words	39.97 (0.83)	4.83 (0.10)	19-48 (0.40-1.00)
	Recall critical lure	4.20 (0.26)	2.85 (0.18)	0-12 (0.00-0.75)
	Recognition critical lure	7.76 (0.49)	4.30 (0.27)	0-15 (0.00-0.94)
RNG		Mean	SD	Range
	Subtest			
	Seriation	33.67	7.12	16-54

This pattern of findings demonstrates that even in a healthy sample of undergraduate students, individual differences in executive functions are related to false recollections. Note again that in the high seriation group heightened levels of false recall and false recognition were not accompanied by an increased accurate recall or recognition. Thus, the link between poor executive function and pseudo-memories cannot be explained in terms of better or poorer encoding.

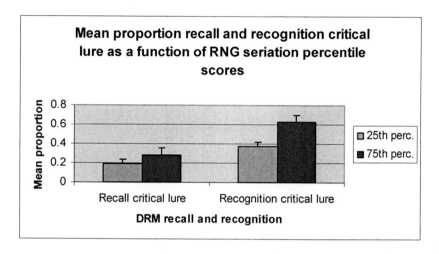

Figure 1. Mean proportion scores of the free recall and recognition of the critical items based on the 25th and 75th seriation percentile scores of the participants ($\underline{n}$ = 70). Error bars indicate SE of mean. A significant differences was found between the 25th percentile and 75th percentile mean proportion scores of the recognition critical lure [$\underline{t}$(36) = 3.15, $\underline{p}$ < 0.01].

Working Memory

Working memory is closely related to the executive functions of the frontal lobe. A recent paper by Reinitz and Hannigan (2004) describes three experiments relating pseudo-memories to working memory capacity. The authors had their participants ($\underline{n}$ = 48) study pairs of compound words, either simultaneously or sequentially. The subsequent recognition test included within-pair and between-pair conjunction foils and true conjunction pairs. Overall, the results indicated that intact working memory is necessary for binding stimulus parts together in episodic memory. Inefficient working memory will lead to binding failures, and subsequent an increase in pseudo-memories.

McCabe and Smith (2002) examined age differences in the ability to suppress pseudo-memories, using the DRM paradigm. In two separate experiments, some younger and older adults were unwarned about the potential pseudo-memories occurring as a result of exposure to the DRM procedure. Others were warned before studying the DRM lists. Still others were warned after studying and before testing. Lists were presented at different rates (4 sec/word or 2 sec/word). Individual difference measures like working memory were also administered. Young adults were better in discriminating between studied words and critical lure words when warned about the DRM effect (either before or after study). Older adults were able to discriminate between studied items and critical lure words when given warnings before study, but not when given warnings after study and before retrieval. As to the individual differences measures, working memory capacity predicted false recognition following study and retrieval warning. That is, reduced working memory capacity was associated with higher rates of false recollections. McCabe and Smith (2002) conclude that discriminating between similar sources of activation critically depends on working memory capacity, which declines with advancing age. This leads to a heightened susceptibility to pseudo-memories.

Inspired by these studies on working memory, we conducted an experiment to examine whether individual differences in working memory capacity in a healthy student sample affect the development of pseudo-memories as measured by the DRM paradigm (Peters, Jelicic, Verbeek, and Merckelbach, *in preparation*). As a measure of working memory capacity we used digit span (forward and backward, which are subtasks of the Wechsler Adult Intelligence Scale; for a Dutch translation, see Stinissen et al., 1970). Recent work shows that this task activates the right dorsolateral prefrontal cortex (DLPFC), the parietal lobes as well as the anterior cingulate (Gerton, Brown, Meyer-Lindenberg, Kohn, Holt, Olsen, and Berman, 2004). A total sample of 60 undergraduate students took part in our experiment. Participants were subjected to a Dutch version of the Deese/ Roediger-McDermott (DRM) paradigm (Deese, 1959; Roediger and McDermott, 1995). Participants were given the digit span task after the recall of the 10th DRM list (and before the recognition part of the DRM paradigm). Series of digits were read aloud (e.g. 2 4 7), each series increasing in length (from 2 digits to 8 digits). After each series, participants were asked to repeat this series orally. The test consisted of 12 series in the normal front to back order (forward) and 12 series in the back to front order (backward). The number of correctly reproduced series was used as a measure of working memory capacity.

The overall probability for recalling or recognizing the critical lure was 0.47 and 0.87 (see table 2). No significant correlations were found between either recall or recognition of the study words and the digit span task scores (all p's > 0.05; two-tailed). Mean proportion of recognition of critical lures was significantly correlated with digit span backward scores (r = -0.40; p < 0.01). Similarly, there was a borderline significant correlation between recall of critical lures and digit span backward (r = -0.23; p = 0.08; two-tailed). Participants who performed poorly on digit span backward more often falsely recognized the critical lure word compared to those who scored high on the backward digit span.

Table 2. Mean proportion scores (including *SD* and Range) of recall and recognition of studied and critical lure words of an undergraduate sample (*n* = 60). Digit Span forward and backward scores are described in overall mean scores

Item type	Mean	SD	Range
Recall studied words	0.61	0.07	0.39
Recall critical lures	0.47	0.19	0.80
Recognition studied words	0.79	0.11	0.47
Recognition critical lures	0.84	0.15	0.60
Digit Span Forward	6.10	1.21	4.00
Digit Span Backward	4.65	1.05	5.00

Multiple linear regression analysis was conducted with the mean proportions of recall and recognition as dependent variables and digit span forward and backward entered as independent variables. The results are shown in table 3. The digit span forward and backward test did not have a significant influence on the recall and the recognition of old (e.g., presented) words (all p's > 0.30). A significant relationship was found between the digit span backwards and the mean recognition proportion of the critical lure words.

Table 3 Summary of Multiple Regression Analysis for variables predicting proportion recall and recognition of critical lure words (*n* = 60)

Variable	*B*	SE *B*	B	T
Recall				
Digit Span forward	3.27	0.02	0.00	0.002
Digit Span backward	-0.04	0.02	-0.23	-1.70*
Recognition				
Digit Span forward	-0.008	0.02	-0.06	-0.51
Digit Span backward	-0.06	0.02	-0.39	-3.10**

Note. R^2 = .051 for Recall; R^2 = .16 for Recognition digit span backward
* borderline significant p = 0.09
** $p < 0.01$

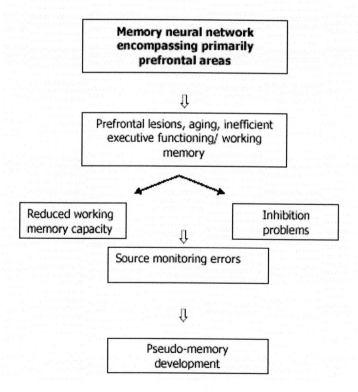

Figure 2. Model on the involvement of prefrontal areas on pseudo-memory development.

The studies described above converge on the notion that individual differences in cognitive inhibition and working memory are related to pseudo-memories. A lack of cognitive inhibition and/or reduced working memory capacity will lead to a liberal criterion setting and a weakened suppression of irrelevant information. As a consequence, source monitoring errors occur, which may ultimately produce pseudo-memories (see figure 2).

FUTURE

A good starting point for further neuropsychological research on the origins of pseudo-memories is the Constructive Memory Framework (CMF) proposed by Schacter and colleagues (Schacter, Norman, and Koutstaal, 1998; Dodson and Schacter, 2002). According to their framework, new experiences are organized in patterns of features that represent different aspects of the experience. For example: The things I did on my birthday, the things I eat on that day, and the various presents I got. These features are encoded across different regions of the brain. The retrieval of this information requires an act of pattern completion, whereby the features belonging to a past experience are activated and the activation spreads along other features (spreading activation). It further proposes that false recollections are modulated by neuropsychological factors operating primarily at encoding or retrieval stages of memory. More specifically, the prefrontal cortex is involved in the updating, suppression, and monitoring of information. There are two problems that have to be solved in order for people to be able to reconstruct accurate memories of past events. First, during the encoding process, features must be connected together to form a "coherent" representation (i.e., the feature binding process). It is also necessary to keep the bound representations separate from each other (pattern separation). Inadequate bindings between features can lead to source memory errors, whereby persons can retrieve specific fragments of an experience, but cannot recall the context of encoding. When, during pattern separation, different experiences overlap, people can sometimes only recall the gist of these experiences. For example, celebrating your birthday is a yearly recurring event. For this reason, connecting the different experiences of this event is preferable. However, the features of your last birthday need to be different from the representations of your previous birthdays. Otherwise you will not be able to distinguish between the different birthday representations.

During retrieval, the memory system must also solve binding and separation problems in order to reconstruct relatively accurate memories of past events. Once memory representations have been retrieved, the memory system faces another problem, referred to by Johnson, Hashtroudi, and Lindsay (1993) as the source monitoring problem. This phase of retrieval involves criterion-setting, which determines whether the memory representation is a veridical recollection of an experienced event or a fantasy. In the case of our birthday example this means that during retrieval, sufficient retrieval cues need to be present to remember an accurate representation of this day. Also specific criteria need to be employed to be certain that the retrieved event is the correct experience rather than the product of a dream or fantasy. Lax criterion setting can lead to remembering an experience that we only imagined to have happened.

Neural substrates implicated by this theory involve the medial temporal lobes that sustain encoding and retrieval of recent experiences and the prefrontal cortex that sustain control and the retrieval of old experiences. The CMF emphasizes that the prefrontal cortex sustains both retrieval focus and criterion-setting. Plainly, both require cognitive inhibition of schema-related material. In our studies (Peters, et al., *submitted*; Peters, et al., *in preparation*), this aspect was tapped by a reduced ability to suppress stereotypical series of digits (e.g., 2, 3, 4) or reduced working memory capacity. Eventually, a lack of cognitive inhibition may lead to liberal criterion setting and an inability to suppress related information, with the potential consequence of source monitoring deficits.

CONCLUSION

We believe that the CMF and especially the role of the prefrontal areas in the origins of pseudo-memories warrant further study. It would not only be worthwhile to examine pseudo-memories in special samples, for example patients with brain damage, but also to address pseudo-memories and their correlates in normal, healthy samples. As said before, in healthy samples, there are a number of traits, notably dissociation and depression (or negative affectivity), that seem to predispose to pseudo-memories (e.g., Candel et al., 2003; Horselenberg, Merckelbach, van Breukelen, and Wessel, 2004). On the other hand, the connection between these traits and pseudo-memories is far from robust. That is, some studies were unable to find a significant correlation between for example dissociation and pseudo-memories (Horselenberg et al., 2000). Perhaps, then, traits like dissociation and depression serve as antecedents of pseudo-memories to the extent that they are accompanied by subtle disturbances in executive functions of the prefrontal areas. Thus, the precise connection between dissociation, depression, and executive functions requires systematic study. Note that there is some tentative evidence that dissociative symptoms go hand in hand with mild executive dysfunctions. For example, relying on a sample of forensic patients, Cima and colleagues (2001) found that high levels of dissociative symptoms were related to poor performance on a 'frontal'task (the Behavioural Assessment of Dysexecutive Syndrome; BADS; Wilson, Alderman, Burgess, Emslie, and Evans, 1996). Likewise, Giesbrecht and co-workers (2004) noted that in a healthy undergraduate sample dissociative symptoms were linked to certain aspects of the RNG task (cf. supra). With these findings in mind, we believe that research on the associations between traditional personality traits (e.g., dissociation), executive functions (e.g., cognitive inhibition, working memory), and pseudo-memories might be informative. Having said this, we also believe that two potential limitations of this research domain deserve some comment. First, the term "executive function" is often used in a broad way and our use of this concept throughout the chapter is no exception to this rule. Clearly, research on the neuropsychology of pseudo-memories would benefit from a more articulated definition of this key concept (see also Miyake, Friedman, Emerson, Witzki, Howerter, and Wagner, 2000; Friedman and Miyake, 2004). Subdividing the concept of "executive function" in different well-defined subcomponents like cognitive inhibition, monitoring, updating, would be a first step. Secondly, the term pseudo-memory has been used in a liberal way too. Thus, increases in subjective confidence, confabulations, and false alarms on recognition tasks have all been treated as manifestations of pseudo-memories. But, again, this domain would benefit from a stricter definition of what counts as a full-blown pseudo-memory (see Smeets et al., in press).

BH AGAIN

Our patient BH had evident signs of right prefrontal damage. Unfortunately, these signs were disregarded by the psychiatrists who treated him. These clinicians were preoccupied by his retrograde amnesia. BH had great difficulties to retrieve accurate and detailed memories about his childhood and, in fact, he was unsure about his identity. Meanwhile, the police required complete information about his age and his place of birth, so as to provide him with legal documents. Encouraged by the police, BH first underwent a series of hypnosis sessions avid subsequently treatment with the "truth serum" pentobarbital. During the hypnosis and pentobarbital sessions, the psychiatrists interviewed him. Their questions were based on the assumption that BH had a military background. Hence, BH was asked about military training, secret missions, parachutes, weapons, the U.S. army, Russia, and many related themes. It is not too farfetched to say that the psychiatrists combined post-hoc misinformation, imagination inflation, and semantic-relatedness techniques during their interviews. That this was not without effect became clear when BH began to uncover memories about his Canadian background and his work as a CIA agent. Although these memories were detailed and compelling, they turned out to be full-blown pseudo-memories. By coincidence, the police was able to establish the real identity of BH. He was born in a Paris suburb and had never been to Canada or the US. One day, he became involved in a fight, during which he was badly injured. To this very day BH prefers to believe that he is a Canadian who worked for the CIA rather than a Parisian who one day decided to visit Amsterdam.

AUTHOR NOTES

This review and the described studies by the first author were supported by a grant from the Dutch organization for scientific research N.W.O. grant number 452-02-006.

REFERENCES

Alexander, K.W., Goodman, G.S., Schaaf, J.M., Edelstein, R.S., Quas, J.A., and Shaver, Ph. R. (2002). The role of attachment and cognitive inhibition in children's memory and suggestibility for a stressful event. *Journal of Experimental Child Psychology, 83,* 262-290.

Anderson, M.C., and Spellman, B.A. (1995). On the status of inhibitory mechanisms in cognition: Memory retrieval as a model case. *Psychological Review, 102,* 68-100.

Baltoa, D.A., Cortese, M.J., Duchek, J.M., Adams, D., Roediger, H.L.III., McDermott, K.B., and Yerys, B.E. (1999). Veredical and false memories in healthy older adults and in dementia of the Alzheimer's type. *Cognitive Neuropsychology, 16,* 361-384.

Bartlett, F. C. (1932). *Remembering.* Cambridge: Cambridge University Press.

Brown, R.G., Soliveri, P., and Jahanshahi, M. (1998). Executive processes in Parkinson's disease: Random Number Generation and response suppression. *Neuropsychologia, 36,* 1355-1362.

Budson, A.E., Sullivan, A.L., Daffner, K.R., and Schacter, D.L. (2003). Semantic versus phonological false recognition in aging and Alzheimer's disease. *Brain and Cognition, 51,* 251-261.

Butler, K.M., McDaniel, M.A., Donburg, C.C., Roediger, H.L.III, and Price, A.L. (2004). Age differences in veridical and false recall are not inevitable: The role of frontal lobe function. *Psychonomic Bulletin and Review, 11,* 921-925.

Caltogirone, C., Zoccolotti, P., Originale, G., Daniele, A., and Mammucari, A. (1989) Autonomic reactivity and facial expression of emotion in brain-damaged patients. In G. Gainotti, and C. Caltagirone (Eds.), *Emotions and the dual brain* (pp. 204-221). Berlin: Springer-Verlag.

Candel, I., Merckelbach, H., and Kuijpers, M. (2003). Dissociative experiences are related to commissions in emotional memory. *Behaviour Research and Therapy, 41,* 719-725.

Ceci, S. J., and Bruck, M. (1993). Suggestibility of the child witness: A historical review and synthesis. *Psychological Bulletin, 113,* 403-439.

Cima, M., Merckelbach, H., Klein, B., Shellbach-Matties, R., and Kremer, K. (2001). Frontal lobe dysfunction, dissociation, and trauma self-reports in forensic psychiatric patients. *The Journal of Nervous and Mental Disease, 189,* 188-190.

Cohen, G., and Faulkner, D. (1989). Age differences in source forgetting: Effects on reality monitoring and on eyewitness testimony. *Psychology and Aging, 4,* 10-17.

Crombag, H.F.M., Wagenaar, W.A., and van Koppen, P.J. (1996). Crashing memories and the problem of "source monitoring". *Applied Cognitive Psychology, 10,* 95-04.

Curran, T., Schacter, D.L., Norman, K.A., and Gallucio, L. (1997). False recognition after a right frontal lobe infarction: Memory for general and specific information. *Neuropsychologia, 35,* 1035-1047.

Dalla Barba, G. (1993). Confabulation: Knowledge and recollective experience. *Cognitive Neuropsychology, 10,* 1-20.

Deelman, B.G., Brouwer, W.H., van Zomeren, A.H., and Saan, R.J. (1980). Functiestoornissen na trauma capitis. [Deficiencies in functioning following trauma capitis] In A. Jennekens-Schinkel (Ed.), *Neuropsychologie in Nederland* [Neuropsychology in the Netherlands]. Deventer: Van Loghum Slaterus.

Deese, J. (1959). On the prediction of occurence of particular verbal intrusions in immediate recall. *Journal of Experimental Psychology, 58,* 17-22.

Delbecq-Derousne, J., Beauvois, M.F., and Shallice, T. (1990). Preserved recall versus impaired recognition. *Brain, 113,* 1045-1074.

Dodson, C. S., and Schacter, D. L. (2002). The cognitive neuropsychology of false memories: Theory and data. In A. D. Baddeley, M. D. Kopelman, and B. A. Wilson (Eds.), *Handbook of memory disorders* (pp. 343-362). Chichester: Wiley and Sons, Ltd.

Draaisma, D. (2000). *Metaphors of memory: A history of ideas about the mind.* Cambridge: Cambridge University Press.

Dywan, J., and Jacoby, L.L. (1990). Effects of aging on source monitoring: Differences in susceptibility to false fame. *Psychology and Aging, 5,* 379-387.

Eisen, M.L., and Lynn, S.J. (2001). Dissociation, memory and suggestibility in adults and children. *Applied Cognitive Psychology, 15,* S49-S73.

Fletcher, P.C., Shallice, T., Frith, C.D., Frackowiak, R.S., and Dolan, R.J. (1998). The functional roles of the prefrontal cortex in episodic memory. II. Retrieval. *Brain, 121,* 1249-1256.

Friedman, N.P., and Miyake, A. (2004). The relations among inhibition and interference control functions: A latent –variable analysis. *Journal of Experimental Psychology: General, 133,* 101-135.

Garry, M., Manning, C. G., Loftus, E. F., and Sherman, S. J. (1996). Imagination inflation: Imagining a childhood event inflates confidence that it occurred. *Psychonomic Bulletin and Review, 3,* 208-214.

Geraerts, E., Smeets, E., Jelicic, M., van Heerden, J. and Merckelbach, H (*in press*). Fantasy proneness, but not self-reported trauma is related to DRM performance of women reporting recovered memories of childhood sexual abuse. *Consciousness and Cognition.*

Gerton, B.K., Brown, T.T., Meyer-Lindenberg, A., Kohn, P., Holt, J.L., Olsen, R.K., and Berman, K.F. (2004). Shared and distinct neurophysiological components of the digits forward and backward tasks as revealed by functional neuroimaging. *Neuropsychologia, 42,* 1781-1787.

Giesbrecht, T., Merckelbach, H., Geraerts, E., and Smeets, E. (2004). Dissociation in undergraduate students: Disruptions in executive functioning. *The Journal of Nervous and Mental Disease, 192,* 567-569.

Ginsburg, N., and Karpiuk, P. (1994). Random Number Generation: Analysis of responses. *Perceptual and Motor Skills, 79,* 1059-1067.

Ginsburg, N., and Karpiuk, P. (1995). Simulation of human performance on a random generation task. *Perceptual and Motor Skills, 81,* 1183-1186.

Gonsalves, B., and Paller, K.A. (2002). Mistaken memories: Remembering events that never happened. *The Neuroscientist, 8,* 391-395.

Greenberg, D. L., and Rubin, D. C. (2003). The neuropsychology of autobiographical memory. *Cortex, 39,* 687-728.

Gudjonsson, G.H., and Clare, I.C.H. (1995). The relationship between confabulation and intellectual ability, memory, interrogative suggestibility and acquiescence. *Personality and Individual Differences, 19,* 333-338.

Horselenberg, R., Merckelbach, H., Muris, P., Rassin, E., Sijsenaar, M., and Spaan, V. (2000). Imagining fictitious childhood events: The role of individual differences in imagination inflation. *Clinical Psychology and Psychotherapy, 7,* 128-137.

Horselenberg, R., Merckelbach, H., van Breukelen, G., and Wessel, I. (2004). Individual Differences in the Accuracy of Autobiographical Memory. *Clinical Psychology and Psychotherapy, 11,* 168-176.

Intons-Peterson, M.J., Rocchi, P., West, T., McLellan, K., and Hackney, A. (1999). Age, testing at preferred or nonpreferred times (testing optimality), and false memory. *Journal of Experimental Psychology: Learning, Memory, and Cognition, 25,* 23-40.

Janowsky, J.S., Shimamura, A.P., and Squire, L.R. (1989). Source memory impairment in patients with frontal lobe lesions. *Neuropsychologia, 27,* 1043-1056.

Johnson, M.K, Hashtroudi, S., and Lindsay, D.S. (1993). Source Monitoring. *Psychological Bulletin, 114,* 3-28.

Kapur, S., Craik, F.I., Jones, C., Brown, G.M., Houle, S., and Tulving, E. (1995) Functional role of the prefrontal cortex in retrieval of memories: A PET study. *Neuroreport, 6,* 1880-1884.

Keefe, R.S.E., Arnold, M.C., Bayen, U.J., and Harvey, P.D. (1999). Source monitoring deficits in patients with schizophrenia; a multinominal modelling analysis. *Psychological Medicine, 29,* 903-914.

Kensinger, E. A., and Schacter, D. L. (1999). When true memories suppress false memories: effects of ageing. *Cognitive Neuropsychology, 16,* 399-415.

Kopelman, M. D. (2002). Disorders of memory. *Brain, 125,* 2152-2190.

Kopelman, M. D. (1999). Varieties of false memory. *Cognitive Neuropsychology, 16,* 197-214.

Kopelman, M.D., Green, R.E.A., Guinan, E.M., Lewis, P.D.R., and Stanhope, N. (1994). The case of the amnesic intelligence officer. *Psychological Medicine, 24,* 1037-1045.

Koriat, A., Goldsmith, M., and Pansky, A. (2000). Toward a psychology of memory accuracy. *Annual Review of Psychology, 51,* 481-537.

Koutstaal, W., and Schacter, D.L. (1997). Gist-based false recognition of pictures in older and younger adults. *Journal of Memory and Language, 37,* 555-583.

Lödvén, M. (2003). The episodic memory and inhibition accounts of age related increases in false memories: A consistency check. *Journal of Memory and Language, 49,* 268-283.

Loftus, E.F. (2003). Our changeable memories: Legal and practical implications. *Nature Neuroscience Reviews, 4,* 231-234.

Loftus, E. F. (1993). The reality of repressed memories. *American Psychologist, 48,* 518-537.

Loftus, E. F., Feldman, J., and Dashiell, R. (1995). The reality of illusory memories. In D. L. Schacter (Ed.), *Memory distortion: How minds, brains and societies reconstruct the past* (pp. 47-68). Cambridge, MA: Harvard University Press.

Loftus, E.F., and Ketcham, K. (1994). *The Myth of Repressed Memory : False Memories and Allegations of Sexual Abuse.* New York: St. Martin's Press.

Loftus, E. F., Miller, D. G., and Burns, H. J. (1978). Semantic integration of verbal information into a visual memory. *Journal of Experimental Psychology: Human Learning and Memory, 4,* 19-31.

Loftus, E. F., and Palmer, J. C. (1974). Reconstruction of automobile destruction: An example of the interaction between language and memory. *Journal of Verbal Learning and Verbal Behaviour, 13,* 585-589.

Markowitsch, H.J. (1996). Organic and psychogenic retrograde amnesia: Two sides of the same coin? *Neurocase, 2,* 357-371.

Marsh, E.J., Baltoa, D.A., and Roediger, H.L. III. (2005). Learningn facts from fiction: The effects of healthy aging and early stage dementia of the Alzheimer's type. *Neuropsychology, 19,* 115–129.

Mayes, A.R., Downes, J.J., McDonald, C., Rooke, S., Sagar, H.J., and Meudell, P.R. (1994). Two tests for assessing remote public knowledge: A tool for assessing retrograde amnesia. *Memory, 2,* 183-210.

McCabe, D.P., and Smith, A.D. (2002). The effect of warnings on false memories in young and older adults. *Memory and Cognition, 30,* 1065-1077.

Melo, B., Winocur, G., and Moscovitch, M. (1999). False recall and false recognition: An examination of the effects of selective and combined lesions to the medial temporal lobe/diencephalons and frontal lobe structures. *Journal of Cognitive Neuropsychology, 16,* 343-360.

Merckelbach, H., and Smith, G.P. (2003). Diagnostic accuracy of the Structured Inventory of Malingered Symptomatology (SIMS) in detecting instructed malingering. *Archives of Clinical Neuropsychology, 18,* 145-152.

Merckelbach, H., and Wessel, I. (1998). Assumptions of students and psychotherapists about memory. *Psychological Reports, 82,* 763-770.

Mitchell, K.J., Johnson, M.K., and Mather, M. (2002). Source monitoring and suggestibility to misinformation: Adult age-related differences. *Applied Cognitive Psychology, 16,* 1-13.

Miyake, A., Friedman, N.P., Emerson, M.J., Witzki, A.H., Howerter, A., and Wager, T.D. (2000). The unity and diversity of executive functions and their contributions to complex "frontal lobe" tasks: A latent variable analysis. *Cognitive Psychology, 41,* 49-100.

Moritz, S., Woodward, T.S., and Ruff, C.C. (2003). Source monitoring and memory confidence in schizophrenia. *Psychological Medicine, 33,* 131-139.

Multhaup, K.S., De Leonardis, D.M., and Johnson, M.K. (1999). Source memory and eyewitness suggestibility in older adults. *Journal of General Psychology, 126,* 74-84.

Neisser, U. (1967). *Cognitive Psychology.* New York: Appleton-Century-Crofts.

Norman, K. A., and Schacter, D. L. (1997). False recognition in young and older adults: Exploring the characteristics of illusory memory. *Memory and Cognition, 25,* 838-848.

Nyberg, L., Cabeza, R., and Tulving, E. (1996). PET studies on encoding and retrieval: The HERA model. *Psychonomic Bulletin and Review, 3,* 135-148.

Ost, J., Vrij, A., Costall, A., and Bull, R. (2002). Crashing memories and reality monitoring: Distinguishing between perceptions, imaginations, and 'false memories'. *Applied Cognitive Psychology, 16,* 125-134.

Parkin, A. J. (1997). The neuropsychology of false memory. *Learning and Individual Differences, 9,* 341-357.

Parkin, A. J., Bindschaedler, C., Harsent, L., and Metzler, C. (1996). Pathological false alarm rates following damage to the left frontal cortex. *Brain and Cognition, 32,* 14-27.

Parkin, A.J., Leng, N.R.C., Stanhope, H., and Smith, A.L. (1988). Memory impairment following ruptured aneurysm of the anterior communicating artery. *Brain and Cognition, 7,* 231-243.

Peters, M.J.V., Jelicic, M., Haas, N., and Merckelbach, H. (*submitted*). Mild executive dysfunctions in undergraduates are related to recollecting words never presented.

Peters, M.J.V., Jelicic, M., Verbeek, H., and Merckelbach, H. (*in preparation*). Differences in working memory capacity influence the recollection of words never presented.

Rapcsak, S.Z., Polster, M.R., Comer, J.F., and Rubens, A.B. (1994). False recognition and misidentification of faces following right hemisphere damage. *Cortex, 30,* 565-583.

Rapcsak, S.Z., Reminger, S.L., Glisky, E.L., Kaszniak, A.W., and Comer, J.F. (1999). Neuropsychological mechanisms of false facial recognition following frontal lobe damage. *Cognitive Neuropsychology, 16,* 267-292.

Read, J.D., and Lindsay, D.S. (1997). *Recollections of trauma: Scientific research and clinical practice.* New York: Plenum Press.

Reed, L.J., Marsden, P., Lasserson, D., Sheldon, N., Lewis, P., Stanhope, N., Guinan, E., and Kopelman, M.D. (1999). FDG-PET analysis and findings in amnesia resulting from hypoxia. *Memory, 7,* 599-612.

Reinitz, M.T., and Hannigan, S. (2004). False memories for compound words: Role of working memory. *Memory and Cognition, 32,* 463-473.

Reitan, R.M. (1958). Validity of the Trail Making Test as an indication of organic brain damage. *Perceptual and Motor Skills, 8,* 271-276.

Reitan, R.M., and Wolfson, D. (1993). *The Halstead-Reitan Neuropsychological Test Battery: Theory and clinical interpretation.* Tucson AZ: Neuropsychology Press.

Roediger, H. L. III., and McDermott, K. B. (1995). Creating false memories: Remembering words not presented in lists. *Journal of Experimental Psychology: Learning, Memory and Cognition, 21,* 803-814.

Sanders, H.I., and Warrington, E.K. (1971). Memory for remote events in amnesic patients. *Brain, 94,* 661-668.

Schacter, D.L. (2001). *The seven sins of memory: How the mind forgets and remembers.* New York: Houghton Mifflin Company.

Schacter, D. L. (1999). The seven sins of memory: Insights form psychology and cognitive neuroscience. *American Psychologist, 54,* 182-203.

Schacter, D. L., Buckner, R. L., Koutstaal, W., Dale, A. M., and Rosen, B. R. (1997). Late onset of anterior prefrontal activity during retrieval of veridical and illusory memories: An event-related fMRI study. *NeuroImage, 6,* 259-269.

Schacter, D. L., Curran, T., Galluccio, L., Milberg, W. P., and Bates, J. F. (1996a). False recognition and the right frontal lobe: A case study. *Neuropsychologia, 34,* 793-808.

Schacter, D.L., Koutstaal, W., and Norman, K.A. (1997). False memories and aging. *Trends in Cognitive Sciences, 1,* 229-236.

Schacter, D. L., Norman, K. A., and Koutstaal, W. (1998). The cognitive neuroscience of constructive memory. *Annual Review of Psychology, 49,* 289-318.

Schacter, D. L., Reiman, E., Curran, T., Yun, L.S., Bandy, D., McDermott, K. B., and Roediger, H. L., III. (1996c). Neuroanatomical correlates of veridical and illusory recognition memory: Evidence from positron emission tomography. *Neuron, 28,* 1166-1172.

Schacter, D.L., Savage, C. R., Alpert, N. M. , Rauch, S. L., and Albert, M. S. (1996b). The role of hippocampus and frontal cortex in age-related memory changes: A PET study. *Neuroreport, 7,* 1165-1169.

Schacter, D.L., and Slotnick, S.D. (2004). The cognitive neuroscience of memory distortion. *Neuron, 44,* 149-160.

Shimamura, A.P. (1995). Memory and the frontal lobe function. In M. Gazzaniga (Ed.), *The cognitive neurosciences* (p. 803-813). Cambridge, MA: MIT Press.

Smeets, T., Merckelbach, H., Horselenberg, R., and Jelicic, M. (*in press*). Trying to recollect past events: Confidence, beliefs, and memories. *Clinical Psychology Review.*

Stadler, M.A., Roediger, H.L.III., McDermott, K.B. (1999). Norms for word lists that create false memories. *Memory and Cognition, 27,* 494-500.

Stinissen, J., Willems, P., Coetsier, P. and Hulsman, W. (1970). *Handleiding bij de nederlandstalige bewerking van de Wechsler Adult Intelligence Scale (WAIS).* Lisse, The Netherlands: Swets en Zeitlinger.

Squire, L.R., and Schacter, D.L. (2002). *Neuropsychology of Memory* (3rd edition). New York: The Guilford Press.

Tranel, D., and Damasio, H. (1994). Neuroanatomical correlates of electrodermal skin conductance responses. *Psychophysiology, 31,* 427-438.

Waldie, B.D., and Kwong See, S.T. (2003). Remembering words never presented: False memory effects in dementia of the Alzheimer type. *Aging Neuropsychology and Cognition, 10,* 281-297.

Ward, J., Parkin, A.J., Powell, G., Squires, E.J., Townshend, J., and Bradley, V. (1999). False recognition of unfamiliar people: "seeing film stars everywhere". *Cognitive Neuropsychology, 16,* 293-315.

Watson, J.M., Baltoa, D.A., and Sergent-Marshall, S.D. (2001). Semantic, phonological, and hybrid veridical and false memories in healthy older adults and in individuals with dementia of the Alzheimer type. *Neuropsychology, 15,* 254-267.

Weinstein, E.A. (1996). Symbolic aspects of confabulation following brain injury: Influence of premorbid personality. *Bulletin of the Menninger Clinic, 60,* 331-350.

Wheeler, M.A., Stuss, D.T., and Tulving, E. (1997). Toward a theory of episodic memory: The frontal lobes and autonoetic consciousness. *Psychological Bulletin, 121,* 331-354.

Williams, M.A., Moss, S.A., Bradshaw, J.L., and Rinehart, N.J. (2002). Random Number Generation in Autism. *Journal of Autism and Developmental Disorders, 32,* 43-47.

Wilson, B.A., Alderman, N., Burgess, P.W., Emslie, H.E., and Evans, J.J. (1996). *Behavioural Assessment of Dysexecutive Syndrome.* Bury St. Edmunds: Thames Valley.

Winograd, E., Peluso, J.P., and Glover, T.A. (1998). Individual differences in susceptibility to memory illusions. *Applied Cognitive Psychology, 12,* S5-S27.

Young, A.W., Flude, B.M., Hay, D.C., and Ellis, A.W. (1993). Impaired discrimination of familiar from unfamiliar faces. *Cortex, 29,* 65-75.

Zoccolotti, P., Scabini, D., and Violani, C. (1982). Electrodermal responses in patients with unilateral brain damage. *Journal of Clinical Neuropsychology, 4,* 143-150

In: Focus on Neuropsychology Research
Editor: Joshua R. Dupri, pp. 185-197

ISBN 1-59454-779-3
© 2006 Nova Science Publishers, Inc.

Chapter 7

THE BENEFICIAL EFFECTS OF POLYPHENOLS IN AGE-RELATED NEUROLOGICAL DISORDERS

Bastianetto Stéphane and Rémi Quirion[*]

Department of Psychiatry, Douglas Hospital Research Centre,
McGill University, 6875 LaSalle Boulevard, Verdun, Québec, Canada H4H 1R3

ABSTRACT

Polyphenols have received particular attention because of their possible beneficial health effects in age-related neurological disorders. In support of this hypothesis, epidemiological studies reported a lower incidence of stroke, Parkinson's disease and dementia in populations that consume beverages or food (i.e. red wine, green tea, fruits, vegetables) enriched in polyphenolic compounds. These findings concur with animal and *in vitro* studies indicating that polyphenols derived from either beverages, fruits (e.g. catechins, resveratrol) or plant extracts (i.e. blueberry, Ginkgo biloba and tea) displayed neuroprotective abilities. For example, our studies and those obtained by other groups indicated that various polyphenols derived from green tea and red wine protected cultured neuronal cells against toxicity induced by free radicals and beta-amyloid (Aß) peptides, whose accumulation likely play a deleterious role in age-related neurological disorders. These effects involved their well-known antioxidant activities, but also their abilities to directly interact with Aß and to modulate intracellular effectors and genes associated with cell death/survival. We overview here epidemiologic and pre-clinical studies that support the role of polyphenols in the beneficial effects of diet in human.

INTRODUCTION

Age-related neurological disorders, particularly Alzheimer's disease (AD), are one of the major health concerns of industrialized countries. Drugs prescribed in the treatment of

---

[*] Corresponding author: Tel.: +1-514-761-6131; ext. 2934; Fax: +1-514-762-3034; E-mail: remi.quirion@douglas.mcgill.ca

dementia (i.e. galantamine, donepezil....) have modest beneficial effects and are not capable of stopping or reversing cognitive deficits in AD patients. It is now conceivable to prevent or delay the development of cognitive symptoms by inhibiting factors that contribute to the deleterious effects of normal and pathological brain aging. The notion that a healthy diet have potential health benefits in the elderly received a great deal of attention following the report that high intake of fruits, vegetable and non-alcoholic beverage such as green tea was linked to a lower incidence of stroke (Keli et al., 1996; Joshipura et al., 1999; Knekt et al., 2000; Johnsen et al., 2003; Sauvaget et al., 2003) and Parkinson's disease (Checkoway et al., 2002; Pan et al., 2003; Tan et al., 2003). Moreover, epidemiological studies reported a lower risk of dementia in the elderly population who moderately consume red wine, and possibly other alcoholic beverages (Orgogozo et al., 1997; Obisean et al., 1998; Leibovici et al., 1999; Ruitenberg et al., 2002; Luchsinger et al., 2004). Numerous *in vitro* and animal studies reported that polyphenols displayed protective abilities in various models of toxicity, supporting a central role for these molecules in the purported beneficial effects of food and red wine (for reviews, see Youdim and Joseph, 2001; Bastianetto and Quirion, 2001, 2002; Han et al., 2005). Besides the well-known radical scavenger and anti-inflammatory properties of polyphenols, recent evidence indicates that a wide spectrum of mechanisms, ranging from the inhibition of neurotoxic agents to the modulation of protein and gene expressions, may also account for their neuroprotective actions (Youdim and Joseph, 2001). We provide here an overview of epidemiologic and pre-clinical studies reporting on the benefits of a healthy diet and of polyphenols in human as well as *in vitro* and animal models of toxicity. Various mechanisms underlying the neuroprotective effects of polyphenols are also discussed as well as future directions in both animal and human studies.

EPIDEMIOLOGICAL STUDIES

Fruits and Vegetables

Accumulating evidence from epidemiological studies suggests that fruit and vegetable intakes decrease the risk of age-related neurological disorders (for review see Renaud, 2001). For example, a longitudinal study showed that elderly who consume 11.5 mg/day and higher of flavonoids have about half the risk to develop dementia, compared with those with lower daily intake (Commenges et al., 2000). In this study, the most important source was fruits (35%) followed by vegetables, wine and tea (Commenges et al., 2000). Other studies found an inverse association between a high dietary intake of polyphenols, derived particularly from fruits and the occurrence of stroke in the old age (Keli et al., 1996; Johnsen et al., 2003). Another longitudinal study performed in individuals aged 34 to 75 years reported that the intake of fruits and vegetables (e.g. cruciferous and green leafy vegetables) was associated with a lower (30%) risk to suffer from a stroke (Joshipura et al., 1999). Finally, a prospective Japanese cohort study demonstrated that individuals who consume green-yellow vegetables and fruits have a lower risk (25-35%) to suffer from stroke, intracerebral hemorrhage, and cerebral infarction mortality, compared with those who eat only vegetables and fruits once or less per week (Sauvaget et al., 2003).

Red Wine

Two 3- and 5-year follow-up studies enrolling elderly subjects reported that moderate red wine drinkers had a lower risk of AD than those who never or hardly ever drank wine (Lindsay et al., 2002; Truelsen et al., 2002). These results are in agreement with previous studies showing that 3-4 glasses of red wine per day (i.e. 250-500 ml) may have beneficial effects (over liquors and beer) against macular degeneration, AD and cognitive deficits (Orgogozo et al., 1997; Obisean et al., 1998; Leibovici et al., 1999; Luchsinger et al., 2004). Moreover, two other studies reported that a light-to-moderate (up to 3 glasses per day) consumption of alcohol, particularly wine, was associated with a lower risk of dementia (Ruitenberg et al., 2002; Huang et al., 2002).

Tea

Keli et al. (1996) have reported that flavonoid intake was inversely correlated to the risk of stroke, with black tea being the major source (about 70%) of flavonoids. In this study, the authors found that the risk of stroke was diminished by 70% in individuals who consumed more than 5 cups of tea per day compared to those who drank less than 2.6 cups/day (Keli et al., 1996). Two other studies suggested that daily tea consumption (from 3 to 5 cups) may decrease the risk of developing PD (Pan et al., 2003; Tan et al., 2003). However, cohort studies regarding a possible relationship between tea consumption and dementia are lacking.

NEUROPROTECTIVE EFFECTS OF POLYPHENOLS: *IN VITRO* AND ANIMAL STUDIES

The main argument for the purported protective effects of natural extracts, fruits, vegetables and beverages (i.e. red wine, tea) is through the presence of their enrichment in various polyphenolic compounds (Table 1). About seven thousands polyphenols have been identified and the most numerous ones belong to the sub-category of flavonoids. The other main group belongs to the class of stilbenes and includes resveratrol found in grape vine.

Flavonoids

Flavonoids are a main group of polyphenols that possess three phenolic structures referred as the A, B and C rings. More than 4000 varieties of flavonoids have been identified and can be divided into various classes according to their oxidation level on the C-ring, including flavones, flavanols (catechins), anthocyanidins, flavones, flavonols, flavanones and isoflavones (Figure 1).

Table 1. Dietary Source of polyphenols

Families of polyphenols	Source
Flavonols (quercetin, myricetin, kaempferol)	Apricot, apple, cranberries, kiwi, strawberries, orange, grape, onion, leek, broccoli, potato, parsley, curly kale, bean, tomato, lettuce, black Tea, red wine, standardized Ginkgo biloba extract
Flavanols (catechin, epicatechin, gallocatechin, epigallocatechin, epicatechin gallate, epigallocatechin gallate)	Chocolate, beans, apricot, cherry, grape, peach, blackberry, strawberries, apple, green tea, black tea, cider
Flavones (apigenin, luteolin)	Celery, parsley, green bell pepper, spinach
Flavanones/flavanonols (naringenin, narigin, fisetin, hesperetin, eriodictyol, taxifolin)	Citrus fruit, citrus peel
Isoflavones (daidzein, genistein)	Soybean, soy milk, tofu, yuba, miso
Anthocyanins (cyanidin, delphidin, malvidin, pelargonidin, peonidin, petunidin)	Berries, cherries, grapes, raspberries, red wine, strawberries, tea, fruit peels with dark pigments
Stilbenes (resveratrol)	Grape, peanuts, red wine

Flavonols

We and other groups have reported that the Ginkgo biloba extract EGb 761 - a well-standardized natural extract that is approved in Europe for the treatment of cognitive impairments seen in AD patients (Le Bars et al., 1997) - protected cultured neurons exposed to either Aß peptides or oxidative stress (Bastianetto et al., 2000a,b; Yao et al., 2001). We demonstrated that these effects were attributable to the presence of 24% of flavonols in the total extract (Bastianetto et al., 2000a,b but see Yao et al., 2001). In both models, the effects of EGb 761 were shared by its flavonoid fraction that essentially contains flavonol-O-glycosides (i.e. quercetin, myricetin and kaempferol) whereas other ingredients such as terpenes failed to exert any protective effects (Bastianetto et al., 2000b). Moreover, using the dichlorofluorescein (DCF) assay, we found that EGb 761 and its flavonoid fraction decreased reactive oxygen accumulation (ROS) produced by either $Aß_{25-35}$ or the NO donor sodium nitroprusside (SNP), supporting the idea that the antioxidant activities of flavonols play a predominant role in the neuroprotective action of the total extract (Bastianetto et al., 2000a,b; Smith et al., 2003). However, antioxidant activities may not the sole mechanism underlying the neuroprotective effects of EGb 761 and its active flavonoids fraction. Considering the deleterious role of the accumulation of Aß peptides (Aß) in the pathogenesis of AD, Ono et al. (2003) investigated *in vitro* anti-amyloidogenic and fibril-destabilizing effects of flavonols. Using thioflavin fluorescent assay, these authors found that myricetin (EC_{50} = 0.3-0.4 µM) was most potent, followed by morin, quercetin and kaempferol, to inhibit the formation of Aß fibrils from $Aß_{1-40}$ and $Aß_{1-42}$ (Ono et al., 2003). Moreover, these polyphenols are capable of destabilizing pre-formed Aß fibrils *in vitro*, myricetin being also the most potent one (EC =1.8 µM). Using non-neuronal HEK 293 cell cultures, Ono et al. (2003) showed that the toxic effects of Aß fibrils were reduced by the most potent flavanol, myricetin (1 µM). Similar protective effects against Aß toxicity was also observed using Hypericum perforatum ethanolic extract, which shared with fractions containing flavonol glycosides and flavonol, the ability to reduce $Aß_{25-35}$-induced cell death in rat cultured hippocampal neurons (Silva et al., 2004). According to these authors, anti-necrotic but not anti-apoptotic effects of polyphenols appeared to be involved in their neuroprotective effects, possibly through their antioxidant activities (Silva et al., 2004).

Using hippocampal neuronal cell cultures, we reported that quercetin strongly protected against toxicity induced by SNP (Bastianetto et al., 2000c). Quercetin was also able to block ROS accumulation and protein kinase C (PKC) activation produced by SNP, suggesting the involvement of at least two mechanisms that may act additively or synergistically (Bastianetto et al., 2000c). The role of quercetin in protecting mouse cortical neuronal cells in various models of toxicity was investigated by Ha et al (2003). Pre- and co-treatment with quercetin (100 µM) inhibited (from 20% to 60%) neurotoxicity produced by either oxygen-glucose deprivation, excitotoxicity or oxidative stress, suggesting that quercetin may protect against neuronal injury associated with cerebral ischemia (Ha et al., 2003). Regarding the possible beneficial role of fruits and vegetables in reducing stroke, Dajas et al. (2003) investigated the effects of quercetin (the best-described flavonol found in abundance in apples, broccoli and onions) in a model of permanent focal ischemia. Quercetin was administered i.p. 30 min after vessel occlusion in lecithin preparations to facilitate brain penetration. The lecithin/quercetin (30 mg/kg) preparation (but not an aqueous administration of quercetin) significantly (by 56%) decreased the size of the ischemic lesion, as did the flavanone fisetin, whereas the flavanol catechin was not effective (Dajas et al., 2003; Rivera et al., 2004). Significant cerebral concentrations of quercetin (509 ng/g) were detected in the brain only following peripheral injection of the liposomal (lecithin) preparations, suggesting that this type of preparations may be critical for the expression of the protective effects of flavonoids in the CNS (Dajas et al., 2003; Rivera et al., 2004). Considering the overall poor daily intake or flavonols (20-35 mg/day on average) and the poor absorption of quercetin in the human body, the genuine beneficial role of flavonols in regards to CNS diseases will require further investigation.

Flavanols

Flavanols, also known as catechins, are polyphenols concentrated in high amounts in berries and beverages such as tea and red wine. Various cell cultures and animal models of toxicity demonstrated the strong neuroprotective abilities of catechins (Sun et al., 1999; Bastianetto et al., 2000c; Choi et al., 2001, 2002; 2004; Lee et al., 2003, 2004; Suzuki et al., 2004). For example, we reported that (+)-catechin was the most potent flavonoid over quercetin and resveratrol to protect hippocampal neurons against toxicity induced by SNP, possibly through its free radical scavenging and iron-chelating properties (Bastianetto et al., 2000c). Many other studies have focused on the most abundant flavanol present in green tea, namely EGCG which represents up to 25% of the total extract (Wang et al., 2000). EGCG (5-10 µM) was shown to protect neuronal cells against excitotoxicity and this effect was likely due to antioxidant and free radical scavenging properties. Catechins and particularly EGCG may also function indirectly as antioxidants by inhibiting certain transcription factors [e.g.

nuclear factor-kappaB (NF kappaB), activator protein-1 (AP1)] and enzymes [inducible nitric oxide synthase, lipoxygenases, cyclooxygenases and xanthine oxidase] or by activating antioxidant enzymes [e.g. glutathione S-transferases and superoxide dismutases] (Lee et al., 2000, 2003, 2004; Choi et al., 2004; Mandel et al., 2004). Levites et coll (2002) found that EGCG may exert neuroprotective effects by inhibiting the induction of pro-apoptotic genes (e.g. bax, bad, gadd45 and fas ligand) or restoring the activities of protective kinases [e.g. PKC, extracellular signal-regulated kinases (ERK1/2)]. Interestingly, two studies reported that EGCG was able to block the deleterious effects of $A\beta_{25-35}$, possibly through its antioxidant activities (Choi et al., 2001) and modulatory effect on PKC activity (Levites et al., 2003). Our data also suggested that EGCG shared with green and black teas the ability to protect hippocampal neurons and to inhibit the formation of Aß oligomers that may be responsible, at least in part, for the neurotoxic effects of Aß peptides (Bastianetto et al., unpublished data). Moreover, animal studies have shown that peripheral administration of grape and green tea extracts (Hong et al., 2002; Suzuki et al., 2004; Hwang et al., 2004) or catechins (Inanami et al., 1998; Lee et al., 2000, 2003, 2004; Nagai et al., 2002; Choi et al., 2004) were shown to protect against neuronal toxicity induced by ischemia, supporting the hypothesis that flavanols (or their metabolites) can cross the blood brain barrier (Suganuma et al., 1998). These studies also suggested that the antioxidant properties of EGCG, and to a lesser extent its modulatory effect on polyamine metabolism, contribute to its neuroprotective effects (Lee et al., 2003, 2004; Choi et al., 2004).

Other Flavonoids

Data on the protective effects of other groups of flavonoids are limited. However, it was recently reported that baicalin and its aglycone baicalein, two flavones that are enriched in the traditional Asian herbal medicine *Scutellaria baicalensis*, can reduce the toxicity induced by Aß peptides in PC 12 cells, possibly by reducing the accumulation of ROS (Heo et al., 2004). Baicalein was able to reduce neuronal death induced by either glutamate or glucose deprivation, whereas baicalin was only effective in preventing glutamate toxicity, suggesting that their underlying mechanisms of action may be distinct (Heo et al., 2004a). Similar protective effects were obtained in neuronal cortical cells as baicalein attenuated both neuronal apoptosis and c-jun protein over-expression induced by $A\beta_{25-35}$ (Lebeau et al., 2001). According to the authors, these results suggested that the inhibitory action of baicalein on 12-lipoxygenase may participate in its anti-apoptotic effect (Lebeau et al., 2001). Another study showed that baicalein (50µM), and especially its oxidized forms, inhibited fibrillation of alpha-synuclein fibrils and disaggregated existing fibrils, indicating that diets rich in flavonoids, and particularly flavones, may be effective in preventing PD (Zhu et al., 2004). The protective effect of naringenin, the major flavanone constituent isolated from Citrus junos, was studied against Aß-induced toxicity in PC12 cells (Heo et al., 2004b). Pre-treatment with naringenin (25-100 µM) prevented both cell death and ROS accumulation induced by $A\beta_{25-35}$ (Heo et al., 2004b). Naringenin (4.5 mg/kg) was also able to reverse the anti-amnestic effect of scopolamine in mice as measured in the passive avoidance test. The action of naringenin may be related, at least in part, to its purported inhibitory effect on acetylcholinesterase activity (Heo et al., 2004c). The effect of 4',5-dihydroxy-3',6,7-trimethoxyflavone from Artemisia asiatica on Aß-induced neurotoxicity was investigated by the same group (Heo et al., 2001). They showed that a pretreatment with 4',5-dihydroxy-3',6,7-trimethoxyflavone prevented various events (cell death, ROS) induced by Aß peptides exposure in PC 12 cells (Heo et al., 2001). Finally, two studies reported that high nM (100nM) and µM (50µM) concentrations of genistein, the most active component of soy isoflavones, protected hippocampal neurons against Aß-induced apoptosis, suggesting a dual mechanism that involved its estrogenic and antioxidant properties, respectively (Zeng et al., 2003). According to Bang et al. (2004), genistein could be an alternative to estrogen in the treatment of AD.

THE STILBENE RESVERATROL

Resveratrol (cis- and trans- 3',4',5 trihydroxystilbene) belongs to the non-flavonoid class of polyphenols known as stilbenes and is mainly present in grapevines and peanuts. Cell cultures studies have shown that resveratrol possesses protective abilities against toxicities induced by oxidative stress, Aß peptides and glutamate. We reported that resveratrol (1-25 µM) was able to block hippocampal neuronal cell death and ROS accumulation (but not PKC activation) produced by SNP, suggesting its antioxidant properties mainly contribute to its neuroprotective effects (Bastianetto et al., 2000c). Similarly, Karlsson and coll. (1999) demonstrated that free radical scavenging properties of resveratrol were responsible for its neuroprotective effects in rat mesencephalic dopaminergic neuronal cultures exposed to the pro-oxidant, tert-butyl hydroperoxide. Han and coll. (2004) reported that resveratrol (20 µM) protected hippocampal neurons against Aß peptides (Aß$_{25-35}$, Aß$_{1-40}$ and Aß$_{1-42}$)-induced toxicity. This effect was shared by the PKC inhibitor GF 109203X - but not by other kinases inhibitors, suggesting a role for PKC in the neuroprotective effect of resveratrol in this model. Similar protective effects against Aß$_{25-35}$–induced toxicity were seen in human neuroblastoma cells and were accompanied by an increase in the level of the antioxidant protein, glutathione (Savaskan et al., 2003). Other studies reported that the neuroprotective effects of resveratrol are not solely due to its antioxidant action but also to its ability to reverse the phosphorylation of stress-activated protein kinase/c-Jun N-terminal kinase (SAPK/JNK) (Nicolini et al, 2003), the activation of caspase 7 (Nicolini et al, 2003) and even heme oxygenase 1 (Zhuang 2003). Resveratrol has also been shown to increase cell survival by stimulating SIRT1-dependent deacetylation of p53 and is considered as a potential calorie restriction mimetic (Howitz et al., 2003). Finally, our data from binding and autoradiography studies suggested the existence of unique [^{3}H]-resveratrol binding site(s) in rat brain that may contribute to its purported effects (Han et al., submitted).

The neuroprotective abilities of peripheral administration of resveratrol in rodent models of ischemia and excitotoxicity were also been reported, indicating that it (or its metabolites) can cross the blood brain barrier. For example, chronic administration of resveratrol partially but significantly protected areas (e.g. olfactory cortex, hippocampus) subjected to either kainic acid (Virgili and Contestabile, 2000; Gupta et al., 2002) or cerebral ischemia (Sinha et al., 2001; Huang et al., 2001; Wang et al., 2002; Inoue et al., 2003) in rodents. Wang et al. (2002) reported that resveratrol could be detected in the brain reaching a peak at 4 hours after its peripheral administration, providing support for its ability to cross the blood brain barrier, at least in rodents. The protective effects of resveratrol were showed to be accompanied by decreases in the levels of malondialdehyde (MDA) and reduced glutathione, supporting its antioxidant properties (Sinha et al., 2002; Gupta et al., 2002). Moreover, Inoue et al. (2003) found that the neuroprotective effects of resveratrol in the middle cerebral artery occlusion model required the expression of the α isotype of peroxisome proliferator-activated receptors (PPARα, a nuclear receptor family of ligand-dependent transcription factor involved in ischemia/reperfusion injury as neuroprotection was not observed in PPARα knockout mice (Inoue et al., 2003). Finally, Sharma and Gupta (2002) reported that a 3 week-treatment with *trans*-resveratrol prevented cognitive impairments induced by streptozotocin in a model of sporadic dementia of Alzheimer's type in rats. This effect was associated with a rise in brain glutathione and decreased levels in MDA (Sharma and Gupta, 2002).

CONCLUSION

During the last decade, epidemiological studies have focused to the health-promoting effects of polyphenols in reducing the risk of neurological disorders in the elderly population. Taken together, these studies suggested a correlation between diet and incidence of these diseases that has yet to be further investigated. Hence, studies regarding consumption of tea (a major source of flavonoids in many countries) have been targeted at its possible cardiovascular and anti-carcinogenic effects and it remains to determine if tea may also reduce the incidence of Alzheimer's disease. Moreover, it has been suggested that data from epidemiologic studies may be biased, particular with respect to the potential role of flavonoids in the occurrence of stroke (Peters et al., 2001). For example, tea consumption has been reported to increase the risk of stroke in Australia, but tends to decrease it in continental Europe (Peters et al., 2001). It is important to include other dietary factors such vitamins C and E, carotenoids, folic acid, fibers and lifestyle that may impact the incidence and to develop new approaches (e.g. validation of biomarkers of polyphenols and their metabolites) to make questionnaire-based assessment more reliable.

Pre-clinical studies strongly suggested that polyphenols are components responsible for the potential benefits of diet in brain aging. Mechanisms of action by which they act are not completely elucidated but include antioxidant properties and modulatory effects on protein and gene expression that play a pivotal role in the cell death/survival. However, since most of the research involved *in vitro* studies and animal models of ischemia, it is difficult to draw definite conclusions about the usefulness of polyphenols in the diet. It is a need to investigate further their *in vivo* distribution in brain areas in order to have a better insight on their metabolism, at least in rodents. It will be also of particular interest to study their effects in various neurotransmitter systems and in models of transgenic rodents that feature AD pathology, in order to have a better insight in their possible beneficial role in Alzheimer's disease.

ACKNOWLEGEMENTS

This work was supported by research grants from the Canadian Institutes of Health Research (CIHR) to R. Quirion.

REFERENCES

Bang, OY; Hong HS; Kim DH; Kim H; Boo JH; Huh K; Mook-Jung I. Neuroprotective effect of genistein against beta amyloid-induced neurotoxicity. *Neurobiol. Dis*, 2004 16, 21-28.

Bastianetto S; Quirion R. Resveratrol and red wine constituents: evaluation of their neuroprotective properties. *Pharm News* 2001 8, 33-38.

Bastianetto S; Quirion R. Natural extracts as possible protective agents of brain aging. *Neurobiol Aging* 2002 23, 891-897.

Bastianetto S; Zheng WH; Quirion R. The ginkgo biloba extract (EGb 761) protects and rescues hippocampal cells against nitric oxide-induced toxicity: involvement of its flavonoid constituents and protein kinase C. *J Neurochem* 2000a 74, 2268-2277.

Bastianetto S; Ramassamy C; Doré S; Christen Y; Poirier J; Quirion R. The ginkgo biloba extract (EGb 761) protects hippocampal neurons against cell death induced by β-amyloid. *Eur J Neurosci* 2000b 12, 1-9.

Bastianetto S; Zheng WH; Quirion R. Neuroprotective abilities of resveratrol and other red wine constituents against nitric oxide-related toxicity in cultured hippocampal neurons. *Br J Pharmacol* 2000c 131, 711-720.

Checkoway H; Powers K; Smith-Weller T; Franklin GM; Longstreth WT Jr; Swanson PD. Parkinson's disease risks associated with cigarette smoking, alcohol consumption, and caffeine intake. *Am J Epidemiol* 2002 155, 732-738.

Choi YT; Jung CH; Lee SR; Bae JH; Baek WK; Suh MH; Park J; Park CW; Suh SI. The green tea polyphenol (-)-epigallocatechin gallate attenuates beta-amyloid-induced neurotoxicity in cultured hippocampal neurons. *Life Sci* 2001 70, 603-614.

Choi JY; Park CS; Kim DJ; Cho MH; Jin BK; Pie JE; Chung WG. Prevention of nitric oxide-mediated 1-methyl-4-phenyl-1,2,3,6-tetrahydropyridine-induced Parkinson's disease in mice by tea phenolic epigallocatechin 3-gallate. *Neurotoxicology* 2002 23, 367-74.

Choi YB, Kim YI, Lee KS, Kim BS, Kim DJ. Protective effect of epigallocatechin gallate on brain damage after transient middle cerebral artery occlusion in rats. *Brain Res* 2004 1019, 47-54.

Commenges D; Scotet V; Renaud S; Jacqmin-Gadda H; Barberger-Gateau P; Dartigues JF. Intake of flavonoids and risk of dementia. *Eur J Epidemiol* 2000 16, 357-363.

Conte A; Pellegrini S; Tagliazucchi D. Synergistic protection of PC12 cells from beta-amyloid toxicity by resveratrol and catechin. *Brain Res Bull* 2003 62, 29-38.

Dajas F; Rivera F; Blasina F; Arredondo F; Echeverry C; Lafon L; Morquio A; Heizen H. Cell culture protection and in vivo neuroprotective capacity of flavonoids. *Neurotox Res* 2003 5, 425-432.

Gupta YK; Briyal S; Chaudhary G Protective effect of trans-resveratrol against kainic acid-induced seizures and oxidative stress in rats. *Pharmacol Biochem Behav* 2002 71, 245-249.

Ha HJ; Kwon YS; Park SM; Shin T; Park JH; Kim HC; Kwon MS; Wie MB. Quercetin attenuates oxygen-glucose deprivation- and excitotoxin-induced neurotoxicity in primary cortical cell cultures. *Biol Pharm Bull* 2003 26, 544-546.

Han YS; Zheng WH; Bastianetto S; Chabot JG; Quirion R. Neuroprotective effects of resveratrol against beta-amyloid-induced neurotoxicity in rat hippocampal neurons: involvement of protein kinase C. *Br J Pharmacol* 2004 141, 997-1005.

Heo HJ; Kim DO; Choi SJ; Shin DH; Lee CY. Potent Inhibitory effect of flavonoids in Scutellaria baicalensis on amyloid beta protein-induced neurotoxicity. *J Agric Food Chem* 2004a 52, 4128-4132.

Heo HJ; Kim DO; Shin SC; Kim MJ; Kim BG; Shin DH.. Effect of antioxidant flavanone, naringenin, from Citrus junos on neuroprotection. *J Agric Food Chem* 2004b 52, 1520-1525.

Heo HJ; Kim MJ; Lee JM; Choi SJ; Cho HY; Hong B; Kim HK; Kim E; Shin DH. Naringenin from Citrus junos has an inhibitory effect on acetylcholinesterase and a mitigating effect on amnesia. *Dement Geriatr Cogn Disord.* 2004c 17, 151-157.

Heo HJ; Cho HY; Hong B; Kim HK; Kim EK; Kim BG; Shin DH. Protective effect of 4',5-dihydroxy-3',6,7-trimethoxyflavone from Artemisia asiatica against Abeta-induced oxidative stress in PC12 cells. *Amyloid* 2001 8, 194-201.

Hong JT; Ryu SR; Kim HJ; Lee JK; Lee SH; Kim DB; Yun YP; Ryu JH; Lee BM; Kim PY. Neuroprotective effect of green tea extract in experimental ischemia-reperfusion brain injury. *Brain Res Bull* 2000 53, 743-749.

Howitz KT; Bitterman KJ; Cohen HY; Lamming DW; Lavu S; Wood JG; Zipkin RE; Chung P; Kisielewski A; Zhang LL; Scherer B; Sinclair DA. *Nature* 2003 425, 191-6.

Huang W; Qiu C; Winblad B; Fratiglioni L. Alcohol consumption and incidence of dementia in a community sample aged 75 years and older, *J Clin Epidemiol* 2002 55, 959-964.

Huang SS; Tsai MC; Chih CL; Hung LM; Tsai SK. Resveratrol reduction of infarct size in Long-Evans rats subjected to focal cerebral ischemia. *Life Sci* 2001 69, 1057-1065.

Hwang IK; Yoo KY; Kim DS; Jeong YK; Kim JD; Shin HK; Lim SS; Yoo ID; Kang TC; Kim DW; Moon WK; Won MH. Neuroprotective effects of grape seed extract on neuronal injury by inhibiting DNA damage in the gerbil hippocampus after transient forebrain ischemia. *Life Sci* 2004 75, 1989-2001.

Inanami O; Watanabe Y; Syuto B; Nakano M; Tsuji M; and Kuwabara M; Oral administration of (-)catechin protects against ischemia-reperfusion-induced neuronal death in the Gerbil. *Free Rad Res* 1998 29, 359-365.

Inoue H; Jiang XF; Katayama T; Osada S; Umesono K; Namura S. Brain protection by resveratrol and fenofibrate against stroke requires peroxisome proliferator-activated receptor alpha in mice. *Neurosci Lett* 2003 352, 203-206.

Johnsen SP; Overvad K; Stripp C; Tjonneland A; Husted SE; Sorensen HT. Intake of fruit and vegetables and the risk of ischemic stroke in a cohort of Danish men and women *Am J Clin Nutr* 2003 78, 57-64.

Joshipura K J; Ascherio A; Manson JE; Stampfer MJ; Rimm EB; Speizer FE; Hennekens CH; Spiegelman D; Willett WC. Fruit and vegetable intake in relation to risk of ischemic stroke. *JAMA* 1999 282, 1233-1239.

Karlsson J; Emgard M; Brundin P; Burkitt MJ. *Trans*-resveratrol protects embryonic mesencephalic cells from tert-butyl hydroperoxide: electron paramagnetic resonance spin trapping evidence for a radical scavenging mechanism. *J Neurochem* 2000 75, 141-150.

Keli SO; Hertog MG; Feskens EJ; Kromhout D. Dietary flavonoids, antioxidant vitamins, and incidence of stroke: the Zutphen study. *Arch Intern Med* 1996 156, 637-642.

Knekt P; Isotupa S; Rissanen H; Heliovaara M; Jarvinen R; Hakkinen S; Aromaa A; Reunanen A. Quercetin intake and the incidence of cerebrovascular disease. *Eur J Clin Nutr* 2000 54, 415-417.

Kreijkamp-Kaspers S; Kok L; Grobbee DE; de Haan EH; Aleman A; Lampe JW; van der Schouw YT. Effect of soy protein containing isoflavones on cognitive function, bone mineral density, and plasma lipids in postmenopausal women: a randomized controlled trial. *JAMA* 2004 292, 65-74.

Le Bars PL; Katz MM; Berman N; Itil TM; Freedman AM; Schatzberg AF. A placebo-controlled, double-blind, randomized trial of an extract of ginkgo biloba for dementia. *JAMA* 1997 278, 327-332.

Lebeau A; Esclaire F; Rostene W; Pelaprat D. Baicalein protects cortical neurons from beta-amyloid (25-35) induced toxicity. *Neuroreport.* 2001 12, 2199-2202.

Lee H; Bae JH; Lee SR. Protective effect of green tea polyphenol EGCG against neuronal damage and brain edema after unilateral cerebral ischemia in gerbils. *J Neurosci Res* 2004 77, 892-900.

Lee SY; Kim CY; Lee JJ; Jung JG; Lee SR. Effects of delayed administration of (-)-epigallocatechin gallate, a green tea polyphenol on the changes in polyamine levels and neuronal damage after transient forebrain ischemia in gerbils. *Brain Res Bull* 2003 61, 399-406.

Lee S; Suh S; Kim S. Protective effects of the green tea polyphenol (-)-epigallocatechin gallate against hippocampal neuronal damage after transient global ischemia in gerbils. *Neurosci.* Lett 2000 287, 191-194.

Leibovici D; Ritchie K; Ledesert B; Touchon J. The effects of wine and tobacco consumption on cognitive performance in the elderly: a longitudinal study of relative risk. *Int J Epidemiol* 1999 28, 77-81.

Levites Y, Amit T; Youdim MB; Mandel S. Involvement of protein kinase C activation and cell survival/ cell cycle genes in green tea polyphenol (-)-epigallocatechin 3-gallate neuroprotective action. *J Biol Chem* 2002 277, 30574-30580.

Lindsay J; Laurin D; Verreault R; Hebert R; Helliwell B; Hill GB; McDowell I. Risk factors for Alzheimer's disease: a prospective analysis from the Canadian Study of Health and Aging. *Am J Epidemiol* 2002 156, 445-453.

Luchsinger JA; Tang MX; Siddiqui M; Shea S; Mayeux R. Alcohol intake and risk of dementia. *J Am Geriatr Soc* 2004 52, 540-546.

Miloso M, Bertelli AA; Nicolini G; Tredici G. Resveratrol-induced activation of the mitogen-activated protein kinases, ERK1 and ERK2, in human neuroblastoma SH-SY5Y cells. *Neurosci Lett* 1999 264, 141-144.

Nagai K; Jiang MH; Hada J; Nagata T; Yajima Y; Yamamoto S; Nishizaki T. (-)-Epigallocatechin gallate protects against NO stress-induced neuronal damage after ischemia by acting as an anti-oxidant. *Brain Res* 2002 956, 319-322.

Nicolini, G., Rigolio R, Scuteri A, Miloso M, Saccomanno D, Cavaletti G, Tredici G. Effect of *trans*-resveratrol on signal transduction pathways involved in paclitaxel-induced apoptosis in human neuroblastoma SH-SY5Y cells. *Neurochem Int* 2003 42, 419-429.

Obisesan TO, Hirsh R; Kosoko O; Carlson L; Parrott M. Moderate wine consumption is associated with decreased odds of developing age-related macular degeneration in NHANES-1. *J Am Ger Soc* 1998 46, 1-7.

Ono K; Yoshiike Y; Takashima A; Hasegawa K; Naiki H; Yamada M. Potent anti-amyloidogenic and fibril-destabilizing effects of polyphenols in vitro: implications for the prevention and therapeutics of Alzheimer's disease. *J Neurochem* 2003 87, 172-181.

Orgogozo JM; Dartigues JF; Lafont S; Letenneur L; Commenges D; Salamon R; Renaud S; Breteler MD. Wine consumption and dementia in the elderly: a prospective community study in the Bordeaux area. *Revue Neurologique* 1997 153, 185-192.

Pan T; Jankovic J; Le W. Potential therapeutic properties of green tea polyphenols in Parkinson's disease. *Drugs Aging* 2003 20, 711-721.

Peters U, Poole C, Arab L. Does tea affect cardiovascular disease? A meta-analysis. *Am J Epidemiol* 2001 154, 495-503.

Renaud S C. Diet and stroke. *J Nutr Health Aging* 2001 5, 167-172.

Rivera F; Urbanavicius J; Gervaz E; Morquio A; Dajas F. Some Aspects of the in vivo Neuroprotective Capacity of Flavonoids: Bioavailability and Structure-Activity Relationship. *Neurotox Res* 2004 6, 543-553.

Ruitenberg A; van Swieten JC; Witteman JC; Mehta KM; van Duijn CM; Hofman A; Breteler MM. Alcohol consumption and risk of dementia: the Rotterdam Study. *Lancet* 2002 359, 281-286.

Sauvaget C; Nagano J; Allen N; Kodama K. Vegetable and fruit intake and stroke mortality in the Hiroshima/Nagasaki Life Span Study. *Stroke* 2003 34, 2355-2360.

Savaskan E; Olivieri G; Meier F; Seifritz E; Wirz-Justice A; Muller-Spahn F. Red wine ingredient resveratrol protects from beta-amyloid neurotoxicity. *Gerontology* 2003, 49, 380-383.

Sharma M; Gupta YK. Chronic treatment with *trans* resveratrol prevents intracerebroventricular streptozotocin induced cognitive impairment and oxidative stress in rats. *Life Sci* 2002 71, 2489-2498.

Silva BA; Dias AC; Ferreres F; Malva JO; Oliveira CR. Neuroprotective effect of H. perforatum extracts on beta-amyloid-induced neurotoxicity. *Neurotox Res* 2004 6, 119-130.

Sinha K; Chaudhary G; Gupta YK; Protective effect of resveratrol against oxidative stress in middle cerebral artery occlusion model of stroke in rats. *Life Sci* 2001 71, 655-65.

Smith JV; Luo Y. Elevation of oxidative free radicals in Alzheimer's disease models can be attenuated by Ginkgo biloba extract EGb 761. *J Alzheimers Dis* 2003 5, 287-300.

Suganuma M; Okabe S; Oniyama M; Tada Y; Ito H; Fujiki H. Wide distribution of [3H](-)-epigallocatechin gallate, a cancer preventive tea polyphenol, in mouse tissue. *Carcinogenesis* 1998 19, 1771-1776.

Sun GY; Xia J; Draczynska-Lusiak B; Simonyi A; Sun AY. Grape polyphenols protect neurodegenerative changes induced by chronic ethanol administration. *Neuroreport* 1999 10, 93-96.

Suzuki M; Tabuchi M; Ikeda M; Umegaki K; Tomita T. (2004) Protective effects of green tea catechins on cerebral ischemic damage. *Med Sci Monit* 2004 10, BR166-174.

Tan EK; Tan C; Fook-Chong SM; Lum SY; Chai A; Chung H; Shen H; Zhao Y; Teoh ML; Yih Y; Pavanni R; Chandran VR; Wong MC. Dose-dependent protective effect of coffee, tea, and smoking in Parkinson's disease: a study in ethnic Chinese. *J Neurol Sci* 2003 216, 163-167.

Truelsen T; Thudium D; Grønbæk M. Amount and type of alcohol and risk of dementia. Neurology 2002 59, 1313-1319.

Virgili M; Contestabile A. Partial neuroprotection of in vivo excitotoxic brain damage by chronic administration of the red wine antioxidant agent, trans-resveratrol in rats. *Neurosci Lett* 2000 281, 123-126.

Wang LF; Kim DM; Lee CY. Effects of heat processing and storage on flavanols and sensory qualities of green tea beverage. *J Agric Food Chem* 2000 48, 4227-4232.

Wang Q; Xu J; Rottinghaus GE; Simonyi A; Lubahn D; Sun GY; Sun AY. Resveratrol protects against global cerebral ischemic injury in gerbils. *Brain Res* 2002 958, 439-447.

Yao Z; Drieu K; Papadopoulos V. The Ginkgo biloba extract EGb 761 rescues the PC12 neuronal cells from beta-amyloid-induced cell death by inhibiting the formation of beta-amyloid-derived diffusible neurotoxic ligands. *Brain Res* 2001 889, 181-190.

Youdim M; Joseph J. A possible emerging role of phytochemicals in improving age-related neurological dysfunctions: a multiplicity of effects. *Free Rad Biol Med* 2001 30, 583-594.

Zeng H; Chen Q; Zhao B. Genistein ameliorates beta-amyloid peptide (25-35)-induced hippocampal neuronal apoptosis. *Free Radic Biol Med* 2004 36, 180-188.

Zhu M; Rajamani S; Kaylor J; Han S; Zhou F; Fink AL. The flavonoid baicalein inhibits fibrillation of alpha-synuclein and disaggregates existing fibrils. *J Biol Chem* 2004 279, 26846-26857.

Zhuang H; Kim YS; Koehler RC; Dore S. Potential mechanism by which resveratrol, a red wine constituent, protects neurons. *Ann. N. Y. Acad. Sci.* 2003 993, 276-283.

In: Focus on Neuropsychology Research
Editor: Joshua R. Dupri, pp. 199-217

ISBN 1-59454-779-3
© 2006 Nova Science Publishers, Inc.

Chapter 8

CURRENT ISSUES IN RESPONSE BIAS DURING NEUROPSYCHOLOGICAL ASSESSMENT: INCOMPLETE EFFORT TO MALINGERING

Thomas M. Dunn[*]

School of Psychological Sciences
University of Northern Colorado, Greeley

ABSTRACT

The purpose of this chapter is to review the recent literature regarding the assessment of biased responding, especially in the context of malingering. It makes the case that biased responding is multifaceted and that clinicians need to be aware of a variety of issues pertaining to effort. The different types of malingering are discussed, as well as the particular situations when patients are likely to feign symptoms. The more common commercially-available tests to assess effort are reviewed, with a discussion of their strengths and weaknesses. Other means of assessing response bias are mentioned, including the use of traditional neuropsychological assessments, as well as the issue of coached malingerers. Finally, specific suggestions for the practicing neuropsychologist are given.

INTRODUCTION

During clinical neuropsychological evaluation, a major concern is whether the patient being assessed is putting forth their best possible effort. The validity of the neuropsychological test results may be suspect when a clinician believes that the patient is not exerting maximum effort. There are a variety of reasons why patients may not try their best. Some of these reasons, while disrupting accurate assessment, are innocuous such as the child

[*] Thomas M. Dunn, Ph.D.; Campus Box 94; 0014 McKee Hall; University of Northern Colorado; Greeley, CO 80639; Thomas.dunn@unco.edu; O: 970.351.1501; F: 970.351.1103

who does not understand the importance of trying hard, or the patient with cognitive deficits who is fatigued after a long test battery (Constantinou and McCaffery, 2003; Uttl, Graf and Cosentino, 2000). Further, there may be situations when the patient is disinterested in the assessment process and will perform with a minimum of compliance to the test directions. Some patients are simply overwhelmed by the testing process and give up trying to do well, responding randomly to test items. Others may not understand the test instructions and perform poorly because they do not ask for clarification. While all of these examples are of patients whose different behaviors will result in response bias, they are united in that these are patients who are not deliberately trying to alter their presentation to attempt to portray themselves as being more impaired than they really are. There are times where response bias is more insidious; such as patients who are trying to feign their presentation for secondary gain.

When a patient manufactures or exaggerates symptoms for secondary gain, the patient is known to be malingering (Rogers, 1997). Malingering is a different presentation than a fictitious disorder, where symptoms are invented for the additional attention of being sick (DSM-IV, 1994). People malinger in a variety of situations and do so with a number of different presentations. In an effort to categorize the different type of malingering, it may be helpful to consider the following categories. **Administrative Malingering** is when people feign illness or injury to achieve relief from an assignment or a particular duty. For example students regularly feign illness to get out of taking an exam or being held accountable for a paper deadline. Soldiers may fake an injury to get out of field maneuvers for the day. In some cases, such malingering can persist for some time, including the sailor who concocts symptoms of an illness or injury that will allow him early discharge from the military. Similarly, inmates may pretend to be sick in order to be admitted to a medical unit whose living unit is more comfortable and the food may be better.

Drug Seeking is a behavior that is commonly seen by physicians by patients who malinger pain symptoms in order to gain access to narcotic medicines for recreational purposes, or to sustain drug dependence. Other medical symptoms may be feigned for other controlled substances, such as faking a generalized tonic-clonic seizure in hopes that they may find a provider who is willing to administer a benzodiazepine in order to treat the seizure.

Medicolegal Malingering is seen when an individual elects to produce medical symptoms that are not there in an effort to earn a lighter sentence or avoid prosecution all together. Such tactics include pretending to be psychotic or developmentally delayed during the proceedings, others will claim to have no memory of the event in question.

When great sums of money are involved, some individuals may engage in **Compensation Seeking Malingering**, where the sole purpose of faking injury or illness is to win a disability award, or a favorable monetary settlement from court proceedings. It has long been though a high percentage of head injury litigants are feigning at least some of their symptoms (Youngjohn, Burrows and Erdal, 1995). While people may malinger for a variety of reasons, perhaps the most common is in the pursuit of money.

Malingering for Basic Needs is better known by its colloquial term, "three hots-and-a-cot. This tactic, often employed by the poor and destitute, is to fake a medical condition in order to admitted to the hospital long enough to get off the street and have a meal. Other patients, for example, will present to a psychiatric intake appointment and lie about their impending plan to commit suicide. Such claims must be taken seriously and often this type of malingering will result in a hospital admission that lasts at least overnight.

When malingering takes the form of neuropsychological symptoms, it has been described as "malingered neurocognitive dysfunction" and involves feigned cognitive symptoms, such as memory loss (Slick, Sherman and Iverson, 1999, p. 545). While people may malinger a variety of presentations, such as pain, sensory loss, or other somatic complaints, neurocognitive malingering is thought to be a commonly feigned condition since lay people tend to understand that amnesia is common feature to head injury (Aubrey, Dobbs and Rule, 1989; Wong, Regennitter and Barrios, 1994), and memory loss in particular is commonly malingered since most people believe their feigning is difficult to detect during testing (Rogers, 1997). Neuropsychological malingering may also be common since settlement awards in these cases commonly approach a half million dollars (West and Knowles, 1991).

While not all clinicians' practices regularly involve cases where large monetary settlements are at issue, it is important that all clinical neuropsychologists consider effort when interpreting test results. Sub-optimal effort can generate a test profile that is not indicative of the patient's true abilities. While many neuropsychologists rely on clinical judgment to assess effort, almost 80% of "expert neuropsychologists" surveyed indicated that they used a specialized malingering measure when assessing patients involved in litigation (Slick, Tan, Strauss and Hultsch, 2004). Other than clinical judgment, many neuropsychologists will use formal malingering measures that are designed to look like memory tests, but instead effort. Further, it has been found that traditional neuropsychological test performance can be evaluated in the context of effort.

BACKGROUND

Examples of malingering can be found in many contexts and date back centuries, ranging from soldiers faking illness to avoid duty, to a suspected murderer feigning mental illness, to a worker pretending to have whiplash to get workers' compensation. Response bias should be viewed along a continuum (see Figure 1). At one end is non-purposeful response bias marked by sub-optimal effort that, in context, is understandable. For example, fatigue and indifference are not unexpected in a long day of neuropsychological testing. When response bias is purposeful –deliberately trying to skew test results for secondary gain— this end of the continuum is malingering. Miller (2001) contends that flagrant malingering also has different characteristics. At one end of this continuum is the patient who exaggerates existing symptoms to make her condition seem worse than it really is. For example, a patient may actually be experiencing intermittent short-term memory problems, but when evaluated, she presents as having constant memory deficits. Further, there is the patient who has recovered fully from neurocognitive deficits, but who continues mimic symptoms as if they are ongoing. Or, such a patient may have had headaches following a brain injury and continue to report their occurrence when the physical symptoms have abated. Some patients will misattribute their symptoms, taking symptoms attributed to one event (such as a skiing injury) and attributing it to another (such as a car accident). At the extreme end of the malingering continuum is the patient who has no neuropsychological symptoms, has never had deficits, and yet manufactures his presentation. An example of this patient is a person who has been in a motor vehicle collision and who maintains that he is unable to speak since the accident. See Table 1 for a summary of the continuum of response bias and suggestions for coping with such patients.

As previously mentioned, non-purposeful response bias may not be due to someone dilberately faking their symptoms, but could be due to fatigue, disinterest, or other benign reasons. Teasing apart non-purposeful from purposeful response bias is a complicated manner, and the clinician may have trouble determining if the response bias is truly in fact in the pursuit of secondary gain (Millis and Volinsky, 2001). In fact, as Slick et al., (2004) note, 12% of expert neuropsychologists never use the term "malingering" and 41% report rarely using the term. Instead, tests results are often reported as inconclusive, performance described as sub-optimal, or incomplete effort was given during the testing. Table 2 summarizes some of the various terms that have been found to describe a response bias in the literature. For the purposes of this chapter, "response bias" will be used to encompass a wide variety of behaviors that span from incomplete effort to outright malingering (see Hom and Denney, 2002).

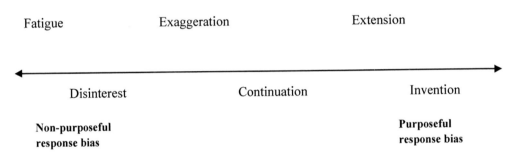

Figure 1.

Table 1. Types of Response Bias

Type of response bias	Possible Management Techniques
Disinterest/apathy in testing process. (May lead to random or irrelevant responding)	Rapport building is critical; reward trying hard; intersperse more tedious tests (E.g., Wisconsin Card Sorting Task) with tasks children tend to enjoy (E.g., Trail Making Test).
Fatigue (May lead to random or irrelevant responding)	Be aware that fatigue is an issue; break testing into several sessions; perform testing early in the day.
Exaggeration of Symptoms	Alert patient that testing is inconclusive since real deficits are being over-shadowed by inconsistent test performance.
Extension of Symptoms/ Misattribution of symptoms	Consider test results in context with other data sources, such as interviews with family, employer, other health care professionals, etc.
Invention of Symptoms	Use at least two malingering measures to supplement traditional test battery; careful medical records review of neuropsychological history, gather information from a variety of sources.
Fake Good (Defensiveness)	Careful review of clinical record and test results.

Note: Including a measure of effort will be helpful in all categories.

Table 2. How many different ways to say response bias?

Description	Citation
Dissimulation	Rogers (1987)
Dysperformance	Mathias, Greve, Bianchini, Houston and Crouch (2002)
Exaggeration	Iverson and Binder (2000)
Feigning	Rogers, Harrell and Liff (1993)
Inadequate Effort	Barrash et al. (2004)
Incomplete Effort	Baker, Donders and Thompson (2000)
Insufficient Effort	Thompson (2002)
Invalid Responding	Frederick, Crosby and Wynkoop (2000)
Malingered Neurocognitive Dysfunction	Slick, Sherman and Iverson (1999)
Noncredible Cognitive Performance	Boone and Lu (2003)
Nonoptimal Test Performance	DiCarlo, Gfeller and Oliveri (2000)
Poor Effort	Barrash, Suhr and Manzel (2004)
Suboptimal Effort	Green, Rohling, Lees-Haley and Allen (2001)
Suspect Effort	Nelson, Boone, Dueck, Wagener, Lu and Grills (2003)

Note: Citations are examples of when a term was noticed in a journal article, not necessarily the first appearance of such a term.

STRATEGIES FOR ASSESSING RESPONSE BIAS

There is a rich literature describing the various means for detecting response bias (for an excellent review, see Rogers, Harrell and Liff, 1993). While many of these strategies are theoretically possible, for practical purposes only a handful of approaches are useful to the clinician. One approach is to design a task that is very easy and that even the most impaired individual should have no little performing well. Another approach is to administer instruments that look as if they are testing memory and instead assess effort. These types of tests, known as symptom validity tests (SVT), rely on binominal probability theory by giving the patient a target item to remember and later pair the target with a distracting item. Patients are asked to select the item they have seen before. Patients who are trying hard typically will get all or almost all of these items correct, even if they have cognitive deficits. Those who have sub-optimal scores are not trying their hardest rather than having true memory problems. Scores falling below 50% are below what would be expected for chance level performance and indicate purposeful response bias. Other techniques rely on an examination of performance plotted across item difficulty. A genuine performance typically shows a steep curve as most easy items are completed without difficulty, percent of items correct decline as the test gets harder. A faked profile will show a flat profile, indicating poor performance across all items. Finally, erratic or unusual responses to test items may also suggest a style that is inconsistent with a patient who is taking the testing seriously. Many scholars have suggested that existing neuropsychological measures can be used to detect response bias (e.g., Larrabee, 2003).

NEUROPSYCHOLOGICAL MEASURES USEFUL
IN ASSESSING RESPONSE BIAS

A variety of traditional neuropsychological measures have been reported to be useful for the detection of response bias by examining results for atypical performance. Using standard neuropsychological instruments to assess possible response bias is advantageous as no additional tests need to be added to the neuropsychological test battery. Examining performance on standard instruments used in prior assessments is also helpful for a retrospective examination of response bias when the patient is no longer assessable. Finally, there has been concern that some patients may be coached to defeat response bias tests (Youngjohn, 1995). As sophistication of some patients grows to measures explicitly designed to detect response bias, examining performance on standard instruments may be helpful as coached patients may not be conscious of the need to make their response bias less flagrant on these measures.

The Wechsler Adult Intelligence Scale, now in its third edition (WAIS-III), is a commonly used assessment of IQ and often an integral part of the neuropsychological test battery (Wechsler, 1997a). The Digit Span subtest of the WAIS-III is of interest when assessing for response bias, since performance on this subtest tends to remain intact even in patients with neuropsychological deficits, and is commonly misperceived as a memory test when it in fact measures attention. Greiffenstein, Baker and Gola (1994) found that a "Reliable Digit Span" (RDS) score could be derived by adding together the longest digits forward and backward scores. When the RDS is less than seven, performance is suspect. This finding has been validated in subsequent studies (e.g., Mathias, Greve, Bianchini, Houston and Crouch, 2002). Mittenberg, Theroux-Fichera, Zielinski and Heilbronner (1995) found that a Digit Span subtest score that was five or more scaled score points below the Vocabulary subtest was an excellent indicator of response bias. This finding has been validated in subsequent studies (Greve, Bianchini, Mathias, Houston and Crouch, 2003; Miller, Ryan, Carruthers and Cluff, 2004).

Often accompanying the WAIS-III is the Wechsler Memory Scale, also in its third edition (WMS-III). As its title implies, the WMS-III is a complementary memory assessment to the WAIS-III that uses norms from the same group as the WAIS-III (Wechsler, 1997b). A number of studies have identified certain specific response patterns on the WMS-III as possible indicators of response bias. Mittenberg, Azrin, Millsaps and Heilbronner (1993) suggested that when patient's Attention/Concentration Scores is lower than their General Memory Index score that such a presentation is so atypical that the only explanation can be response bias. Killgore and DellaPietra (2000) derived a "Rarely Missed Index" from the Logical Memory Delayed Recall (LMDR) subtest of the WMS-III. This subtest requires the patient to answer yes or no questions about a story read to them earlier in the test. Some of these items are so rarely missed, even by people who have never heard the story before, that getting these items incorrect may indicate response bias.

The Faces subtest of the WMS-III may also help provide a clue about response bias. Faces is a forced choice measure where the patient looks at a series of 24 faces and then is shown 48 faces, half of which were in the series before. The patient gives a yes/no response to each stimulus, making the Faces subtest a forced choice measure, allowing it to be used as an SVT. Glassmire, Bierley, Wisniewski, Green, Kennedy and Date (2003) found that scoring below a raw score of 31 was extremely atypical and suggests response bias. Finally, Langeluddecke and Lucas (2003) found that 80% of the malingering patients in their sample could be identified either by raw scores below 43 on the Auditory Recognition – Delayed subtest of the WMS-III, or by a raw score of less than 18 on the Word List II – Recognition subtest.

Another common memory assessment instrument, the California Verbal Learning Test (CVLT, Delis, Kramer, Kaplan and Ober, 1987) has been identified as having some promise as a tool to measure response bias. Millis, Putnam, Adams, and Ricker (1995) found that a discriminant function based on performance across the word list trials 1 – 4 could detect response bias. While this formula had high sensitivity and specificity, a later study found that using the CVLT may have an inordinately high false positive rate which suggests using caution when evaluating performance on this instrument for response bias (Baker, Donders and Thompson, 2000).

While not initially designed to be used as a test of response bias, the Warrington Recognition Memory Task (WRMT) contains two subtests (verbal and non-verbal) that employ a two-item, forced choice design (Warrington, 1984). The forced choice design easily allows for a symptom validity testing paradigm and has become widely known as a test of response bias. Millis (1992) found that a cutoff score of less than 32 indicated biased responding. Other studies have validated this finding (Millis and Putnam, 1994; Iverson and Franzen, 1998). In the 2004 survey of expert neuropsychologists, Slick, et al. reported that half of their respondents used the WRMT.

In addition to memory assessment, many neuropsychological test batteries include the Trail Making Test (Parts A and B) as it is quick to administer and is very sensitive to cognitive dysfunction (Reitan and Wolfson, 1993; Lezak, 1995). Ruffolo, Guilmette and Willis (2000) found that performance errors and extended time to completion scores may suggest response bias. Another study found that Trail Making Scores falling below the 5th percentile were highly suspect (Iverson, Lange, Green and Franzen, 2002). Roberts and Horton (2003) found similar findings when the Trail Making Test was used to detect malingering in a sample of substance abusers. Despite this support, Iverson et al. (2002) suggest caution when using Trails as the sole measure of response bias, as the Trail Making Test has low sensitivity to deliberate exaggeration. Instead, they suggest that atypically poor performance on Trails be a "red flag for the clinician," rather than providing definitive proof of response bias (Iverson et al., 2002, p. 405). This is good advice for any of the instruments discussed.

There are other neuropsychological instruments that are reported in the literature as helpful in detecting response bias, but will not be fully discussed here in the interests of brevity. Some examples are listed in Table 3.

MEASURES DESIGNED TO DETECT RESPONSE BIAS

While traditional neuropsychological instruments may be helpful in detecting response bias, there are also measures that are specifically designed to assess effort. There are a number of these tests that are commercially available. The major instruments will be reviewed.

Table 3. Other common neuropsychological tests that may be useful when examining for response bias

Test/Subtest	Feature	Citation
Cognitive Behavioral Driver's Inventory (CBDI)	Extreme Scores	Ray, Engum, Lambert, Bane, Nash and Bracy (1997)
Memory Assessment Scales (MAS)	Atypically Low Scores	O'Bryant, Duff, Fisher and McCaffrey (2004)
Auditory Verbal Learning Test – Expanded Version (AVLTX)	Profile with additional subtest	Barrash, Shur and Manzel (2004)
Minnesota Multiphasic Personality Inventory -2nd Edition (MMPI-2)*	Numerous profiles	Ross, Millis, Krukowski, Putnam, and Adams (2004)
Rey-Osterrieth Complex Figure (ROCFT)	Atypically low scores	Lu, Boone, Cozolino, Mitchell (2003)
Halstead Category Test	Errors on Subests I and II	Forrest, Allen and Goldstein (2004)
Finger Tapping Test	Atypically Low Scores	Ginger (2005)
Wisconsin Cart Sorting Task (WCST)	Several features	Greve, Bianchini, Mathias, Houston and Crouch (2002); King, Sweet, Sherer, Curtiss and Vanderloeg (2002)

*Not a neuropsychological test, but commonly part of a neuropsychological test battery

Rey 15-Item Memory Test (RMT)

One of the oldest tests of response bias is the Rey 15-Item Memory Test which was reportedly developed to assure insurance companies that head injured patients were not faking their presentation (Lezak, 1995; Frederick, 2002a). This test consists of five rows, ABC; 1 2 3; a b c; I II III; and a circle, square and triangle. The patient is instructed to look at the items for 10 seconds and is then asked to recall the items after a 15 second delay (Lezak, 1995). Even cognitively impaired patients typically perform quite well on this test, and recall of less than nine items is typically viewed as biased responding (Goldberg and Miller, 1986; Bernard and Fowler, 1990), although scholars have debated this cutoff score (see Taylor, Kreutzer and West, 2003).

Frederick (2002a) points out that the RMT has several advantages. It is in the public domain, so it is free to generate and reproduce at will. It can be given in less than a minute, is scored in seconds, and is sensitive to response bias. The RMT is noteworthy for the wealth of literature discussing it. However, as Rogers et al. (1997) observe, it is quite transparent, and a sophisticated patient may quite well see that it is a test of effort and perform well on it despite biased responding on other measures. Low scores on the RMT should be of interest to the neuropsychologist, however, high scores do not rule out response bias.

Portland Digit Recognition Test (PDRT)

The Portland Digit Recognition Test is typically an example of a measure that employs symptom validity testing, where a patient is given an item to remember and then has to later select that item from two choices (Binder and Pankratz, 1987; Binder, 1993a). The test has 72 items, 36 classified as easy, 36 classified as hard. While some experimental, computerized versions of the PDRT do exist, this test is administered by an examiner (Binder, 2002). Some clinicians have complained that the PDRT takes too long to administer, as its administration may sometimes last longer than an hour.[1] Binder (1993b) has also published an abbreviated version that takes about 20 minutes to complete, but is designed for use with patients who are performing well. The research about reliability, validity, sensitivity and specificity is based on the PDRT and not on the abbreviated version (Binder, 2002).

Since the PDRT is a forced choice measure, chance level performance is 50% correct (or, on the PDRT, a raw score of 36). Less than chance level performance is highly indicative of response bias. Binder (1993a) suggests a raw cutoff score of 39 items as indicating response bias. The PDRT has good psychometric properties, with acceptable reliability and validity scores (Binder and Willis, 1991). The PDRT has been favorably reviewed by Sweet (2000) and is reported to be used by more than 40% of expert neuropsychologists (Slick et al., 2004).

Computerized Assessment of Response Bias (CARB)

The Computerized Assessment of Response Bias is another example of a symptom validity test, as the instrument presents a string of five-digit numbers and then asks the patient to select the item that they have seen before (Allen, Conder, Green, and Cox, 1997). The patient makes his or her selection from a computer keyboard. Administration takes less than a half-hour and will terminate early if the patient's effort is good. A variety of results are printed, including response time, which may also indicate response bias (Rose, Hall and Szalda-Petree, 1995). The CARB is a remarkably easy one to accomplish, and even patients with a severe traumatic brain injury (TBI) tend to get 97% or better of the items correct (Allen, et al., 1997). The CARB is truly a test of effort and not one of ability. Patients who score below a 70% overall are not putting forth adequate effort.

On Slick's et al. (2004) survey of expert neuropsychologists, more than two thirds of the respondents stated that they "never" used the CARB. This may be due to a number of reasons. First, when the test first was published, it was one of the first to be given entirely on computer. The traditional neuropsychologist, being accustomed to instruments administered by an examiner, may have been more comfortable with tests that not given on computer (such as the PDRT). Secondly, the test is also published by a small firm called "CogniSyst" and not a major test being produced not by a major test publisher. This may have resulted in its not being widely known. Finally, the test primary developer is not an academic clinician and

---

[1] Binder (2002) notes that most patients who are putting forth reasonable effort can finish this test in about ¾ of an hour. However, it should be noted that the PDRT may be take too long for some clinicians to include in their test battery as a standard instrument. When it is included, it is often because the neuropsychologist has questions of response bias. When a patient's effort is suboptimal, this test can take can take an hour to administer, making it unpopular with examiners and making an comprehensive test battery even longer to complete.

neuropsychologists may prefer to use tests published by academics (such as Binder and his PDRT).

Word Memory Test (WMT)

Like the PDRT and CARB, the Word Memory Test is an instrument that also relies on the assumptions of symptom validity testing. It is described as a test of verbal learning and memory and requires the patient to learn a list of 20 word pairs presented on a computer screen, although it can be modified to be given without the computer (Green, Allen and Astner, 1996). The patient matches the stem word to its match (against a distractor) in both an immediate and delayed (30-minute interval) subtest. Many of these words are obvious conceptual pairs, such as "dog" and "cat." Even someone who has never seen the original word test would likely get many of the pairs correct. The immediate and delayed recall subtests, as well as the consistency between the two, are known as "effort measures" and are followed by measures of memory ability, multiple choice, paired associates, and free recall sections (Green, Lees-Haley and Allen, 2002). Poor scores on the effort measures can only be the result of response bias.

A study of head-injured patients was shown that these subjects had excellent performance on the effort measures, indicating that such measures are not sensitive to cognitive dysfunction (Allen and Green, 1999). The entire test takes less than an hour to administer. The test is scored by a computer and output includes scores, graphs, and response time to test items. Half of the expert neuropsychologists in the Slick et al. (2004) study reported using the WMT. This test is efficient, sensitive, and provides straightforward results. Another nice feature is that it will run on older computers with slower processors, allowing a neuropsychologist to let the patient take the WMT on an out-dated machine rather than having a patient use the clinician's computer.

Test of Memory Malingering (TOMM)

The test of Memory Malingering employs a symptom validity testing paradigm using pictures that are shown to a patient by an administrator. The test was reportedly designed to be sensitive to response bias, while being insensitive to cognitive dysfunction, through the recall of line drawings (Tombaugh, 1996; Tombaugh, 2002). There are two learning trials of 50 drawings of common objects, followed by a recall trial where the patient tries to pick a previously seen picture from two choices. There is also a delayed retention trial after a 15 minute interval. Validation testing found that the TOMM was insensitive to age, education and brain impairment, but quite sensitive to effort (Tombaugh, 2002). Poor performance on the TOMM indicates response bias.

The TOMM is cited as the most widely used instrument for detecting response bias in Slick's et al. (2004) survey. Like the WMT, it is efficient, provides straightforward results, and is known to be sensitive to response bias. The TOMM test booklets resemble other neuropsychological tests, such as the Boston Naming Test, and it is administered by an examiner. There are a plethora of other studies about the TOMM in the literature. Some of the notable studies include Rees, Tombaugh and Boulay's (2001) observation that the TOMM is insensitive to depression. Constantinou and McCaffrey (2003) report that the TOMM can be effectively used to evaluate suboptimal effort of children during neuropsychological testing. Finally, Weinborn, Orr, Woods, Conover and Feix (2003) discuss the use of the TOMM in forensic settings.

Victoria Symptom Validity Test (VSVT)

Slick, Hopp, Strauss and Thompson's (1997) Victoria Symptom Validity Test, as the name implies, is a symptom validity test that requires patients to identify a previously-seen string of numbers from a two choices. The VSVT is presented by computer, showing a number string followed by a blank screen, and finally a "recognition trial" where the patient makes his or her selection from the two choices. Forty-eight items are displayed, in blocks of 16, with the intervening blank screen interval lengthening from five seconds, to ten seconds, to 15 seconds. The 48 items are also divided evenly into easy and difficult items based on whether the numbers in the distractor are in common with the target number (Slick, et al., 1997). The VSVT can be completed in less than 30 minutes. The test is scored automatically and gives percent of items correct, response latency, and proportion of responses made from the left and right side of the keyboard. Cut scores are used to classify patients into "valid, invalid," and "questionable" categories (Thompson, 2002).

Strauss, Hultsch, Hunter, Slick, Paltry and Levy-Bencheton (2000) found that the VSVT was quite effective in discriminating between simulated malingerers and a group asked to do their best. Similar results were found when using the VSVT to discriminate between compensation seeking subjects and non-compensation seeking groups (Grote, Kooker, Garron, Nyenhuis, Smith and Mattingly, 2000). Grote, et al. (2000) urge caution when trying to determine response bias based solely on item response latency. If the Slick et al. (2004) survey is a valid indicator, the VSVT is not popular among expert neuropsychologists with about 80% of their sample reporting "never" using this instrument.

Validity Indicator Profile (VIP)

The Validity Indicator Profile is different from many of the symptom validity tests that have been discussed. The VIP consists of two subtests, a forced choice vocabulary test (VIP-V) and 100 picture matrix problems (VIP-NV) that tap a variety of cognitive processes (Frederick, 1997). On the VIP-V, patients are required to find an analogous word for a target word. On the VIP-NV, patients negotiate matching, decision making, simple math and abstraction problems. Both subtests plot performance on a performance curve across item difficulty (Fredrick, Crosby and Wynkoop, 2000). Patients whose performance curve differs from the norm are suspected of responding in a biased fashion. The VIP is a pencil and paper based test that can be scored by computer and generate a graphic output (Frederick, 2002b). Roughly a third of practitioners responding to the Slick et al. (2004) survey report using this instrument.

Other Measures f Response Bias

While the traditional neuropsychologist is limited to assessing response bias with standard neuropsychological measures and response bias detection instruments, some interesting studies have emerged in the last several years regarding the detection of deceptive presentations using electrophysiological and radiographic measures. For example, Tardif, Barry, Fox and Johnstone (2000) designed a study examining performance of simulated malingerers on the WRMT while recording event-related potentials (ERPs). While the malingering condition had significant differences from the control condition on the WRMT, the groups were equivalent on ERP data. This suggested that the malingering group was recognizing previously seen stimuli and therefore capable of performing better on the memory task than their scores indicate (Tardif, et al., 2000).

Another study used functional magnetic resonance imaging (fMRI) to examine cerebral activity during feigned memory impairment on a symptom validity test (Lee, et al., 2002). Assuming that it is impossible to control cerebral functions detectable by the fMRI, Lee, et al. (2002) scanned six male, native Chinese (Mandarin) speakers while they faked memory impairment on the Hiscock and Hiscock (1989) symptom validity test. They found participants who were feigning impairment had significantly different fMRI scans, indicating a possible existence of a "prefrontal-parietal-sub-cortical circuit" involved in deception (Lee, et al., 2002, p. 162).

A similar study by Ward, Oakley, Frackowiak and Halligan (2003) used positron emission tomography (PET) scanning to examine the cortical activity of 12 "normal, hypnotized" subjects, half of whom had the suggestion that their left leg was paralyzed, the other half were instructed to feign paralysis (p. 295). When obtaining a PET scan for the participants' brains during the instructed task, the patients who were told to fake paralysis had significantly different cortical activity than the other group. The authors conclude that PET may be effective in differentiating patients who are feigning neurological impairment (Ward, et al., 2003).

While the evidence from these physiological and radiological studies are interesting, and may lead to further study, these findings provide few practical tools for the neuropsychologist who does not typically have such measurement devices at their disposal. Further, such instruments are not used in the typical neuropsychological workup.

Multimodal Assessment of Response Bias

Whether a neuropsychologist uses an instrument specifically designed to detect response bias, or examines traditional measures for suboptimal performance, it is clear that making a definitive decision about malingering is best done using a multimodal approach. Examination for response bias begins with a thorough review of the patient's medical, occupational and educational records. The test results should be taken in context of the patient's injury or illness. Atypical performance on traditional measures may give the clinician reason to examine the test results more closely for biased responding (Iverson, et al., 2002). The test battery can then be supplemented with a malingering measure. However, to truly guard against response bias, using two measures designed to measure effort is better than one (Gervais et al., 2004; Iverson and Binder, 2000; Lynch, 2004)

Other Concerns

In recent years, there has been some concern in the literature that some patients may undertake sophisticated preparation in order to perform convincingly poorly on neuropsychological measures (see Lees-Haley, 1997). In fact, Youngjohn (1995) confirms an attorney admitting that he had coached his client how to perform during assessment. There have been a number of studies examining how sensitive instruments measuring response bias are to coaching. Other studies have examined the effect on such measures by patients who are educating themselves about neuropsychological symptoms.

DiCarlo, Gfeller and Oliveri (2000) examined the effects of coaching on detecting feigned cognitive impairment on the Category Test (Defilipis and McCampbell, 1979). They found that coached malingering simulators performed better than un-coached simulators, but still performed in a range that suggested response bias. A 2002 study by Cato and colleagues (Cato, Brewster, Ryan and Giuliano) found that the RWMT and RMT were somewhat susceptible to coaching strategies aimed at making simulators look more authentic. Suhr (2002) found that the Auditory Verbal Learning Test (AVLT) was robust in its ability to detect coaching malingerers when examining the responses in the context of the serial position effect. Similar effects were found when examining the "Exaggeration Index" (Barrash, Suhr and Manzel, 2004) on an extended version of the AVLT (Suhr, Gunstad, Greub and Barrash, 2004). Dunn, Shear, Howe and Ris (2003) examined coaching simulated malingerers to perform less flagrantly on the CARB and WMT. They found that while coached participants performed more authentically than un-coached participants, they still performed in a range that suggested response bias.

While some measures appear to be robust against deliberate coaching to defeat malingering measures, some measures may be susceptible to sophisticated patients who may be aware of measures designed to detect response bias. As mentioned above, the most effective way to guard against such patients is a thorough clinical interview, close inspection of the neuropsychological profile for atypical responses, and the use of multiple measures that are designed to detect response bias (Millis and Volinsky, 2001).

Practical Suggestions for the Practicing Neuropsychologist

Response bias is detrimental to valid neuropsychological testing whether it is purposeful or non-purposeful. An assessment of effort should be part of any comprehensive neuropsychological test battery. Some other suggestions follow:

- The term "malingering" should be used with great caution. Response bias can be non-purposeful and better effort can be elicited by building rapport, including more frequent breaks during testing, and being sure that the patient is vested in the process. Declaring someone a malingerer may haunt the clinical record for years and may result in a patient getting substandard care by health care professionals who will never take the patient seriously.
- Get information from a wide range of sources, including patient care records, educational sources, employment records, and interviews with family.
- Attempt several observations of the patient, in more than one visit.

- With highly suspicious patients, use a variety of methods to assess effort, as some people truly malingering will perform differently on different measures (Gervais, Rohling, Green and Ford, 2004).

REFERENCES

Allen, L.M., Conder, R.L., Green, P. and Cox, D.R. (1997). *CARB-97 manual for the Computerized Assessment of Response Bias*. Durham, NC: CogniSyst.

Allen, L.M. and Green, P. (1999). Performance of neurological patients on the Word Memory Test (WMT) and the Computerized Assessment of Response Bias (CARB). *Supplement to the Word Memory Test and the CARB '97 Manuals*. Durham, NC: CogniSyst.

American Psychiatric Association. (1994). *Diagnostic and Statistical Manual of Mental Disorders* (4th ed.). Washington, D.C.: Author.

Aubrey, J.B., Dobbs, A.R. and Rule, B.G. (1989). Laypersons' knowledge about the sequelae of minor head injury and whiplash. *Journal of Neurology, Neurosurgery, and Psychiatry, 52*, 842 – 846.

Baker, R., Donders, J. and Thompson, E. (2000). Assessment of incomplete effort with the California Verbal Learning Test. *Applied Neuropsychology, 7*, 111 – 114.

Barrash, J., Suhr, J. and Manzel, K. (2004). Detecting poor effort and malingering with an expanded version of the Auditory Verbal Learning Test (AVLTX): Validation with clinical samples. *Journal of Clinical and Experimental Neuropsychology, 26*, 125 – 140.

Bernard, L.C. and Fowler, W. (1990). Assessing the validity of memory complaints: Performance of brain-damaged and normal individuals on Rey's task to detect malingering. *Journal of Clinical Psychology, 46*, 432 – 436.

Bernard, L.C., Houston, W. and Natoli, L. (1993). Malinginering on neuropsychological memory tests: Potential objective indicators. *Journal of Clinical Psychology, 49*, 432 – 436.

Binder, L.M. (1993a). *Portland Digit Recognition Test Manual*, 2nd Ed. Beaverton, OR: Author.

Binder, L.M. (1993b). An abbreviated form of the Portland Digit Recognition Test. *The Clinical Neuropsychologist, 7*, 104 – 107.

Binder, L.M. and Pankratz, L. (1987). Neuropsychological evidence of a factitious memory complaint. *Journal of Clinical and Experimental Neuropsychology, 9*, 167 – 171.

Binder, L.M. and Willis, S.C. (1991). Assessment of motivation after financially compensable minor head trauma. *Assessment, 3*, 403 – 409.

Binder, L.M. (2002). The Portland Digit Recognition Test: A Review of Validation Data and Clinical Use. *Journal of Forensic Neuropsychology, 2*, 27 – 41.

Boone, K.B. and Lu, P. (2003). Noncredible cognitive performance in the context of severe brain injury. *The Clinical Neuropsychologist, 17*, 244 – 254.

Cato, M.A., Brewster, J., Ryan, T. and Giuliano, A.J. (2002). Coaching and the ability to simulate mild traumatic brain injury symptoms. *The Clinical Neuropsychologist, 16*, 524 – 535.

Constantinou, M. and McCaffrey, R.J. (2003). Using the TOMM for evaluating children's effort to perform optimally on neuropsychological measures. *Child Neuropsychology, 9,* 81 – 90.

Defilippis, N.A. and McCampbell, E. (1979). *The Booklet Category Test: Research and clinical form.* Manual. Odessa, Fl: Psychological Assessment Resources.

Delis, D.C., Kramer, J.H., Kaplan, E. and Ober, B.A. (1987). *The California Verbal Learning Test: Adult version manual.* San Antonio: Psychological Corporation.

DiCarlo, M.A., Gfeller, J.D. and Oliveri, M.V. (2000). Effects of coaching on detecting freighted cognitive impairment with the Category Test. *Archives of Clinical Neuropsychology, 15,* 399 – 413.

Dunn, T.M., Shear, P.K., Howe, S. and Ris, M.D. (2003). Detecting neuropsychological malingering: Effects of coaching and information. *Archives of Clinical Neuropsychology, 18,* 121 – 134.

Forrest, T.J., Allen, D.N. and Goldstein, G. (2004). Malingering Indexes for the Halstead Category Test. *The Clinical Neuropsychologist, 18,* 334 – 347.

Frederick, R.I. (1997). *Validity Indicator Profile Manual.* Minnetonka, MN: NCS Assessments.

Frederick, R.I. (2002a). A review of Rey's strategies for detecting neuropsychological impairment. *Journal of Forensic Neuropsychology, 2,* 1 – 25.

Frederick, R.I. (2002b). Review of the Validity Indicator Profile. *Journal of Forensic Neuropsychology, 2,* 125-145.

Fredrick, R.I., Crosby, R.D. and Wynkoop, T.E. (2000). Performance curve classification of invalid responding on the Validity Indicator Profile. *Archives of Clinical Neuropsychology, 15,* 281 – 300.

Gervais, R.O., Rohling, M.L., Green, P. and Ford, W. (2004). A comparison of WMT, CARB, and TOMM failure rates in non-head injury disability claimants. *Archives of Clinical Neuropsychology, 19,* 475-487.

Ginger, A., Boone, K.B., Lu, P., Dean, A., Wen, J., Nitch, S. et al. (2005). Sensitivity and specificity of Finger Tapping Test scores for the detection of suspect effort. *Clinical Neuropsychologist, 19,* 105 – 120.

Glassmire, D.M., Bierley, R.A., Wisniewski, A.M., Greene, R.L., Kennedy, J.E. and Date, E. (2003). Using the WMS-III faces subset to detect malingered memory impairment. *Journal of Clinical and Experimental Neuropsychology, 25,* 465 – 481.

Goldberg J.O. and Miller, H.R. (1986). Performance on psychiatric inpatients and intellectually deficient individuals on a task that assesses the validity of memory complaints. *Journal of Clinical psychology, 42,* 792 – 795.

Green, P., Allen, L.M. and Astner, K. (1996). *Manual for Computerised Word Memory Test.* Durham: CogniSyst.

Green, P., Lees-Haley, P.R. and Allen, L.M. (2002). The Word Memory Test and the validity of neuropsychological test scores. *Journal of Forensic Neuropsychology, 2,* 97 – 124.

Green, P., Rohling, M.L., Lees-Haley, P.R. and Allen, L.M. (2001). Effort has a greater effect on test scores than severe brain injury in compensation claimants. *Brain Injury, 15,* 1045 – 1060.

Greiffenstein, M. F., Baker, W. J. and Gola, T. (1994). Validation of malingered amnesia measures with a large clinical sample. *Psychological Assessment, 6,* 218 – 224.

Greve, K.W., Bianchini, K.J., Mathias, C.W., Houston, R.J. and Crouch, J.A. (2002). Detecting malingered performance with the Wisconsin Card Sorting Task: A preliminary investigation in traumatic brain injury. *The Clinical Neuropsychologist, 16,* 179 – 191.

Greve, K.W., Bianchini, K.J., Mathias, C.W., Houston, R.J. and Crouch, J.A. (2003). Detecting malingered performance on the Wechsler Adult Intelligence Scale validation of Mittenberg's approach in traumatic brain injury. *Archives of Clinical Neuropsychology, 18,* 245 – 260.

Grote, C.J., Kooker, E.K., Garron, D.C., Nyenhuis, D.L., Smith, C.A.and Mattingly, M.L. (2000). *Journal of Clinical and Experimental Neuropsychology, 22,* 709 -719.

Hisock, M. and Hiscock, C.M. (1989). Refining the forced-chioice method for the detection of malingering. *Journal of Clinical and Experimental Neuropsychology, 11,* 967 – 974.

Hom, J. and Denney, R.L. (Eds.). (2002). *Detection of Response Bias in Forensic Neuropsychology.* Preface. New York: Haworth Medical Press.

Horton, A.M. and Roberts, C. (2003). Trail Making Test cut-offs for malingering among cocaine, heroin, and alcohol abusers. *International Journal of Neuroscience, 113,* 223 – 231.

Iverson, G.L. and Binder, L.M. (2000). Detecting exaggeration and malingering in neuropsychological assessment. *Journal of Head Trauma Rehabilitation, 15,* 829 – 585.

Iverson, G.L. and Franzen, M.D. (1998). Detecting malingered memory deficits with the Recognition Memory Test. *Brain Injury,12,* 275 – 282.

Iverson, G.L., Lange, R.T., Green, P. and Franzen, M.D. (2002). Detecting exaggeration and malingering with the Trail Making Test. *The Clinical Neuropsychologist, 16,* 398 – 406.

Killgore, W.D.S. and DellaPietra, L. (2000). Using the WMS-III to detect malingering: Empirical validation of the rarely missed index (RMI). *Journal of Clinical and Experimental Psychology, 4, 49 – 64.*

King, J.H., Sweet, J.J., Sherer, M., Curtiss, G. and Vanderploeg, R.D. (2002). Validity indicators within the Wisconsin Card Sorting Test: Application of the new and previously researched multivariate procedures in multiple traumatic brain injury samples. *The Clinical Neuropsychologist, 16,* 506 – 523.

Langeluddecke, P.M. and Lucas, S.K. (2003). Quantitative measures of memory malingering on the Wechsler Memory Scale-Third Edition in mild head injury litigants. *Archives of Clinical Neuropsychology, 18,* 181 – 197.

Larrabee, G.J. (2003). Detection of malingering using atypical performance patterns on standard neuropsychological tests. *The Clinical Neuropsychologist, 17,* 410 – 425.

Lee, T.M.C., Liu, H., Tan, L., Chan, C.C.H., Mahankali, S., Feng, C. et al. (2002). *Human Brain Mapping, 15, 157 – 164.*

Lees-Haley, P.R. (1997). Attorneys influence expert evidence in forensic psychological and neuropsychological cases. *Assessment, 4,* 321 – 324.

Lezak, M.D. (1995). *Neuropsychological Assessment.* (3rd ed.). New York: Oxford.

Lu, P.H., Boone, K.B., Cozolino, L. and Mitchell, C. (2003). Effectiveness of the Rey-Osterrieth complex figure test and the Meyers and Meyers recognition trial in the detection of suspect effort. *Clinical Neuropsychologist, 17,* 426 – 440.

Lynch, W.J. (2004). Determination of effort level, exaggeration and malingering in neurocogntive effort. *Journal of Head Trauma Rehabilitation, 19,* 277 – 283.,

Mathias, C.W., Greve, K.W., Bianchini, K.J., Houston, R.J. and Crouch, J.A. (2002). Detecting malingered neurocognitive dysfunction using the reliable digit span in traumatic brain injury. *Assessment, 9*, 301 – 308

Miller, L. (2001). Not just malingering: Syndrome diagnosis in traumatic brain injury litigation. *NeuroRehabilitation, 16*, 109 – 122.

Miller, L.J., Ryan, J.J., Carruthers, C.A. and Cluff, R.B. (2004). Brief screening indexes for malingering: A confirmation of Vocabulary minus Digit Span from the WAIS-III and the Rarely Missed Index from the WMS-III. *The Clinical Neuropsychologist, 18*, 327 – 333.

Millis, S.R. (1992). The Recognition Memory Test in the detection of malingered and exaggerated memory deficits. *Clinical Neuropsychologist, 6*, 406 – 414.

Millis, S.R. (2002). Warrington's Recognition Memory Test in the detection of response bias. *Journal of Forensic Neuropsychology, 2, 147 – 166.*

Millis, S.R. and Putnam, S.H. (1994). The Recognition Memory Test in the assessment of memory impairment after financially compensable mid head injury: A replication. *Perceptual and Motor Skills, 79*, 384 – 386.

Millis, S.H., Putnam, S.H., Adams, K.M. and Ricker, J.H. (1995). The California Verbal Learning Test in the detection of incomplete effort in neuropsychological evaluation. *Psychological Assessment, 7*, 463 – 471.

Millis, S.R. and Volinsky, C.T. (2001). Assessment of response bias in mild head injury: Beyond malingering tests. *Journal of Clinical and Experimental Neuropsychology, 23*, 809 – 828.

Mittenberg, W., Azrin, R., Millsaps, C. and Heilbronner, R. (1993). Identification of malingered head injury on the Wechsler Memory Scale – Revised. *Psychological Assessment, 5*, 34 – 40.

Mittenberg, W., Theroux-Fichera, S., Zielinski, R.E. and Heilbronner, R.L. (1995). Identification of malingered head injury on the Wechsler Adult Intelligence Scale – Revised. *Professional Psychology: Research and Practice, 26*, 491 – 498.

Nelson, N.W., Boone, K., Dueck, A., Wagener, L., Lu, P. and Grills, C. (2003). Relationships between eight measures of suspect effort. *The Clinical Neuropsychologist, 17*, 263 – 272.

O'Bryant, S.E., Duff, K., Fisher, J., McCaffrey, R.J. (2004). Performance profiles and cut-off scores on the memory assessment scales. *Archives of Clinical Neuropsychology, 19*, 489 – 496.

Ray, E.C., Engum, E.S., Lambert, E.W., Bane, G.F., Nash, M.R. and Bracy, O.L. (1997). Ability of the Cognitive Behavioral Driver's Inventory to distinguish malingerers from brain-damaged subjects. *Archives of Clinical Neuropsychology, 12*, 491 – 503.

Rees, L.M., Tombaugh, T.N., and Boulay, L. (2001). Depression and the Test of Memory Malingering. *Archives of Clinical Neuropsychology, 16*, 501 -506.

Reitan, R.M. and Wolfson, D. (1993). *The Healstead-Reitan Neuropsychological test battery: Theory and clinical interpretations.* Tucson, AZ: Neuropsychology Press.

Rose, F.E., Hall, S. and Szalda-Petree, A.D. (1995). Portland Digit Recognition Test—Computerized: Measuring response latency improves the detection of malingering. *Clinical Neuropsychologist, 9*, 124 – 134.

Ross, S.R., Millis, S.R., Krukowski, R.A., Putnam, S.H. and Adams, K.M. (2004). Detecting incomplete effort on the MMPI-2: An examination of the fake-bad scale in mild head injury. *Journal of Clinical and Experimental Neuropsychology, 26*, 115 – 124.

Rogers, R.R. (1984). Towards and empirical model of malingering and deception. *Behavioral Sciences and the Law, 2, 93 - 111.*

Rogers, R.R. (1997). Current status of clinical methods. In R.R. Rogers (Ed.). *Clinical assessment of malingering and deception* (2nd ed.), (pp 373 – 397). New York: Guilford.

Rogers, R., Harell, E. and Liff, C. (1993). Feigning neuropsychological impairment: A critical review of methodological and clinical considerations. *Clinical Psychology Review, 13,* 255 – 274.

Ruffolo, L.F., Guilmette, T.J. and Willis, W.G. (2000). Comparison of time and error rates on the Trail Making Test among patients with head injuries, experimental malingerers, patients with suspect effort on testing, and normal controls. *The Clinical Neuropsychologist, 14,* 223 – 230.

Slick, D.J., Sherman, E.M.S. and Iverson, G.L. (1999). Diagnostic criteria for malingered neurocognitive dysfunction: Proposed standards for clinical practice and research. *The Clinical Neuropsychologist, 13,* 545 – 561.

Slick, D.J., Tan, J.E., Strauss, E.H., and Hultsch, D.F. (2004). Detecting malingering: A survey of experts' practices. *Archives of Clinical Neuropsychology, 19,* 465 – 473.

Slick, D., Hopp, G., Strauss, E. and Thompson, G.B. (1997). *Victoria Symptom Validity Test, Version 1.0 Professional Manual.* Odessa, TX: Psychological Assessment Resources.

Strauss, E., Hultsch, D.F., Hunter, M., Slick, D.J., Paltry, B. and Levy-Bencheton, J. (2000). Using intraindividual variability to detect malingering in cognitive performance. *The Clinical Neuropsychologist, 14,* 420 – 432.

Suhr, J.A. (2002). Malingering, coaching, and the serial position effect. *Archives of Clinical Neuropsychology, 17,* 69 – 77.

Suhr, J.A., Gunstad, J., Greub, B. and Barrash, J. (2004). Exaggeration Index for an expanded version of the Auditory Verbal Learning Test: Robustness to coaching. *Journal of Clinical and Experimental Neuropsychology, 26,* 416 – 427.

Sweet, J.J. (2000). Malingering: Differential diagnosis. In J.J. Sweet (Ed.), *Forensic Neuropsychology* (pp. 255 – 285). Lisse: Swets and Zeitlinger.

Tardif, H.P., Barry, R.J., Fox, A.M. and Johnstone, S.J. (2000). Detection of feigned recognition memory impairment using the old/new effect of the event-related potential. *International Journal of Psychophysiology, 36,* 1 – 9.

Taylor, L.A., Kreutzer, J.S. and West, D.D. (2003). Evaluation of malingering cut-off cores for the Rey 15-Item Test: A brain injury base series. *Brain Injury, 17,* 295 – 308.

Thompson, G.B. (2002). The Victoria Symptom Validity Test: An enhanced test of symptom validity. *Journal of Forensic Psychology,* , 43 – 67.

Tombaugh, T.N. (1996). *The Test of Memory Malingering (TOMM).* Toronto: Multi-Health Symptoms.

Tombaugh, T.N. (2002). The Test of Memory Malingering (TOMM) in forensic psychology. *Journal of Forensic Psychology, 2,* 69 – 96.

Uttl, B., Graf, P., and Cosentio, S. (2000). Exacting assessments: Do older adults fatigue more quickly? *Journal of Clinical and Experimental Neuropsychology, 22,* 496 – 507.

Ward, N.S., Oakley, D.A., Frackowiak, R.S.J. and Halligan, P.W. (2003). Differential brain activations during intentionally simulated and subjectively experienced paralysis. *Cognitive Neuropsychiatry, 8,* 295 – 312.

Warrington, E. K. (1984). *Recognition Memory Test.* Windsor: NFER-Nelson.

Wechsler, D. (1997a). *WAIS-III administration and scoring manual.* San Antonio: The Psychological Corporation.

Wechsler, D. (1997b). *WMS-III administration and scoring manual.* San Antonio: The Psychological Corporation.

Weinborn, M., Orr, T., Woods, S.P., Conover, E. and Feix, J. (2003). A validiation of the Test of Memory Malingering in a forensic psychiatric setting. *Journal of Clinical and Experimental Neuropsychology, 25,* 979 – 990.

West, M.A. and Knowles, D.R. (1991). Estimating cost of health care and economic loss in brain injury. In, D.O. Hans and A.S. Carlin (Eds.), *Forensic Neuropsychology: Legal, and Scientific Bases* (pp. 214 – 227). New York: Guilford.

Wong, J.L, Regennitter, R.P. and Barrios, F. (1994). Base rate and simulated symptoms of mild injury among normals. *Archives of Clinical Neuropsychology, 9,* 411 – 425.

Youngjohn, J.R. (1995). Confirmed attorney coaching prior to neuropsychological evaluation. *Assessment, 2,* 279 – 283.

Youngjohn, J. R., Burrows, L. and Erdal, K. (1995). Brain damage or compensational neurosis? The controversial post-concussive syndrome. *Clinical Neuropsychologist, 9,* 112–123.

INDEX

D

E

F

Q

R